AF795780

Reproduction and the Maternal Body in Literature and Culture

This book examines a selection of texts to discuss how midwifery, obstetrics and women's bodies were constructed during the (long) eighteenth century and how these material-discursive entanglements between science, medicine, literature and culture have shaped society's views of pregnancy, childbirth and reproduction.

Drawing on theories from disciplines such as feminist new materialism, this book traces the history of both the reproductive body and the pluralistic medical knowledges that attended to pregnancy and childbirth during the Enlightenment and early Romanticism in Britain. It identifies the significance of literary and cultural artefacts in this knowledge formation, including the materiality of the female reproductive body itself, and raises awareness of myths about pregnancy and childbirth that persist today. This book features chapters exploring Jonathan Swift's *Gulliver's Travels*, John Cleland's *Fanny Hill*, Laurence Sterne's *Tristram Shandy*, Eliza Fenwick's *Secresy, Or: The Ruin on the Rock*, Mary Wollstonecraft's *Maria, Or: The Wrongs of Woman* and Mary Shelley's *Frankenstein.*

Reproduction and the Maternal Body in Literature and Culture is an innovative and interdisciplinary contribution to the medical humanities and feminist philosophy of science and will interest scholars from a range of backgrounds, including literature and cultural studies, midwifery, medicine and history.

Jennifer S. Henke is a literary and cultural studies scholar, with a PhD from the University of Bremen, Germany, and a *Venia Legendi* for Anglophone Literary and Cultural Studies from the University of Bonn, Germany.

Routledge Advances in the Medical Humanities

Medical Education, Politics and Social Justice
The Contradiction Cure
Alan Bleakley

Poetry in the Clinic
Towards a Lyrical Medicine
Alan Bleakley and Shane Neilson

Critical Humanities and Ageing
Forging Interdisciplinary Dialogues
Edited by Marlene Goldman, Kate de Medeiros and Thomas Cole

Palliative Care Nursing as Mindfulness
Embodying a Relational Ethic through Strong Emotion, Uncertainty and Death
Lacie White

From Loneliness to Solitude in Person-centred Health Care
Stephen Buetow

Ageism and Person-Centred Care
Rehabilitating Bias for Age-Friendly Practice
Stephen Buetow

Metacognition, Metahumanities, and Medical Education
Thinking without the Box
Alan Bleakley, Quentin Eichbaum and Rachel Ellaway

Reproduction and the Maternal Body in Literature and Culture
Bodies of Knowledge, 1726–1818
Jennifer S. Henke

For more information about this series visit: www.routledge.com/Routledge-Advances-in-the-Medical-Humanities/book-series/RAMH

Reproduction and the Maternal Body in Literature and Culture

Bodies of Knowledge, 1726–1818

Jennifer S. Henke

Routledge
Taylor & Francis Group
LONDON AND NEW YORK

First published 2025
by Routledge
4 Park Square, Milton Park, Abingdon, Oxon OX14 4RN

and by Routledge
605 Third Avenue, New York, NY 10158

Routledge is an imprint of the Taylor & Francis Group, an informa business

© 2025 Jennifer S. Henke

The right of Jennifer S. Henke to be identified as author of this work has been asserted in accordance with sections 77 and 78 of the Copyright, Designs and Patents Act 1988.

All rights reserved. No part of this book may be reprinted or reproduced or utilised in any form or by any electronic, mechanical, or other means, now known or hereafter invented, including photocopying and recording, or in any information storage or retrieval system, without permission in writing from the publishers.

Trademark notice: Product or corporate names may be trademarks or registered trademarks, and are used only for identification and explanation without intent to infringe.

British Library Cataloguing-in-Publication Data
A catalogue record for this book is available from the British Library

ISBN: 9781032741703 (hbk)
ISBN: 9781032742229 (pbk)
ISBN: 9781003467977 (ebk)

DOI: 10.4324/9781003467977

Typeset in Times New Roman
by codeMantra

For my mother and for everyone else who supported me relentlessly, believed in this project, and never stopped cheering me on (you know who you are, thank you).

Contents

Part I

Mapping the Field

1.1 Introduction

In the Delivery Room

1.1.1 Birth Pangs, Or: The Initial Spark

A few years ago, I accompanied a pregnant friend on a maternity ward tour of the hospital *DIAKO Ev. Diakonie-Krankenhaus* in the north of Germany. Never actually allowed into the 'secret' chambers of the delivery room, we were permitted to stand in the lobby listening to the obstetrician's detailed explanation of the birthing process in his hospital. Still surprised about not being permitted to enter the spaces we were most interested in, my friend and I wondered about the power constructs involved. Why were we not granted access to the birthing rooms? Why were we rendered 'outsiders' to this knowledge space that was especially relevant to my pregnant friend? Who owned the discursive power in this situation? To whom did the obstetric 'bodies of knowledge' belong? We could only assume that the doctor's aim was not to trouble the listeners with the possible sight of an overtly medicalised environment in which the pregnant women would undergo what seemed to us a relatively risk-free process: birth.

As the obstetrician continued, however, he proffered additional information regarding the hospital's Caesarean section rate. He told us that one in three women gave birth via C-section, a procedure that is medically necessary in cases of emergency but is known to be highly invasive and not without risk.[1] This percentage is reflected in the current data of the *DIAKO*'s hospital guide for the region; in 2021, over a third of all births in the area were delivered via C-section. The statistics also confirm this rate nationwide.[2] But how does this severe medical intervention work precisely?

A Caesarean section involves several steps, such as inserting a catheter to remove urine from the woman's bladder (sometimes the catheter remains in the body for another day postpartum or even longer if necessary) and anesthetising the woman's body from the waist down. The surgeon then cuts through the abdomen and into the uterus to remove the infant. After this major operation, the incisions in the uterus have to be carefully stitched together to avoid complications during future births. While recovering from a C-section usually only takes a few days, it can take up to weeks with mild-to-severe post-operative pain including possible bleeding. The chances are that the woman will have to undergo another C-section for her next birth, depending on the healing process of the scars on her uterus.[3]

DOI: 10.4324/9781003467977-2

In view of these medical details, it seems surprising that one in three women ask for,[4] agree to or might be advised to consent to this major medical intervention. Although some C-sections are indeed necessary, they should be the last resort after having exhausted all other options. This procedure can only be performed in a hospital, but it is not only women anticipating C-section births who enter a hospital's maternity ward in Germany – women in Europe generally prefer the clinic: As much as 99% give birth in a hospital (Jouhki et al. 2017, 35). Moreover, worldwide, roughly 60%–80% of birthing women receive epidural anaesthesia (EA).[5] Although this treatment can effectively manage birth pangs, women are exposed to the risk of more medical intervention during parturition, such as the use of forceps or a vacuum extractor, or the need to be treated with more drugs like oxytocin (Newnham et al. 2021, 435, 440). Despite the fact that women also actively choose EA for very individual and personal reasons, these numbers might lead to the conclusion that nearly all births require constant supervision and medical intervention. This seems understandable given the culturally widespread trope of the delivering woman's pains and struggles during birth, which are, of course, also a part of the reality. However, the assumption that birth as such is almost always a life-threatening event, although such cases certainly exist, seems to contradict the maternal mortality rate in Western Europe, i.e. the number of maternal deaths per 100,000 live births, which is close to zero.[6]

At the same time, the rate of maternal mortality is much higher in some countries outside of Western Europe. While the ratio is currently 10–100,000 live births in the UK compared to 4 in Germany, which adds up to 0.01%–0.02%, it is as high as about 1,200 (1.2%) in countries like South Sudan.[7] In addition, the maternal mortality ratio for Black women is more than twice as high in the US (Hoyert 2022, 1).[8] As Joseph et al. also point out, "recent reports from England reveal maternal death rates among Black women that are fivefold higher than those among White women," despite the NHS's provision of free health care, whereas reasons for this would be "racism including […] social determinants of health such as income, social status, […] social supports, […] and culture" (Joseph et al. 2021, 769). The roots of such disparities are undoubtedly complex, and this issue urgently requires further investigation. This book, however, is based on the premise that pregnancy and birth, though complications can and do occur and must be treated professionally in these cases, can generally be regarded as rather low-risk bodily processes.

Yet, numerous examples in literature, film and popular culture corroborate the impression that giving birth is a dangerous bodily process. As Sarah Fox stresses in *Giving Birth* (2022), "[w]e are culturally trained to think of childbirth as painful," although, as she claims with reference to Barbara Duden,[9] "precise descriptions of the sensations of birthing range from pain to discomfort through to pleasure" (Fox 2022, 14). Nonetheless, pregnancy and childbirth today are medicalised or pathologised conditions to the degree that only the hospital seems to be considered a safe space for bearing children, although home births are also still available in many European countries. It was the experience of not being allowed into the delivery rooms, the surprisingly high C-section rates and the gendered discrepancies in discursive power regarding the (male) doctor's denial of access to the 'knowledge spaces' in the maternity ward that initially sparked my interest in pregnancy and childbirth and their respective medical procedures.

Despite the spatial restrictions in the hospital, it was possible to take a quick look into one of the 'secret' birthing rooms as we passed it; the delivery bed resembling an oversized gynaecological chair ready for the pregnant body's inspection; the foetal cardiotocograph to monitor the unborn child's heart rate; the infusion stand to administer pain killers or hormones like oxytocin to accelerate the birth process; the smell of disinfectant; the idea of inserting long epidural needles into the woman's spine and the overall impression of medical surveillance, seriousness and pathology evoked an atmosphere of an inaccessible or 'secret' laboratory.

At the time, I could not but notice parallels of this in my view eerie overmedicalised space to Mary Shelley's *Frankenstein* (1818 [2022]),[10] a Gothic novel about the megalomanic scientist and anatomist Victor Frankenstein who fabricates a creature by stitching together parts of dead bodies in his secret lab. During my research, I was especially struck by Ellen Moers' pivotal article "Female Gothic: The Monster's Mother" and her reading of the narrative as a "birth myth" (Moers [1976] 2012, 319, 2022, 462). In Moers' view, the overachiever and prototype of the mad scientist, Victor Frankenstein, who fantasises about 'birthing' a human being without the help of a female body, can be understood as the obstetrician who reduces his 'patient,' the Creature, to a conglomerate of inert body parts, an object to be studied by the (male) medical gaze. Moers argues that *Frankenstein* not only addresses rogue science in general but also childbirth, fatal births, the loss of children and especially the treatment of pregnancy and birth by medical men.[11]

Having already sifted through early-modern anatomy books, such as Vesalius' *De Humani* (1543) and the eighteenth-century obstetrical atlases of William Smellie and William Hunter, I was drawn to both the represented and actual *materiality* of the pregnant body. This led me to wonder about its role in the medical and cultural history of childbirth. Moers' reading of *Frankenstein* as a birth myth certainly is a classic approach to the topics of pregnancy, childbirth and medicine in British literature and culture, and her ground-breaking text has been quoted countless times. Nevertheless, it still serves as an excellent introduction and lays the foundation for my original exploration of this topic. Indeed, this book is the first to reconsider the maternal body through a *new materialist* framework, arguing that the pregnant body is entangled with past and present medical as well as cultural practices. It therefore distinguishes itself significantly from both classic and contemporary studies.

Seeing some historical connections between the high rates of C-sections in the twenty-first century and the literary, cultural and medical history of the (female) reproductive body, I thus began to investigate when, why and how pregnancy and childbirth became pathologised to the degree that now only the hospital seems to be the appropriate space for birthing women. As a literature and cultural studies scholar, I was not interested merely in the history of childbirth but especially in the question of what cultural artefacts can tell us about the entanglement of medicine, science and the female reproductive body. These questions led to a larger research project – the 'ward' if you like – on which this book was born.

1.1.2 Parturition: Positioning & Toolbox

This project is primarily situated in the *medical humanities*, more precisely in what Anna Whitehead and Angela Woods have coined the "second wave" or the *critical medical humanities* (Whitehead/Woods 2016, 1; see also Bleakley 2020). As opposed to the "first wave or mainstream medical humanities," which focusses on the doctor–patient relationship in the context of the clinic and the communication between the two by means of narrative while disregarding other aspects such as gender, race, class, sexuality, or culture and history, the second wave shifts attention towards the latter (Whitehead/Woods 2016, 1–2). It also addresses issues relating to knowledge production or "non-human objects" such as the laboratory or the literary text and thus aims at a "widening of focus" (Whitehead/Woods 2016, 2).

Interestingly enough, the critical medical humanities are less interested in the clinical gaze, a well-researched and often applied concept of the first wave, and are more invested in the concept of *entanglement* that moves beyond questions of ethics, education and experience so common for the mainstream medical humanities (Whitehead/Wood 2016, 3). Although medical ethics, empathy, illness narratives and the doctor-patient relationship remain important, the second wave does not want to yield new or more binaries such as "patient/doctor, illness/disease, medicine/humanities"; it rather asks about the "function and status of the literary text, and what kind of evidence it represents" and includes other forms of representation as well, such as visual texts, which is also what this book does especially in Chapter 1.2 (Whitehead/Woods 2016, 4–5).

With recourse to the Frankfurt School and some of its proponents including Michael Foucault, Judith Butler and Bruno Latour, Whitehead and Woods argue that the value of the term 'critical' in conjunction with the medical humanities lies in its potential to bring about actual social, political and structural change by challenging the "apparent neutrality and objectivity of [biomedical] science" (Whitehead/Woods 2016, 5). Furthermore, the work of philosophers like "Sara Ahmed, Donna Haraway, [and] Susan Sontag," whose ideas continue to inform the critical medical humanities, underscore the global aspect of this project (Whitehead/Woods 2016, 6). In addition, Whitehead and Woods emphasise the importance of a historical perspective in order to challenge dominant discourses of biomedicine: These offer "alternative vantage points" of "critique" by not only focussing on "sites of transformation" in the history of science and medicine but also offering "different ways of sensing our world – that were important in the past and that may remain with us today" (Whitehead/Woods 2016, 6–7).

In this context, Whitehead and Woods acknowledge the strong influence of feminist thought on the critical medical humanities, as "this intellectual tradition […] has engaged […] attentively with, amongst others, questions of the medical, the gaze, the body, affect, power and resistance" (Whitehead/Woods 2016, 8). Finally, they add that one concept has proven particularly useful for challenging medical oppositions and binaries – *entanglement* – a notion that helps to understand that the "critical medical humanities [are] based in mobility, fluidity, movement: a creative boundary-crossing in and through which new possibilities can emerge" (Whitehead/Woods 2016, 8).

In fact, the concept of entanglement that emerged in the scope of the material turn and focussed on "nature, bodies and things" nicely "resonat[es] with the critical medical humanities" and especially with the more "recent" and radical theoretical field of feminist materialism, which is why it is perfectly suited for the current investigation of the female reproductive body and its material discursiveness (Whitehead/Woods 2016, 13–14). In short, the concept of entanglement enables to "think beyond the boundaries that have so far characterised the medical humanities" and "rethink [...] the category of the human" as such by "unsett[ling] and complicat[ing]" it (Whitehead/Woods 2016, 10). The current investigation especially deals with the epistemology of childbirth and its cultural and medical practices. It traces the complex, discursive *entanglement(s)* of pluralistic bodies of knowledge and aims at merging the history of science and medicine with questions of how representations of the reproductive body in literature and culture shaped – and were shaped by – gender discourses during the eighteenth century in Britain.

At the heart of this study thus lies the female reproductive body. The novel aspect of this project is that it extends beyond a traditional (Foucauldian) discourse analysis by bringing matter – in this case the body's materiality – to the fore. This investigation is therefore equally situated in the field of *material cultures* or *material feminisms* (Alaimo/Hekman 2008). In this context, this study shall move beyond the 'passive' body to be acted upon by combining discourse analysis with a *new materialist* framework based on established scholarship by N. Katherine Hayles (1999), Donna Haraway ([1985] 2000), Stacy Alaimo and Susan Hekman (2008), Karen Barad (2007, 2008, 2018), Karen Harvey (2010, 2018) and others. These scholars' mostly *material-discursive* approach is based on the premise that matter and thus the body have agency. It does not assume a sense of 'conscious' or subjective (material) agency – rather, this approach builds on the conviction that matter is discursively entangled with its representations. Such a material-discursive maxim therefore avoids a binary hierarchy between representation and represented, signifier and signified as well as image and object.

Especially Karen Barad's theory of *agential realism*, mainly based on ideas developed in quantum physics but also gender and queer studies, proves to be a useful tool to think with or rather, as I argue, *through* the body. In a nutshell, Barad critically examines representationalism and its assumed hierarchy of words over objects. More specifically, Barad, who uses they/them pronouns[12], rejects any form of hierarchical relationship between representation and what is represented, i.e., between mind and matter. In line with feminist science studies, Barad argues that representationalism is a mere by-product of the seemingly overcome Cartesian dualism that privileges mind over matter. While they claim that social constructivists still implicitly accept this hierarchical dualism in favour of the word, Barad is more interested in the question of "how discursive practices produce material bodies" in the first place (Barad 2008, 127).

It is important to note that Barad does *not* reject discourse altogether. Instead, they suggest "[posthuman-]performative alternatives to representationalism" by acknowledging matter's agency (Barad 2008, 122). The aim is rather to "sharpen the theoretical tool of performativity for [...] feminist [...] endeavours" (Barad 2008, 122). In this respect, the very term '(re)production' comes in handy for this book's methodological framework. It can be used as a metaphor to describe how both the discursive and material reproductive body are constantly (re)produced in or *through* literature, culture and medicine in a never-ending cycle of (re)presentation and (re)materialisation. In other words, discourse (re)produces matter while matter simultaneously (re)produces discourse.

This insight is not necessarily new to the humanities. In *Representation: Cultural Representations and Signifying Practices* (1997), the cultural theorist Stuart Hall, for instance, though focussing primarily on language as "central to meaning and culture," acknowledges that "even objects" contribute to the production of (shared) meaning(s) (Hall 1997, 1). He states: "we give things meaning by how we use them, or integrate them into our everyday practices" (Hall 1997, 2). Hall expands these cultural practices or "systems of representation" by not just restricting meaning to spoken or written language – he also addresses the "language of the body," thus already implying that bodies equally have the ability to "say something" (Hall 1997, 4–5). In other words, bodies 'speak.' Hall proceeds: "These elements – sounds, words, notes, gestures, expressions, clothes [and bodies] – are part of our material world; but their importance for language is not what they *are* but what they *do*" (emphasis in the original, Hall 1997, 5). Though Hall still privileges the word over the object, he does, to a certain degree, admit that 'things', such as bodily gestures and hence bodies, do not just exist a priori as passive objects but indeed 'act.' Put simply, they *function*.

Hall also reminds his readers that things do not have meaning "*outside* of how they are represented" (emphasis in the original, Hall 1997, 5). Their meaning is not given and then just 'read.' Instead, meaning is to be understood as a process: "meaning is thought to be *produced* – constructed – rather than simply 'found'" (emphasis in the original, Hall 1997, 5). This "social constructionist approach" to meaning therefore regards representation (as part of meaning-making) "not merely a reflection of the world" (Hall 1997, 6). Hall here seems to already suggest that representations are *entangled* with the world that naturally includes (material) things, objects and bodies. This becomes clear when he describes representation as a "slippery customer": "It is therefore never finally fixed"; "always putting off or 'deferring' its rendezvous with Absolute Truth"; "always negotiating and *inflected*" (emphasis added, Hall 1997, 9–10).

Furthermore, as Hall points out, "representations *interact* with one another [...] displacing one another along an unending chain": The process of meaning-making between "speaker and hearer" is therefore "always *interactive*" (emphasis added, Hall 1997, 10). What Hall seems to ignore, however, is the significance of the material object in this dialogic process. If matter *does* or 'acts' – if it 'speaks' – we need different and more accurate terms to avoid a hierarchy between (active) meaning and (passive) material. This is precisely where *material culture* comes into play: Terms such as *entanglement* not only deny a one-way process of meaning-making but also make matter matter by allowing it agency. In other words, the concept of entanglement does not negate representation – on the contrary, it *amplifies* it by merging the material with the discursive. Ultimately, representation is not only "inflected," to refer back to Hall's term, but rather "diffracted" to use Barad's words – it 'int*ra*-acts' with both the material and the discourses it is entangled with (Barad 2007, 71, 2008, 122). What can be said for sure is that we need different terms and approaches to adequately discuss haptic 'things' such as bodies.

A so-called *material-discursive* approach to the female reproductive body offers a way out of the still widely accepted hierarchical dichotomy of mind over materiality, representation over reality and meaning over matter. Karen Barad's *onto-epistem-ological* approach to matter and meaning questions one crucial aspect of matter and meaning-making in particular: causality. Put simply, according to this theory, matter and meaning do not produce each other in a linear way. On the contrary, both produce one another *simultaneously*. Matter and meaning are therefore, according to Barad, *entangled* in what they call an ongoing process of the "world's becoming" (Barad 2008, 122).

Barad builds on relevant works produced by philosophers such as Michel Foucault, Judith Butler, Donna Haraway and others. The novelty of Barad's highly interdisciplinary approach is that it also utilises insights from the Danish physicist and quantum theorist Niels Bohr. By doing so, Barad amalgamates discourse theory, gender performativity, material culture and posthumanist approaches into a theory of *agential realism* that will be further outlined in Chapter 1.3. The point Barad wants to make is that both representation and matter are to be understood as a 'doing,' a performative act. The term *entanglement* enables us to talk about discourse *and* matter; it avoids a one-sided reading of representation that excludes the haptic dimension of our world.

1.1.3 Dates of Birth: Times, Texts & Place

This project centres on the British Enlightenment or the Age of Reason, lasting from the late seventeenth century to the early nineteenth. I focus on texts produced in the first half of the eighteenth up to the turn of the century and into the early nineteenth. Concentrating on this time frame has proven useful, as it has been acknowledged as an era "decisive in the making of modernity" (Porter 2001, 3) with its vast array of revolutions in the fields of politics, industry and culture; it also witnessed major developments in the realms of science, technology, anatomy and medicine.

The rapid innovations during the eighteenth century inevitably led to a shift in (gendered) knowledges and cultural practices of birth assistance, some of which will be discussed in Chapter 1.2: The professional field of *midwifery*, a more traditional and female-connoted knowledge space, was annexed by *obstetrics*, the institutionalised sphere of (male-dominated) medicine, as the prevalent practice concerned with childbirth and the reproductive body. From a literary and cultural perspective, focussing on the (long) eighteenth century makes further sense as it also saw the rise of the novel and the explosion of other literary and cultural forms such as periodicals, newspapers, medical manuals or (satirical) illustrations. Many of those texts negotiated new scientific and medical developments and changed attitudes towards gender, class and power. Some of these cultural products explicitly or implicitly dealt with questions of childbirth, the role of the medical practitioner or the reproductive body in general.

The medical historian Mary E. Fissell, for instance, traces the history of the reproductive body in early-modern texts such as newspapers, ballads, witchcraft pamphlets, popular medical manuals, prayer books and other forms of print with the aim to uncover the "mysteries of reproduction" that were inextricably linked with cultural, political and economic concerns (Fissell 2009, 1). In this context, Fissell draws a direct connection between "bodies and politics" by referring to the well-known analogy of the 'body politic' "in which the king represents the state's head or heart and the peasants its feet" (Fissell 2009, 2). In terms of childbirth, it was especially the female reproductive body that served as a "microcosm of relations between men and women"; since the man was regarded as the 'head' of the family in analogy to the state's sovereign, the 'opposite sex' had to be equally controlled, particularly in terms of generation, thus rendering the female reproductive body a symbol of power (Fissell 2009, 2).[13] Fissell locates the renegotiations of the reproductive body not only in social and political events like the Protestant Reformation that apprehended pregnancy and childbirth in "deeply religious terms," but she also makes "[c]hanges in the representations of reproduction" responsible for "gender trouble" (Fissell 2004, 10–11). In terms of embodiment, she concludes that "[b]odies are good to think with, but they are also embedded in social practices" (Fissell 2004, 11).

Fissell's approach differs from earlier studies by scholars such as Michael Foucault and shifts the focus from men's to "women's reproductive bodies" in particular (Fissell 2004, 12). She thus dismisses the common critique regarding the absence of male bodies from such studies and emphasises the obvious by stating that "women's bodies are 'about' men as well as women" (Fissell 2004, 13). The literary scholars Andrew Mangham and Greta Depledge confirm the irrelevance of this objection. Like Fissell, they state that an investigation of the female reproductive body's medical history – especially in connection with the ascendence of obstetrics – always already involves male matters: "medical writing is, primarily, a discourse *between* men and, secondly, a discourse *about* women" (emphasis added, Mangham/Depledge [2011] 2012, 3).

Yet, how the female reproductive body's materiality is entangled with both discourse and practice remains unsolved in these studies. What this valuable body of work needs is a way to talk about discourse *and* matter to avoid a one-sided reading of 'representations of reproduction' that excludes the body's materiality. This book aims to fill this gap by adopting a *material-discursive* approach to reproduction. The issues of how knowledge about reproduction was (re)produced (and for whom) or how these 'bodies of knowledge' came into existence through the entanglement of medicine, literature, culture and the (material) body serve as leading questions throughout this study.

This project's corpus primarily consists of the following text types: novels and medical handbooks, including selected medical illustrations and graphic satires that, taken together, form a powerful set of both verbal and visual cultural products dealing with reproduction and the body. This manuscript is divided into three main parts that are not only devoted to novels or fiction but also to 'non-fictional' literary genres consisting of both midwifery and medical manuals or obstetrical atlases. Of course, these medical texts contain words as well, but what distinguishes them is their use of powerful (visual) images of pregnancy and childbirth. What is more, these images significantly contributed to the shift from midwifery to obstetrics by reducing the female pregnant woman to inert body parts. The historian Adrian Wilson confirms that the increasing practice of opening up (dead) human bodies on the dissection table during the long eighteenth century also added to the mother's "depersonalization" by rendering the female reproductive body a "mere materiality," thus detaching it or her from personhood (Wilson 1995a, 4).

When selecting novels, I aimed at gender parity for reasons of equality by choosing three narratives written by male authors and three written by female authors. The selection criteria were as follows: All novels must either explicitly or implicitly address questions of (female) reproduction. These include descriptions, representations and negotiations of conception (e.g., Laurence Sterne's *Tristram Shandy*, 1759), primary as well as secondary reproductive organs including female breasts (e.g., Jonathan Swift's *Gulliver's Travels*, 1726), maternity and abortion (e.g., Eliza Fenwick's *Secrecy*, 1795, and Mary Wollstonecraft's *Maria*, 1798), 'monstrous' births (e.g., Mary Shelley's *Frankenstein,* 1818 [2022]) or avoid pregnancy altogether despite its obvious inescapability, while resorting to gendered metaphors to address sexual acts and organs (e.g., John Cleland's *Fanny Hill*, 1749).

Taken together, these examples also point to the presumed problem of eighteenth-century novels in terms of representing childbirth; to my knowledge, no novel from this period offers detailed descriptions of the actual birth process with all its bodily phenomena. This gap is all the more surprising given that especially early eighteenth-century fiction(s), satirical texts in particular, tend to include page-long and highly detailed descriptions of bodies, body parts and bodily functions as a result of the Enlightenment's revolutions in science, medicine and anatomy among others. From a literary and cultural perspective, however, this problem becomes an advantage as the omittance of graphic pregnancies, abortions or birth processes opens up possibilities for discussing pregnant metaphors in a double sense. Gender parity regarding both the obstetrical atlases and the satirical illustrations was not possible for the simple reason that there existed no female obstetricians (midwives excluded) or female graphic satirists at the time. Nevertheless, the chosen text types significantly improve an understanding of the entanglement of science, history, medicine, culture and the reproductive body in the eighteenth century.

In terms of geographical boundaries, this study pays special attention to the historiography of the reproductive body in Britain. Although, as the historian of early-modern medicine Adrian Wilson recalls, the "medicalization of childbirth" began in France at the end of the eighteenth century, the actual shift from midwifery to obstetrics started in London, not Paris, which is why Wilson claims childbirth to have "its own, distinctive [British] history" (Wilson 1995, 4–5). The historian Lisa Forman Cody affirms this claim and understands the development of midwifery to obstetrics as a "uniquely British domestic revolution" (2008, 4; cf. Fox 2022, 4).[14] Of course, comparable developments and shifts in the field of assisted childbirth were simultaneously taking place in other European countries, including Germany, Holland, and France, and a few aspects regarding these regions are also considered in this book. This study's main focus, however, lies on the history of the female reproductive body in British literature and culture of the eighteenth century.

1.1.4 First Words: Questions & Steps

The general questions of this study are two-fold. On the one hand, they address the history of childbirth and the rise of obstetrics: How, where and with whom did women deliver their children before the institutionalisation of medicine and the birth of the clinic? How and why did the shift from midwifery to obstetrics occur? In order to discuss these questions, it is indispensable to turn to the historiography of reproduction in greater detail, especially with regard to the actual practice of midwifery. Therefore, the deliberately extensive chapter PART I addresses major, mainly historical works in this field (Foucault 1976; Laqueur/Gallagher 1987; Schiebinger 1987; Jordanova 1989; Martin [1987] 1993; Newman 1996; Wilson 1995; Murphey-Lawless 1998; McGrath 2002; Cody [2005] 2008; King 2007; Waddington 2011; Laqueur 2012; Lieske 2012; Mangham/Depledge [2011] 2012; Williams 2012; Buckley 2017; Deutscher 2017). It traces history of sex and sexuality, maternal myths and medical metaphors, the shift from midwifery to obstetrics, the question of female agency, and tackles first problems with regard to (the limits of) representationalism. This chapter's aim is to sketch out possible reasons for why obstetrics rendered itself a higher order of knowledge in contrast to traditional practices of childbirth. Its goal is also to shed light on the implications of this shift in terms of sex, gender and power that will increase an understanding of when, how and why pregnancy and childbirth were pathologised.

On the other hand, this study asks about how these developments were both negotiated in and at the same time shaped by contemporary artefacts: What was the effect of these shifts on literary and cultural production? Conversely, how did these artefacts influence medical discourses of reproduction? More precisely, this book investigates not only in what way medical, literary and cultural texts about pregnancy and birth communicate(d) with but also how they were (and still are) *entangled* with one another. In order to avoid a hierarchy between representation and the body or between meaning and matter, this book draws on theories and concepts from the fields of (feminist) bodies studies, posthumanism and (new) material culture (Hayles 1999; Haraway [1985] 2000; Alaimo/Hekman 2008; Barad 2007, 2008, 2018; Schwennesen/Koch 2009; DeMello 2014; Hillman/Maude 2015; Hoppe/Lemke 2015; Sheehan 2015; Shilling 2016; Richards 2018; Runia 2018). It tackles the question of what 'bodies of knowledge' emerged out of the visual and verbal representations of the reproductive body and how these texts (still) contribute to the globalised fear around childbirth. This study thus asks about the historical link between medicine, gender and reproduction; it also seeks to investigate how an analysis of the female reproductive body in literary and cultural artefacts can contribute to a historiography of reproduction.

PART II turns to selected and exemplary cultural analyses of literary artefacts produced by male and female authors during the eighteenth century. It investigates two canonised satirical texts – Jonathan Swift's *Gulliver's Travels* (1726) and Laurence Sterne's *Tristram Shandy* (1759) – that frame a still under-analysed novel, John Cleland's *Fanny Hill* (1749). PART II then continues with three novels that largely adhere to the Gothic mode: Fenwick's lesser-known *Secresy, Or: The Ruin on the Rock* (1795), Wollstonecraft's *Maria, Or: The Wrongs of Woman* (1798), and finally, Mary Shelley's *Frankenstein, Or: The Modern Prometheus* (1818). Each of the six analysis chapters provides a general introduction to the text followed by a contextualising subchapter, and a section that mainly focusses on the text before ending with a concluding part. PART III 'stitches the pieces together' and further offers an outlook as to how we can possibly conceptualise the female reproductive body in the future.

This book uses the term *(re)production* as an overarching metaphor for pregnancy and birth, literature and culture as well as science and medicine. Following previous scholarship, it utilises this metaphor to investigate the "impact of women's surgery, gynaecology, and obstetrics on literary production" (Mangham/Depledge 2012, 1). It also contradicts the idea of "trickle-down science" and explores the implications literary and cultural artefacts had on midwifery and obstetrics (Fissell 2004, 6). In particular, this book acknowledges the complexity of this grand narrative of childbirth, science and the body that is "still in the making" (Fissell 2004, 6–7).[15] In this context, Andrew Mangham and Greta Depledge identify "literature as a key player in the formation of our current understandings of the female body," and they investigate the "ways in which science draws upon, modifies, and learns from [...] metaphors, myths, and narrative patterns" (Mangham/Depledge 2012, 1). It is essential to note, however, that knowledge formations in literature and science are not to be understood as two-way processes – they are, to use Barad's terms, rather *entangled* in a non-linear and ongoing int*ra*-action of becoming and unbecoming. As Mangham and Depledge also seem to imply: "Literature has not only been inspired by medicine but it has also, in turn, *inspired* medicine" (emphasis in the original, Mangham/Depledge 2012, 2). What these scholars generally emphasise throughout their research is the importance of literature and culture as a "part of reading the complex theoretical history of the female body" (Mangham/Depledge 2012, 4). How, then, are medical, literary and cultural material discourses entangled with each other?

First, I claim that themes of reproduction (in the sense of generation or procreation) are either explicitly or implicitly present in all of the texts within the corpus. In the further course of this study, it is therefore essential not only to address the more or less direct references to pregnancy, birth and the female reproductive body but also the indirect allusions. What is left out is equally important in order to grasp the full picture of reproduction in medical, literary and cultural eighteenth-century artefacts. This project thus also turns to ellipses and blanks in terms of representations of the material-discursive female reproductive body in textual artefacts.

Second, I trace the ways these allusions to reproduction can potentially function as a critique of dominant scientific or medical (material) practices and cultural discourses. Most importantly, as critics of material culture studies have previously expressed, adopting a posthumanist material-discursive approach to the reproductive body does *not* lead to a dissolution of the individual and a resulting release from responsibility. On the contrary, recognising how representations and the material are entangled with one another opens up the opportunity to accept liability for the way bodies and, ultimately, subjects are treated. This is one of the common misunderstandings regarding the field of material cultures: It in no way seeks to dissolve or eradicate the individual and thus responsibility; rather, such investigations raise awareness for scholars,' artists,' scientists' and medical practitioners' accountability, here with regard to the female reproductive body.

Third, I contend that the selected verbal and visual examples achieve their critique of medical practices by exhibiting dismembered 'bodies.' They do so both with respect to the represented physical forms *and* in terms of their narrative structures, the latter holding especially true for the epistolary novel, one of the most popular genres of the eighteenth century. The function of this form of *fragmentation* is to bring hidden *bodies of knowledge* about reproduction to the surface where they can be deconstructed, 'dissected' and criticised. In short, by paying special attention to fragmented bodies, literary forms and dominant (gendered) knowledges, it is possible to acknowledge the discursive complexity of reproduction as well as its medical, social and cultural implications in the eighteenth century and beyond.

To further clarify my use of the word '(re)production'; it serves as a metaphorical umbrella term for reproductive issues ranging from conception to pregnancy to birth to abortion, but it also operates as a keyword for literary, cultural and medical knowledge production. The concept of 'fragmentation,' however, functions as a leitmotif: It points to the fragmented representation and thus objectification and pathologisation of the reproductive body in visual and verbal art forms as well as to the fragmented narrative structures of the chosen texts. Moreover, both the overarching metaphor of (re)production and the leitmotif of fragmentation speak of the simultaneous creation and dispersion of knowledge(s) surrounding pregnancy and childbirth. The pervasiveness of fragmented knowledges concerning reproduction becomes clear if one considers still proliferating myths about childbirth, its alleged risks, and the fears and (mis)information regarding these bodily processes.

1.1.5 Postpartum, Or: A Short Synopsis

This book investigates the still widely under-researched epistemology of midwifery and obstetrics in a newly compiled corpus of textual and visual representations produced during the Age of Enlightenment and early Romanticism in Britain. The study specifically focusses on the pathologisation of the maternal body that seems to have peaked around 1800. Triggered by a paradigm shift, an initially 'female' body of knowledge – *midwifery* – was gradually taken over by the medical field of (male-dominated) *obstetrics* that reduced the maternal patient to her body parts, thus stigmatising pregnancy as an illness to be 'cured' by science. This form of objectification was both influenced by and impacted the way medical illustrations constructed the reproductive body. The discursive shift was also negotiated in cultural artefacts such as novels and graphic satire, of which a certain proportion emphasised society's scepticism towards new scientific practices emerging during the Age of Enlightenment. This book's overall objective is to demonstrate how complex discursive entanglements between science, medicine, literature and culture have shaped society's views on (female) reproduction, birth and the maternal body.

The term reproduction opens up a vast array of associations: It can simply be read as the birthing of humans, but it can also be understood as the (re)production of citizens since children have (always) been viewed as the wealth of the (British) nation. The term further alludes to the (re)production of verbal and visual texts in the form of manuals, novels or illustrations that proliferated during the ongoing printing revolution in the eighteenth century. It equally refers to reproductive myths that, in some instances, influenced the way both lay people and medical experts understood pregnancy and birth. 'Reproduction' thus has multiple senses: It describes the (re)production not only of medical knowledges surrounding pregnancy and childbirth but also the literary and cultural (re)production of these knowledge discourses.

By utilising selected older and newer theories within feminist discourses, this book seeks to (a) trace the history of both the reproductive body and medical knowledges of pregnancy and birth; (b) carve out the significance of literary and cultural artefacts, including the very materiality of the female reproductive body itself, for this knowledge formation; and (c) raise awareness of the myths and misunderstandings around childbirth that are still very much alive today. This investigation is thus situated in the fields of the *critical medical humanities* while also tackling questions raised in the areas of *material culture*.

To retrace the epistemology of what we know today as *obstetrics*, this study centres on the eighteenth century. This period not only saw the emergence of new ideas of democracy, gender and power, but in the scope of the still ongoing Scientific Revolution, it also yielded new ideas of the human and the body in the fields of anatomy and medicine. To grasp the full dimension of these shifts and struggles for authority, this book uses literary and cultural artefacts as a bridge to the past to carve out how they (still) produce the present. It thus also hopes to contribute to a better understanding of current knowledge formations surrounding pregnancy, childbirth and the reproductive body. Moreover, this investigation is not an analysis of *all* texts of the chosen period that dealt with questions of reproduction to a larger or smaller degree. Due to the explosion of literary and cultural products during the eighteenth century, listing and investigating all visual and verbal texts of the time would be impossible. Some readers might therefore miss chapters on other renowned eighteenth-century authors and novels.[16] The reason for their omission is not only that a vast amount of fine scholarly literature already exists on canonised texts of the period: This study also wants to include non-canonised artefacts to demonstrate how both well- and lesser-known texts of the eighteenth-century negotiated questions of reproduction. This inclusion will hopefully provide a fuller picture and inspire other scholars to continue this project by turning to similar corpora.

Finally, this project aims at a historicised cultural materialist approach that can be applied to all selected texts including both (non-narrative) visual and (narrative) verbal texts. It is by no means exhaustive and offers but a small glimpse into the rich and overtly complex history of reproduction and the bodies of knowledge created during the British Enlightenment. The study's political agenda is also quite clear: To further raise awareness for the historicity of the reproductive body and its implications for the handling of childbirth today. Because literature and culture have the potential to frame expectations of and discussions about health, analysing their artefacts can contribute to recognising (and perhaps interrupting) potentially harmful practices based on assumptions that, in turn, are generated through these very (material) discourses. What needs to be stressed in any case is that the role of matter and materiality in shaping all kinds of discourses is still far from being solved. This book hence does not offer an ultimate solution – it rather seeks to push the boundaries of matter and meaning's entanglement just a little further in the hopes to facilitate future scholarly debates in this field.

Notes

1 Cf. https://www.nhs.uk/conditions/caesarean-section/risks/.

2 See the Bremen Hospital Guide for regional and supra-regional data on C-sections: https://www.bremer-krankenhausspiegel.de/qualitaetsergebnisse-a-z/geburtshilfe/anteil-an-kaiserschnitten. Last access: September 2024.

3 For more information on the risks and benefits of C-sections, see Keag OE, Norman JE, Stock SJ (2018) "Long-term risks and benefits associated with cesarean delivery for mother, baby, and subsequent pregnancies: Systematic review and meta-analysis." *PLoS Med* 15(1): e1002494. https://doi.org/10.1371/journal.pmed.1002494.

4 Certainly, women also actively seek a C-section for various reasons, such as "[f]ear of birth," "most commonly as a result of a previous traumatic birth experience that prompted a preference for a planned cesarean to avoid a repetition of the trauma," while others feared they were at high risk due to "having a narrow pelvis," and yet other primiparas (first-time mothers) "requested a planned cesarean based on a deep-seated fear since their early teens, accompanied by alienation towards the idea of giving birth" (Eide et al. 2019: 1).

5 See Seijmonsbergen-Schermers et al. (2020): "Variations in use of childbirth interventions in 13 high-income countries: A multinational cross-sectional study." *PLoS Med* 17(5): e1003103. https://journals.plos.org/plosmedicine/article?id=10.1371/journal.pmed.1003103. Last access: November 2020.

6 See World Health Organization, UNICEF, United Nations Population Fund and The World Bank: *Trends in Maternal Mortality*: 2000 to 2017. WHO, Geneva, 2019. https://data.unicef.org/topic/maternal-health/maternal-mortality/. Last access: November 2020.

7 See World Health Organization, UNICEF, United Nations Population Fund and The World Bank: *Trends in Maternal Mortality: 2000 to 2020* WHO, Geneva, 2023. https://data.unicef.org/topic/maternal-health/maternal-mortality/. Last access: July 2023.

8 See Hoyert, Donna L (2022): *Maternal Mortality Rates in the United States, 2022.* www.cdc.gov/nchs/data/hestat/maternal-mortality/2022/maternal-mortality-rates-2022.htm. Last access: July 2023.

9 See Barbara Duden's *The Woman Beneath the Skin* ([1987] 1988).

10 See also my other publications that deal with reproduction, medicine and literature in *Frankenstein* and other cultural artefacts (2018, 2022, 2023, 2024, 2025).

11 Moers' thesis makes sense if one considers the novelist's own biography. Mary Shelley, who wrote her masterpiece at the tender age of 18, was not only constantly pregnant from the age of 16–21 but also lost most of her children postpartum. In addition, her own mother, Mary Wollstonecraft, died shortly after giving birth to her daughter due to what scholars believe to have been medical malpractice, performed by (male) obstetricians (Gordon 2015, 356; Hunter 2022, xiii;).

12 Barad prefers they/them pronouns as documented on their online university profile: https://philosophy.ucsc.edu/faculty/index.php?uid=kbarad.

13 After the beginning of the print revolution in the fifteenth century, literature of all kind including pamphlets and midwifery manuals "exploded the marketplace" (Fissell 2009, 4). It was especially cheap print, produced by medical authors like Nicholas Culpeper, in which "reproductive bodies became the stuff of political ideas" (Fissell, 2009, 4). Though one of the first to write about midwifery in a reader-friendly manner, Culpeper "belittled women's own ideas about their bodies" and promoted "faith in the male science of anatomy," thus rendering female embodiment "inferior" (Fissell 2009, 4).

14 In addition, specific socio-cultural factors such as class set this development apart: "Mother's choosing male rather than traditional female midwives dramatically broke with the past, and critics quickly charged that this revolutionary alteration upturned not only the British household, but also even the broader social order" (Cody 2008, 3–4). By the second half of the eighteenth century, man-midwives "had successfully begun to displace traditional female attendants among urban, aristocratic, and middling families" (Cody 2008, 3).

15 With reference to Monica Green, Helen King and Patricia Crawford's studies on the history of sex and sexuality, Fissell states that the early print revolution did not, as one might assume, contribute to "broadening medical discourse about women's reproductive bodies," but "actually limited it" (Fissell 2009, 7). What is more, the shift from "orally shared sexual knowledge towards a privileging of textual forms of that knowledge […] tilt[ed] the playing field" in terms of gender and power, shifting it towards the field of (male-dominated) obstetrics (Fissell 2009, 7).

16 Daniel Defoe's *Moll Flanders* (1922), for instance, would equally lend itself to an analysis of pregnancy and childbirth. However, since the current book is based on a German habilitation or post-doctoral thesis that had to be submitted at some point, I will reserve this novel for a future publication.

References

Ahmed, Sara. 2010. *The Promise of Happiness*. Durham, NC: Duke University Press.

Alaimo, Stacy, and Susan Hekman, eds. 2008. *Material Feminisms*. Bloomington: Indiana University Press.

Barad, Karen. 2007. *Meeting the Universe Halfway: Quantum Physics and the Entanglement of Matter and Meaning*. Durham, NC: Duke University Press.

Barad, Karen. 2008. "Posthumanist Performativity: Toward an Understanding of How Matter Comes to Matter." *Signs* 28 (3): 801–31.

Barad, Karen. 2018. "Diffracting Diffraction: Cutting Together-Apart." In *Diffracted World – Diffracted Readings: Onto-Epistemologies and the Critical Humanities*, edited by Birgit Mara Kaiser and Kathrin Thiele, 1–24. Abingdon: Routledge.

Bleakley, Alan (ed). 2020. *Handbook of the Medical Humanities*. Abingdon: Routledge.

Buckley, Jenifer. 2017. *Gender, Pregnancy and Power in Eighteenth-Century Literature: The Maternal Imagination*. Basingstoke: Palgrave Macmillan.

Cleland, John. 1749. *Memoirs of a Woman of Pleasure*. Edited by Peter Sabor. Oxford: Oxford University Press, 2008.

Cody, Lisa Forman. 2008. *Birthing the Nation: Sex, Science, and the Conception of Eighteenth-Century Britons*. Oxford: Oxford University Press. 2005.

Defoe, Daniel. 2003. *Moll Flanders*. New York: Norton.

DeMello, Margo. 2014. *Body Studies: An Introduction*. Abingdon: Routledge.

Deutscher, Penelope. 2017. *Foucault's Futures: A Critique of Reproductive Reason*. New York: Columbia University Press.

Duden, Barbara. 1988. *The Women beneath the Skin: A Doctor's Patients in Eighteenth-Century Germany*. Cambridge, MA: Harvard University Press.

Eide, Kristiane Tislevoll et al. 2019. "Maternal Reasons for Requesting Planned Cesarean Section in Norway: A Qualitative Study." *BMC Pregnancy and Childbirth* 19 (1): 1–11.

Fenwick, Eliza. 1795. *Secresy*. Edited by Isobel Grundy. Peterborough, ON: Broadview Press, 1998.

Fissell, Mary Elizabeth. 2009. *Vernacular Bodies: The Politics of Reproduction in Early Modern England*. Oxford: Oxford University Press.

Foucault, Michel. 1976. *The History of Sexuality*. New York: Pantheon.

Fox, Sarah. 2022. *Giving Birth in Eighteenth-Century England*. London: University of London Press.

Haraway, Donna J. [1985] 2000. "A Cyborg Manifesto: Science, Technology and Socialist Feminism in the Late Twentieth Century." In *The Cybercultures Reader*, edited by David Bell and Barbara Kennedy, 292–324. New York: Routledge.

Haraway, Donna J. 2007. *When Species Meet*. Minneapolis; London: University of Minnesota Press.

Hayles, N. Katherine. 1999. *How We Became Posthuman: Virtual Bodies in Cybernetics, Literature, and Informatics*. Chicago, IL; London: University of Chicago Press.

Henke, Jennifer S. 2018. "In the Flesh – The Politics of Abortion in Ireland." *Hard Times* 102 (2): 114–126. In *Gender Today*, edited by Anke Bartels, Irmgard Maassen, and Ingrid von Rosenberg. Potsdam: Universität Potsdam, Institut für Anglistik und Amerikanistik.

Henke, Jennifer S. 2022. "Mary Wollstonecraft, *Maria: Or, The Wrongs of Woman* (1798)." In *Handbook of the British Novel in the Long Eighteenth Century*, edited by Katrin Berndt and Alessa Johns, 449–466. Berlin; Boston, MA: De Gruyter.

Henke, Jennifer S. 2023. "Contesting Spaces of Knowledge: Reproduction, Medicine and Literature." In *Contradiction Studies: Mapping the Field/Inaugural Conference on Concepts of Contradiction in the Humanities*, edited by Kerstin Knopf, Gisela Febel, and Martin Nonhoff. Heidelberg: Springer.

Henke, Jennifer S. 2024. "'Fruits Which That Unknown Orchard Bore': Practices of Abortion in the 19th Century." *Journal for the Study of British Cultures* 31 (2). Edited by Sarah Wegener and Wolfgang Funk. Heidelberg: Winter, 219–236.

Henke, Jennifer S. 2025. "Matters of Interest: Entangling the Maternal Body." In *Undue Burdens: Reproductive Rights and Bodily Autonomy in the Long Eighteenth Century*, edited by Fiona Brideoake, Ula Lukszo Klein, and Nicole Garret. Charlottesville/VA: University of Virginia Press.

Hillman, David, and Ulrika Maude, eds. 2015. *The Cambridge Companion to the Body in Literature*. New York: Cambridge University Press.

Hoppe, Katharina, and Thomas Lemke. 2015. "Die Macht der Materie: Grundlagen und Grenzen des agentiellen Realismus von Karen Barad." *Soziale Welt* 66 (3): 261–280.

Jouhki, Maija-Riitta, Tarja Suominen, and Päivi Åstedt-Kurki. 2017. "Giving Birth on Our Own Terms: Women's Experience of Childbirth at Home." *Midwifery* 53: 35–41.

Joseph, K. S. et al. 2021. "Maternal Mortality in the United States." *Obstetrics and Gynecology* 137 (5): 763–771.
Jordanova, Ludmilla J. 1989. *Sexual Visions: Images of Gender in Science and Medicine between the Eighteenth and Twentieth Centuries*. Madison: University of Wisconsin Press.
Keag, O. E., J. E. Norman, and S. J. Stock. 2018. "Long-Term Risks and Benefits Associated with Caesarean Delivery for Mother, Baby, and Subsequent Pregnancies: Systematic Review and Meta-Analysis." *PLoS Medicine* 15 (1): e1002494.
King, Helen. 2007. *Midwifery, Obstetrics and the Rise of Gynaecology: The Uses of a Sixteenth-Century Compendium*. London: Routledge.
Laqueur, Thomas, and Catherine Gallagher. 1987. *The Making of the Modern Body: Sexuality and Society in the Nineteenth Century*. Berkeley: University of California Press.
Laqueur, Thomas. 2012. "The Rise of Sex in the Eighteenth Century: Historical Context and Historiographical Implications." *Signs: Journal of Women in Culture and Society* 37 (4): 802–813.
Lieske, Pam. 2012. "'Made in Imitation of Real Women and Children': Obstetrical Machines in Eighteenth-Century Britain." In *The Female Body in Medicine and Literature*, edited by Andrew Mangham and Greta Depledge, 16–33. Liverpool: Liverpool University Press.
Mangham, Andrew, and Greta Depledge, eds. 2011. *The Female Body in Medicine and Literature*. Liverpool: Liverpool University Press.
Martin, Emily. 1993. *The Woman in the Body: A Cultural Analysis of Reproduction*. Buckingham: Open University Press. 1987.
McGrath, Roberta. 2002. *Seeing Her Sex: Medical Archives and the Female Body*. Manchester: Manchester University Press.
Moers, Ellen. 2012. "Female Gothic: The Monster's Mother." In *Frankenstein: The 1818 Text, Contexts, Criticism*, edited by Mary Shelley and J. Paul Hunter, 213–218. New York: Norton.
Moers, Ellen. 2022. "From Female Gothic: The Monster's Mother." In *Frankenstein: The 1818 Text, Contexts, Criticism*, edited by Mary Shelley and J. Paul Hunter, 3rd ed., 214–219. New York: Norton.
Murphey-Lawless, Jo. 1998. *Reading Birth and Death: A History of Obstetrics Thinking*. Bloomington: Indiana University Press.
Newman, Karen. 1996. *Fetal Positions: Individualism, Science, Visuality*. Stanford, CA: Stanford University Press.
Newnham, Elizabeth C. et al. 2021. "Comparison of Labour and Birth Outcomes between Nulliparous Women Who Used Epidural Analgesia in Labour and Those Who Did Not: A Prospective Cohort Study." *Women and Birth* 34: 435–441.
Porter, Roy. 2001. *Enlightenment: Britain and the Creation of the Modern World*. London: Penguin.
Runia, Robin, ed. 2018. *The Future of Feminist Eighteenth-Century Scholarship: Beyond Recovery*. New York: Routledge.
Schiebinger, Londa. 1987. "Skeletons in the Closet: The First Illustrations of the Female Skeleton in Eighteenth-Century Anatomy." In *The Making of the Modern Body: Sexuality and Society in the Nineteenth Century*, edited by Thomas Laqueur and Catherine Gallagher, 42–82. Berkeley: University of California Press.
Schwennesen, Nete, and Lene Koch. 2009. "Visualizing and Calculating Life: Matters of Fact in the Context of Prenatal Risk Assessment." In *Contested Categories: Life Science in Society*, edited by Susanne Bauer and Ayo Wahlberg, 69–87. Farnham: Ashgate.
Seijmonsbergen-Schermers, A. E., T. van den Akker, E. Rydahl, K. Beeckman, A. Bogaerts, L. Binfa et al. 2020. "Variations in Use of Childbirth Interventions in 13 High-Income Countries: A Multinational Cross-Sectional Study." *PLoS Medicine* 17 (5): e1003103.

Sheehan, Paul. 2015. "Posthuman Bodies." In *The Cambridge Companion to the Body in Literature*, edited by David Hillman and Ulrika Maude, 45–59. New York: Cambridge University Press.

Shelley, Mary. 1818. *Frankenstein.* Edited by J. Paul Hunter. 3rd ed. New York: Norton, 2022.

Shilling, Chris. 2016. *The Body: A Very Short Introduction*. Oxford: Oxford University Press.

Sontag, Susan. 1979. *Illness as Metaphor*. New York: Random House.

Sterne, Laurence. 1759. *Tristram Shandy*. Edited by Judith Hawley. New York: Norton, 2019.

Swift, Jonathan. 1726. *Gulliver's Travels*. Edited by Albert J. Rivero. New York: Norton, 2002.

Waddington, Keir. 2011. *An Introduction to the Social History of Medicine: Europe since 1500*. London: Red Globe Press.

Whitehead, Anne, and Angela Woods, eds. 2016. *The Edinburgh Companion to the Critical Medical Humanities*. Edinburgh: Edinburgh University Press.

Wilson, Adrian. 1995a. *The Making of Man-Midwifery: Childbirth in England, 1660–1770*. Cambridge, MA: Harvard University Press.

Wollstonecraft, Mary. [1798] 2009. *Mary and the Wrongs of Woman*. Edited with an introduction by Gary Kelly. Oxford: Oxford University Press.

1.2 Context

Historicising the Reproductive Body

1.2.1 On the Dissection Table

This chapter puts the eighteenth-century reproductive body on the dissection table. Though certainly not unexplored, research on the body in conjunction with the medical historiography of reproduction and childbirth remains comparatively scarce. This does not mean, however, that the history of birth and medicine is uncharted territory. On the contrary, there is a solid but manageable amount of scholarly literature devoted to the history of reproduction, though many of these studies focus on the shift from midwifery to obstetrics. Still, the majority of these books are written by historians with relatively few references to literary and cultural artefacts. One further aim of this study, therefore, is to contribute to closing this gap.

The following sections intend to offer an extensive but non-exhaustive literature overview of selected major studies published on the history of reproduction with special attention to the (female) body. It thus provides but a glimpse into the histor*ies* of pregnancy and birth from different scholarly perspectives – social, medical, feminist, literary, cultural, and visual: It merges research results produced in these disciplines by combining older and newer studies in thematically compiled sections. The aim is to sketch out different reproductive discourses that will subsequently be discussed in relation to the selected case studies. Without a doubt, theories of reproduction have a very long history and reach back to classical antiquity. Since a comprehensive historiography of reproduction is simply impossible in the scope of this investigation, the following section selectively refers to older (ancient) discourses but mostly centres upon those discourse formations produced from the beginning of the British Enlightenment onwards.

That said, how was the body generally regarded during the eighteenth century? In *Flesh in the Age of Reason* (2004), the medical historian Roy Porter deals with this question and extends it by asking what discourses of the body can tell us about ourselves, our identities and culture(s). He identifies a vast amount of sometimes very contradictory attitudes towards corporeality during this period, mainly due to the still prevailing Cartesian dualism between body and mind.[1] As the historian Simon Schama outlines in his preface to Roy Porter's study, dominant eighteenth-century discourses revolved around the belief that it was the mind in

DOI: 10.4324/9781003467977-3

which the 'soul' or 'identity' resided; the mind was the "place [...] where consciousness, sentiment and memory dwelled; the lodging-house, in fact, of humanity" (Schama 2004, ix).[2] Against the backdrop of the flesh, however, Porter asks the "most demanding question" of all: How can we know ourselves – and what does the body have to do with it (Schama 2004, x)?

Porter stresses that it was especially the Age of Enlightenment that changed the way we regard our bodies. One practice significantly contributed to this shift: dissection. Though diseased and decaying corporeality still posed a potential and very real threat to society during this period, the (male) human body was simultaneously celebrated as the "model of all things" due to both the revival of "classical aesthetics" during the Renaissance and advancements in the field of anatomy and medicine; these included new dissection techniques that had previously been invented by the Flemish anatomist, physician and writer Andreas Vesalius (Porter 2004, xiii) (Figures 1a and b).[3]

His sixteenth-century work was not only revolutionary in that it offered anatomists a glimpse into the human body, but the eighteenth century experienced a reinvigoration of his works; with the rise of the anatomy theatre, the dead body was no longer sacrosanct, and "carnal knowledge was no longer forbidden" (Porter 2004, xiii).[4] As a result, studies in the fields of philosophy, science, medicine and theology started to deal with the 'fleshiness' of the "body in question" (Porter 2004, xiv). Sacred theories such as the "body politic" or the theory of the "king's two bodies" as well as the theory of the 'four humours' were increasingly scrutinised and refuted as "vulgar errors" (Porter 2004, xiv). Most importantly, in the scope of the Scientific Revolution as well as the Industrial Revolution, the human body came to be understood as a machine and evoked a "new mechanical philosophy" (Porter 2004, xiv). It is safe to say that a multitude of bodily concepts circulated during the Age of Reason; it was a time that can be understood as a "melting pot" for simultaneously existing body discourses (Porter 2004, xv).

Despite new developments in anatomy, medicine or dissection, however, flesh remained "deeply problematic" as both a "source of pleasure" and a "throughout nuisance, in constant need of care, attention and apology" (Porter 2004, 25). As Porter outlines, this 'body trouble' equally concerned literary and creative artists:

> To a degree that is hard to imagine today, visible, tangible flesh was all too often experienced as ugly, nasty and decaying, bitten by bugs and beset by sores; it was rank, foul and dysfunctional; for all of medicine's best efforts, it was frequently racked with pain, disability and disease; and death might well be nigh. Letters and diaries – to say nothing of Swift's satires or the cartoons of Hogarth and Gillray – document at length and with passion the intense repugnance people so frequently felt towards their own noisome flesh and that of others. That in part explains why [...] the period brought such an earnest raising of the thresholds of embarrassment and shame, so as to hide, deodorize, cleanse, purge, exclude and expel those multitudinous aspects of the flesh and of bodily functions experienced as psychosocially threatening, disgusting and dangerous.
>
> (Porter 2004, 25)

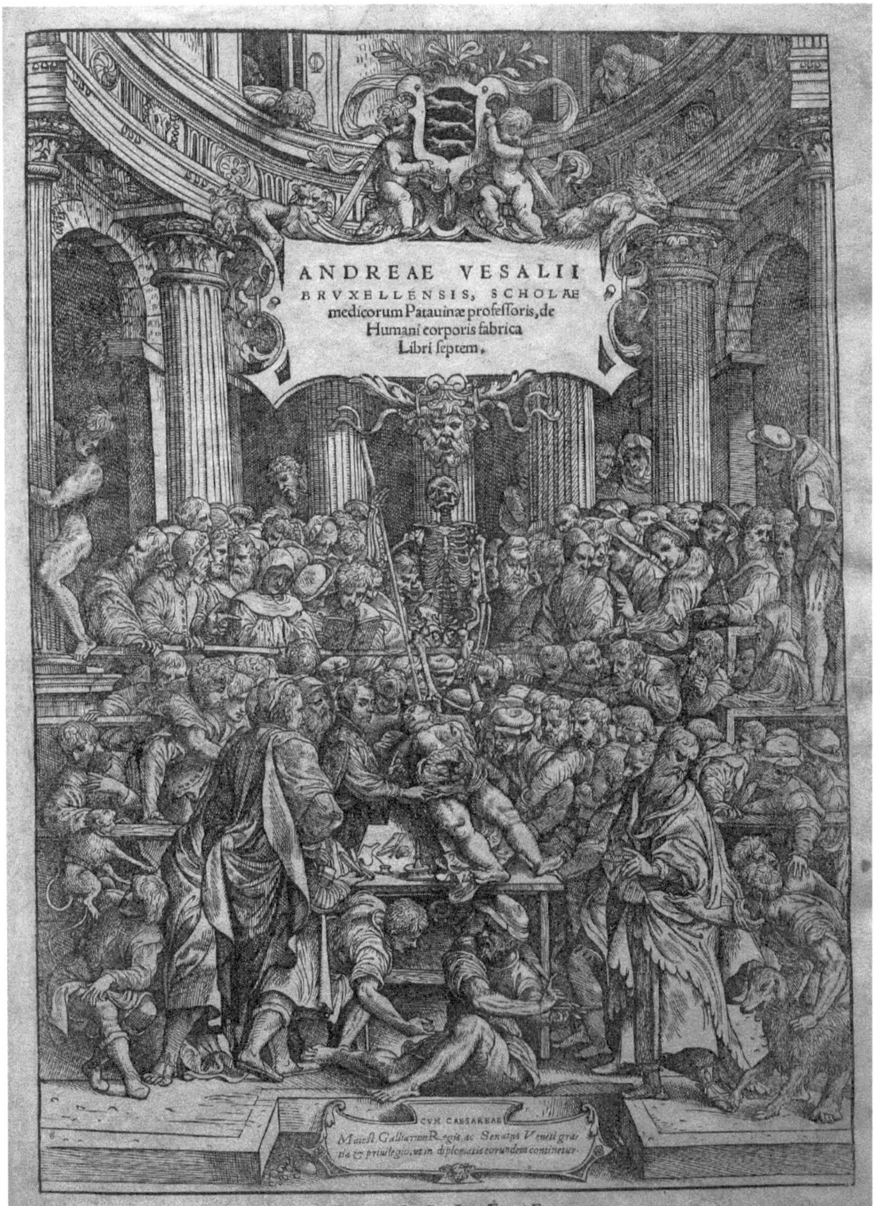

Figure 1a Frontispiece (woodcut) of Vesalius' *De Humani Corporis Fabrica Libri Septem* (1543). It displays Vesalius in the middle of an anatomical theatre, dissecting a *female* cadaver (digital collection of the Münchener Digitalisierungszentrum, open access; see also Saunders/O'Malley 1973, 43).

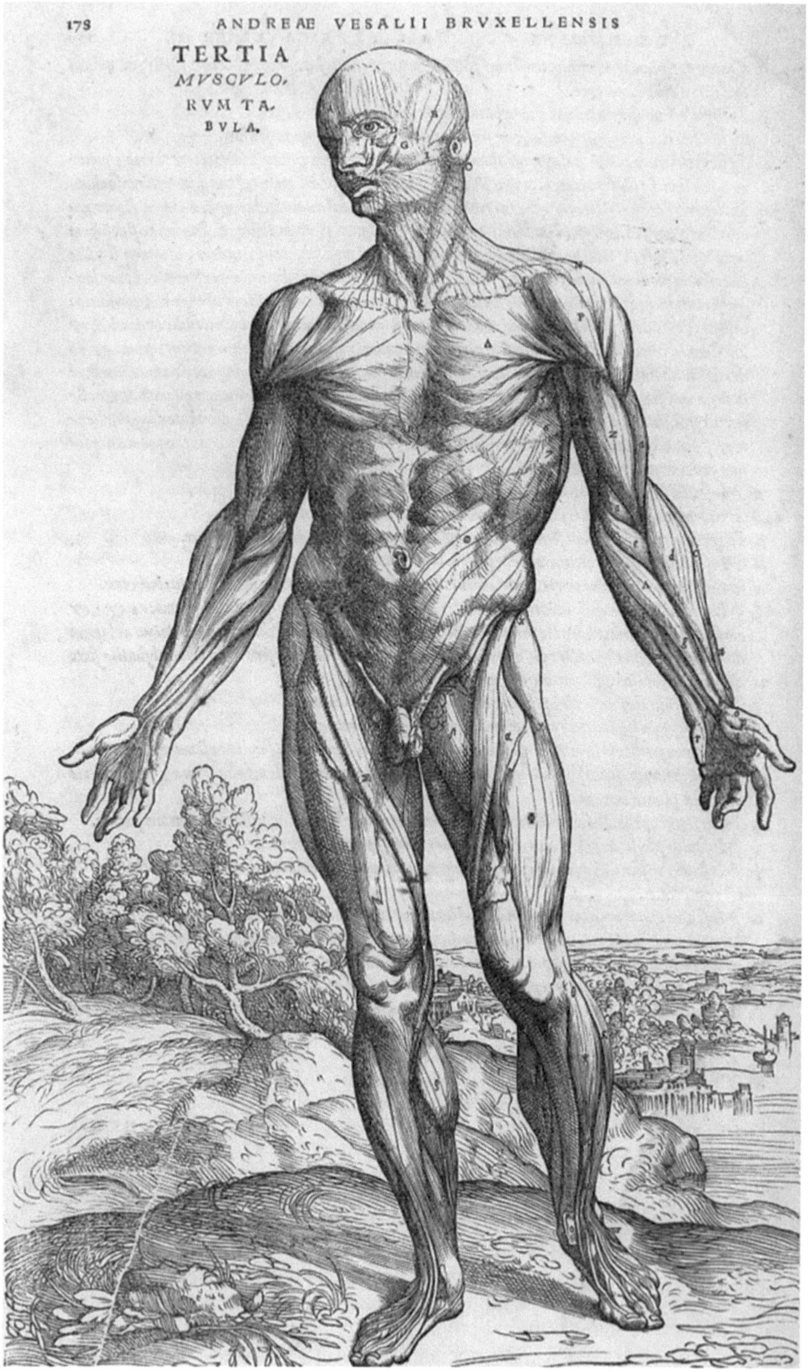

Figure 1b Excerpts from Vesalius' *De Humani*. Almost all illustrations show male bodies as the normative model of the human physique (digital collection of the Münchener Digitalisierungszentrum, open access; see also Saunders/O'Malley 1973, 95, 99).

This "gross corporeality" was one of the reasons why the Cartesian dualism or the "doctrine of mind over matter" continued to flourish (Porter 2004, 26). While to us, as Porter continues, processes of the mind seem to be more easily accessible, we cannot see or feel "what is going on inside" the body without the aid of dissection or autopsy, the latter a word that literally means "to look into one's self" (Porter 2004, 44). Bodies, or the internal parts and processes thereof, thus needed to be "mediated" through scientific and medical ideas, a practice that is as old as classical antiquity (Porter 2004, 44). Though theories of the body were "in flux" during the Enlightenment and often contradicted one another, in reality, many natural philosophers simply poured "old wine into new bottles" (Porter 2004, 54).[5] What can be said for sure is that René Descartes' philosophy certainly contributed to the rise of the individual and its autonomy; however, it achieved this at the cost of the body by "reducing [it] to [a] mere 'extension'" of the soul, thus "creat[ing] more problems than it solved" (Porter 2004, 60). Furthermore, the rise of individualism did not pertain to all individuals. It was highly gendered and mainly applied to men.

Therefore, the 'body trouble' Porter implies especially seems to hold true for the female body, reproductive in particular. Not only does the division between body and mind pose a general problem from a feminist perspective as the philosopher and physicist Evelyn Fox Keller has argued,[6] but in light of Porter's observations it is the female body – due to femininity's association with corporeality – that is rendered a 'mere extension' of the masculine connoted mind. Ironically, femininity's 'downgrade' to flesh also manifests itself in powerful myths such as the 'maternal imagination,' the idea that the mother is able to influence her unborn child's body (which is in turn part of herself). Contrary to the Cartesian dualism, this myth reconnects the mind with the body while simultaneously denying female reason or rationality that is reserved for (medical) men only. At the same time, the association between women and nature or body also offers a certain degree of agency, as scholars like Jenifer Buckley (2017) have argued. As opposed to the sphere of myth, for instance, in the field of eighteenth-century medicine and reproduction, the mind and body were considered separately. Moreover, the maternal subject began to be erased by displaying it not as an autonomous person but as a collection of fragmented and inert body parts. In order to understand this erasure of embodiment, it is necessary to take a closer look at the history of sex and sexuality.

1.2.2 Histories of Sex & Sexuality

The history of reproduction needs to be read against the backdrop of shifting understandings of sex and sexuality. One of the best-known scholars to deal with this issue is the French philosopher and historian Michel Foucault. In the first volume of his study *History of Sexuality – The Will to Knowledge* ([1976] 1978), Foucault discounts the hitherto dominant hypothesis that people of the Western world had mainly repressed their sexuality from the seventeenth until the twentieth century.

On the contrary, he argues that especially the eighteenth and nineteenth centuries were characterised by a heightened interest in sex and sexuality because of new developments in the fields of science and medicine (Foucault [1976] 1978, 30; see also Waddington 2011, 3). Foucault, however, does not participate in a discussion of how the history of sexuality was (and still is) entangled with discursive formations of the reproductive body. This is all the more surprising given the fact that his main focus is on power as a means to control and thus discursively create bodies in the first place.

The cultural and science historian Thomas Laqueur first attempts to close this gap in *The Making of the Modern Body* (1987). In this volume, Laqueur and his co-author, the historian and Victorianist Catherine Gallagher, equally acknowledge the body's historicity while also taking into account discursive constructions of the (female) reproductive body.[7] Laqueur extends his thoughts on the reproductive body, both male and female, in his subsequent and well-known monograph *Making Sex: Body and Gender from the Greeks to Freud* ([1990] 1992). He highlights that especially the eighteenth century saw a "radical [...] reinterpretation of the female body" through the gradual replacement of the so-called "one-sex model" by the "two-sex model," acknowledging the existence of (at least) more than one sex (Laqueur 1992, 4, 8). This seemingly revolutionary insight, however, was not as new as commonly assumed. In order to even further emphasise pluralistic (and dualistic) discourses of the body and reproduction, we need to take a brief step back and shed light on previous periods.

Different theories of reproduction already proliferated in classical antiquity and were revived in the following centuries. As the literary scholar Carolyn D. Williams points out, while Aristotle claimed that the "male provided seed" and the "female only a growth medium," Hippocrates expressed that "both sexes contribute seed to the child" (Williams 2012, 17). Although Galen took up the idea, this "two-seed [or two-soul] theory" actually ignored the fact that both parental units "contribut[ed] equally" to reproduction by comparing semen to an (active) "great sculptor" in the (passive) womb (Williams 2013, 17). Throughout the seventeenth century, ideas emerged about how all "life emerged from eggs in the mother's body," thus enabling the "theory later known as 'ovarism' or 'ovism'" (Williams 2012, 17). This theory, however, did not contribute to the elevation of the female reproductive body. Instead, it fostered the Aristotelian belief that the "mother contributed only matter, while the father provided form and spirit" (Williams 2012, 17). Interestingly, in the seventeenth century, Dutch scientists claimed to have "discovered living creatures in spermatic fluid" that they called "*animalculi* (little animals)" or "*homunculi* (little men)" (Williams 2012, 18). Thus, the two conflicting belief systems of the *ovists* and *animalculists* emerged, while their agents fought over discursive power.

To return to Laqueur and the body as a whole, he argues that until the eighteenth century, both natural philosophers and medical experts believed in the existence of one (default) sex only – the male – whereby the female reproductive organs were regarded as an inwardly reversed and thus inferior version of "the

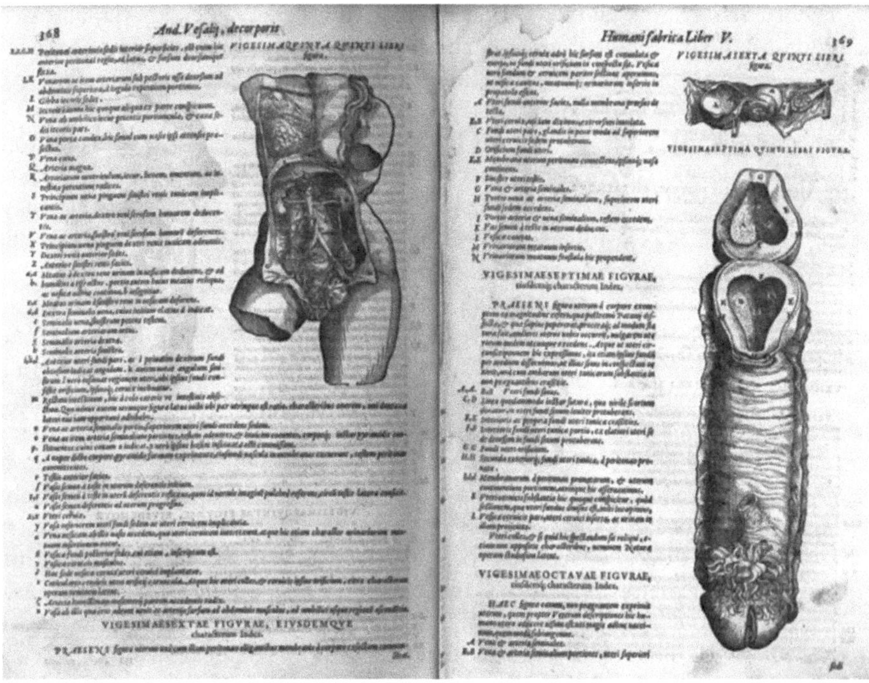

Figure 2 One of the very few illustrations in Vesalius's *De Humani* displays a female torso (left) and a vagina (right) that confirms the one-sex model elaborated by Laqueur and others (digital collection of the Münchener Digitalisierungszentrum, open access; see also Saunders/O'Malley 1973, 171, 173).

same genitals" (Laqueur 1992, 4). By the turn of the century, anatomists and all kinds of authors had (again) accepted a more dualistic understanding of the sexes, which also resulted in a "radical reframing of sexuality" (Laqueur 2012, 806; see also Laqueur 1992, 5) (Figure 2). (Un)Surprisingly, this shift did just as little to advance equality between the sexes: Since the female orgasm had been rendered superfluous for conception in the course of these new insights as opposed to earlier discourses, the main responsibility for becoming pregnant – or avoiding pregnancy altogether – was placed with women "whose [sexual] desires knew no bounds" (Laqueur 1992, 4; see also Laqueur 1987).

In her pivotal book with the telling title *The One-Sex Body on Trial: The Classical and Early Modern* (2013), the medical historian and classical scholar Helen King, however, heavily criticises Laqueur's theory of a shift from a one- to a two-sex model in the eighteenth century. She claims not only that Laqueur ignores or "omits" sources but also that, through a "selective use of 'evidence'," his "model reduces complexity to simplicity" and is therefore "misleading in many ways" (King 2013, xi, 1). For example, according to King, he focussed too much on the idea, first expressed by the Greco-Roman physician Galen (2 AD) and later taken up by the bishop of Emesa, Nemesius (4 AD), that "women had the same genitals as men," while ignoring that "in fact, this is a relatively isolated reference" (Laqueur [1990] 1992, 4; King 2013, 2;).

In general, King criticises Laqueur for "dismissing apparent divergences" from this one-sex model in the centuries preceding the eighteenth (King 2013, 3–4). She goes so far as to argue that, by quoting Katharine Park and Robert A. Nye's review of *Making Sex* titled "Destiny is Anatomy" (1991), "a more complete reading of the sources shows that there was never a one-sex model in Laqueur's sense" (Park and Nye 1991, 54; King 2013, 7). King explains that the "book's main attraction lies in what Stephanie Browner's [book] review calls its 'simple and compelling argument'" (Browner 1992, 221; King 2013, 14;). She adds with reference to Dror Wahrman's article on gender history in the seventeenth and eighteenth centuries, that Laqueur's book is a "seductively straightforward narrative" due to its "two-stage narrative" of "before" and "after" this (alleged) paradigm shift that "contrasts powerfully with the more complex – and thus more difficult to grasp – approach" to the history of the sexed body (Wahrman 2008, 586; King 2013, ix, 14).

Throughout the decades since the publication of *Making Sex*, Laqueur's admittedly not unproblematic theory seems to have enjoyed unbroken popularity at least until the late 2000s, with scholars continuing to praise his work as transformative (King 2013, 5). It thus comes as no surprise that even colleagues like Susan Greenfield and Carol Barash uncritically adopt Laqueur's thesis of a more or less sudden shift between two models in their introduction to the edited volume *Inventing Maternity* (1999). In line with Laqueur, they argue that "whereas women were once seen as being physically analogous (though inferior) to men, [...] in the eighteenth century reproductive organs became the 'foundation of incommensurable difference'" (Laqueur 1990, 149; Greenfield/Barash 1999, 5).

Laura Gowing's book *Common Bodies* (2003), however, which focusses on seventeenth-century England, does acknowledge that "Galen's model, powerful and far-reaching as it was, was never the only way of understanding the body," and that the "comparison of women's bodies to men's was part of a heterogeneous corpus of ideas and arguments" (Gowing 2003, 19). Almost a quarter of a century after Laqueur published *Making Sex*, Helen King refuted this indeed quite seductive narrative of 'before' and 'after' once and for all by means of a monograph devoted entirely to putting the one-sex model, and not least Laqueur, on trial.

To gain an even more comprehensive view of how the reproductive body was understood during the eighteenth century, it is also necessary to ask what kind of language was used to describe pregnancy, birth and reproduction in general. Around the time Laqueur and Gallagher released *The Making of the Modern Body*, the feminist anthropologist of science Emily Martin published *The Woman in the Body – A Cultural Analysis of Reproduction* ([1987] 1993). This extraordinary study, devoted entirely to female experiences and the reproductive body, specifically emphasises the importance of medical metaphors regarding the understanding of issues like menstruation, pregnancy and childbirth.[8]

In her section on birth, Martin stresses the influence of seventeenth- and eighteenth-century medical metaphors on the understanding of pregnancy and childbirth. As outlined in the previous chapter by reference to Porter, especially during the Enlightenment, the "body became to be regarded as a machine" (Martin 1993, 54). This "mechanical metaphor" had a major impact on the still developing field of obstetrics that viewed female reproductive organs such as the womb as a machine or "mechanical pump" (Wertz and Wertz 1977 in Martin 1993, 54). The metaphor was combined with "actual [material] mechanical devices (such as forceps)," thereby exchanging "female midwives' [feeling] hands by male [mechanical] hands using tools" (Martin 1993, 54). In particular, Martin highlights not only the "metaphor of body as machine" but also the idea of the "doctor as mechanic" (Martin 1993, 56). Needless to say, such associations strengthened perceptions of the (reproductive) body as a passive object to be disassembled, investigated and put together again by active repairmen.

Martin also reveals how the metaphor of "production" potentially rendered the doctor or obstetrician a "factory supervisor" and the woman a "'labo[u]rer' whose 'machine' (uterus) produces the 'product,' babies" (Martin 1993, 57). This is, in fact, Martin's main critique – she questions the language used in those medical texts that justified and promoted intervention during the birth process in order to 'boost' productivity while simultaneously erasing the mother: "If the uterus is a machine being held to certain standards of efficient work, what is the woman's role? [...] she is seen as a passive host for the contracting uterus" (Martin 1993, 59, 61). As a result, the woman was reduced to an object in need of medical supervision. The Caesarean section, therefore, was introduced to secure the "best product" – the child – thus rendering the latter a mere commodity (Martin 1993, 64, 67). It is thus safe to say that the language, rhetoric and metaphors used to describe pregnancy, birth and reproduction portrayed the maternal body as a passive object or machine and the male practitioner as the active mechanic responsible for the best outcome – a healthy child.

The studies on sex and sexuality produced by scholars such as Foucault, Laqueur and Martin demonstrate the discursive historicity of the human body. Regarding Foucault, however, it comes as a surprise that although he traces the history of sex and sexuality, he does not pay much attention to the history of pregnancy and birth, as Penelope Deutscher correctly observes in *Foucault's Futures: A Critique of Reproductive Reason* (2017). It is even more astonishing that Foucault also seems to neglect the reproductive body in his earlier work *The Birth of the Clinic: An Archaeology of Medical Perception* ([1963] 1994). In this study, he reconstructs the history of the hospital and develops the concept of the clinical or medical gaze, but does not trace the 'birth of the birth clinic.'

Laqueur, however, puts significantly more emphasis on reproduction. His study is remarkable as it includes numerous visual images of the reproductive body from the sixteenth century onwards. Yet, Laqueur fails to discuss the problematic relationship between representation and reality in his visual analyses and mainly concerns himself with what is represented on the page. The same holds true for

Martin's ideas on mechanical metaphors. Though she makes a point in claiming that such metaphors reduced the female reproductive body to an object, she equally remains on the level of language only. One has to factor in, however, that science and especially medicine, were – and still are – also exceptionally *material* practices that involve the procurement of bodies (or parts thereof), the dissecting of cadavers and the arrangement of limbs and organs.

In other words – bodies needed to be properly prepared for those who wanted to represent them in drawings or other forms of illustration. Anatomists and artists had to make (material) choices, which culminated in specific visual images; this begs the question of how the bodies' own materiality influenced the way they were finally represented but also how these representations affected the way the (material) body was understood. Regrettably, both Foucault and Laqueur disregard the meaning of matter in their purely discursive studies. As a result, these studies distinctly lack the acknowledgement that the material and the discursive cannot be separated. They mostly focus on certain (quasi-)medical discourses that contributed to both the distrust in and objectification of the body, the female reproductive one in particular, as the following chapters further elaborate.

1.2.3 Maternal Myths & Monstrous Mothers

This chapter seizes on the 'suspect' female reproductive body in particular. It explores the entangled distrust in maternal minds and bodies with long-lasting reproductive myths that reach back to ancient times. We must not, however, think of these discourses in strictly linear terms: Theories or rather beliefs like *ovism* or *animalculism*, for example, that emerged in classical antiquity and were revived during the eighteenth century, existed alongside other myths that all fed into the idea that women and their reproductive bodies were irrational and thus inferior or even suspect. In order to understand the maternal myths that circulated in the eighteenth century and that, as recent scholarship has argued (e.g., Buckley 2017), have survived until today, it is necessary to take another step back and consider selected quasi-medical attitudes to female reproduction that dominated in the sixteenth century and beyond. One text the romanticist scholar and translator Janis L. Pallister describes as both "scientific and literary," and that significantly contributed to maternal myths of the eighteenth century, is *Des Monstres et Prodiges* (1573) (Pallister 1983, xv).[9] This treatise was published by the French anatomist and surgeon Ambroise Paré who, according to Pallister, was not only a fundamental Catholic but also a "philosopher, […] historian, […] storyteller, […] critic, […] philologist, […] moralist" and "demonologist" (Pallister 1983, xv).

Paré was a typical Renaissance surgeon with interests in a vast variety of fields from anatomy to "astronomy and philosophy" (Pallister 1983, xv). He mainly focussed on anatomical "accidental anomalies and disorders, including unusual size and proportion, irregularity, and rare or strange phenomena, in short, all its 'monsters and marvels'" (Pallister 1983, xv). Though the history of describing "monsters and deformities" is also as old as classical antiquity, by the end of the Renaissance "treatises on monsters had become a veritable genre" (Pallister 1983, xxii). As Pallister stresses, *Des Monstres* is to be considered as "*the* book on 'monsters'" and represents a "considerable [...] contribution" to the field of "teratology," the study of physical abnormalities in all living beings, including humans, animals and plants (emphasis in the original, Pallister 1983, xvi, xxi, xxiii). But what can this treatise tell us about the female reproductive body?

In the 1570s Paré became increasingly interested in "human reproduction" and its 'monstrous' outcomes that sparked his "'scientific' inquiry" (Pallister 1983, xxiii). To be more precise, he concerned himself not just with the 'products' of human reproduction but was especially interested in the causes of such deformities. In fact, as Pallister emphasises, Paré's didactic aim was not sensationalism but rather to "naturalize monsters" and the "idea of variety" (Pallister 1983, xxvii). Yet, especially the powerful illustrations added to his four-part treatise that he had 'borrowed' from other studies attracted considerable attention and were labelled "grossly indecent," "immoral," "blemish" and "vulgar" by many of his contemporaries (Pallister 1983, xx, xxiv). However, Paré's noticeable "vacillation between [...] vulgar and the technical terminology [was] not so surprising", as his audience largely consisted of "less[er] educated barbers and surgeons" who were used to such registers (Pallister 1983, xxix–xxx). In addition, the "technical medical language was [also] still unfixed at this period" (Pallister 1983, xxx). In fact, Paré was one of the first to attempt a classification of what we would today call birth defects.

In Pallister's translation of the preface, Paré aims at the following definition of 'monsters' that he juxtaposes with 'marvels':

> Monsters are things that appear outside the course of Nature (and are usually signs of some forthcoming misfortune), such as a child who is born with one arm, another who will have two heads, and additional members over and above ordinary. [...] Marvels are things which happen that are completely against Nature as when a woman will give birth to a serpent, or to a dog, or some other thing that is totally against Nature, as we shall show hereafter through several examples of said monsters and marvels, which examples I have gathered along with the illustrations from several authors [...] who will be quoted as deemed appropriate.
>
> (Paré 1983, 3)

Paré here seems to distinguish between 'un-' or supernatural phenomena such as 'monsters' or "Demons and Devils" as a result of God's "wrath" – and 'marvels' resulting from the "narrowness or smallness of the womb" or "corrupt seeds" (Paré 1983, 3). However, in the following list of 13 and "other causes," he fails to clearly differentiate between the two and also adds causes such as the "imagination" or the "artifice of wicked spital beggars"; this in turn results in his quasi-medical treatise regressing to a collection of myths mingled with anatomic observations (Paré 1983, 3). What follows are selected examples of his 'monsters and marvels' that are relevant against the backdrop of reproduction and the 'suspect' female reproductive body.

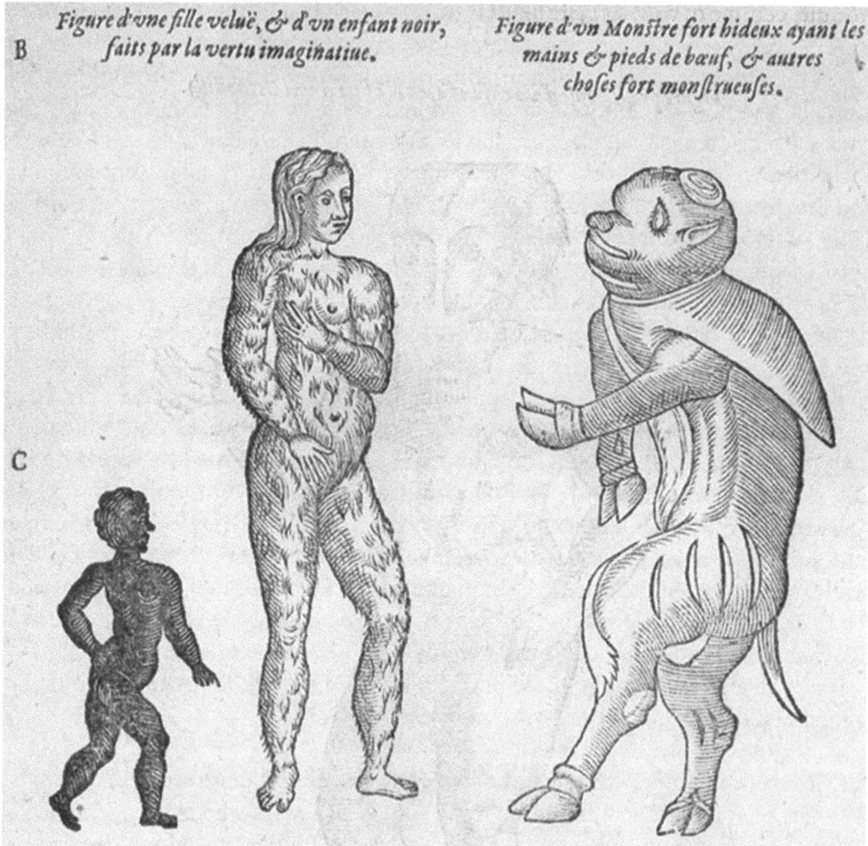

Figure 3 Illustration of 'monstrous progeny' in Paré. The caption relating to the two images on the left reads: "Two figures, one of a furry girl, and the other of a child that was black because of the imagination of their parents." The caption relating to the image on the right reads: "Figure of a very hideous monster having the hands and feet of an ox, and other very monstrous things" (see Paré 1983, 39–40).

In chapter four, for instance, the birth of conjoined twins, as Paré claims, can be traced back to "too great a quantity of seeds [both male and female]" (Paré 1983, 8–23). The same cause holds true for multiple births and "hermaphrodites" as described in chapters five and six (Paré 1983, 23–31). A "lack in the quantity of seed," however, results in a lack of the child's limbs (Pallister 1983, 33–37). Other causes for deformed or missing limbs range from the mother "having remained seated too long, having had her legs crossed" or the "mingling" of human with animal seed (Paré 1983, 43, 67) (Figure 3).

There are two specific examples in Paré's treatise that deserve special attention as they tie in with the myth of maternal imagination that significantly contributed to the 'suspect' female reproductive body. In chapter nine, Paré describes "an example of monsters that are created through the imagination" and mentions that such "causes for monstrous children" were already taught by Greek philosophers like Aristotle and Hippocrates (Paré 1983, 38–42). Paré, however, mingles these apparent reports with religious myth and writes that such occurrences are ascribed to

> the ardent and obstinate imagination [impression] that the mother might receive at the moment she conceived – through some object, or fantastic dream – of certain nocturnal visions that the man or woman have at the hour of conception. This is even verified by the authority of Moses (Chap. 30 [of Genesis]) when he shows how Jacob deceived his father-in-law Laban and enriched himself with the livestock by having rods barked and putting them in the watering trough, so that when the goats and ewes looked at these rods of various colors, they might form their young spotted in various colors: because the imagination has so much power over seed and reproduction that the stripe and character of them remain [imprinted] on the thing bred.
>
> (brackets in the original, Paré 1983, 38)

Paré continues with a concrete example (or rather anecdote as he never provides any sources for his cases) of how Hippocrates "saved a princess accused of adultery, because she had given birth to a child as black as a Moor [sic], her husband and she both having white skin"; he explains that the cause for this wondrous birth had been a "portrait of a Moor [sic], similar to the child which was customarily attached to her bed" (Paré 1983, 39).

Since Paré's main aim is to educate his readers, he advises women "not to be forced to look at or to imagine monstrous things" during conception or until the child is "completely formed" (Paré 1983, 39–41). In another example, the cause for a child "having the face of a frog" was that a woman who "had gone to bed" with a "frog in her hand," and during conception, "by the power of her imagination, this monster had thus been produced" (Paré 1983, 40–41). As a result, the woman is blamed for the child's alleged physicality. This as well as the next case render both the female mind and body suspect.

In chapter 22, Paré reports on an encounter his brother Jehan, also a surgeon, had with a beggar woman "who pretended to have a canker on her breast" (Paré 1983, 74–75). According to Paré, his brother

> saw a fat, plump hedge-whore and beggar begging at the door of a temple [Protestant church?] one Sunday who pretended to have a canker [cancerous ulcer] on her breast, which was a very hideous thing to see, because of a great amount of foul matter which seemed to flow out onto a linen cloth that she had on her front.
>
> (brackets in the original, Paré 1983, 74)

The crux of the matter here is not just the – from a modern perspective – derogatory language Paré uses to describe the beggar woman, but that the focus of this chapter is on the word "imposture" that he uses five times in this short chapter: He continues to describe how his brother suspects the woman to be a liar from the beginning and eventually reveals that her "canker was artificial" as she later confesses (Paré 1983, 75). Paré explains that the woman, as ordered by her "master-beggar," had used a "sponge, soaked and imbued with animal blood and with milk mixed together" that she had "conducted through fake holes in her ulcerated canker, flowing into the linen" (Paré 1983, 75). Jehan had reported her to the magistrate, and once this "monstrous and hideous" hoax was revealed, the "slut" was "condemned [...] to get the whip [...] as one did at the time" and was "banished out of the country" (Paré 1983, 75).

This chapter seems odd for the following reasons: Though the example does describe a 'monstrous and hideous' phenomenon on the woman's breast, the case actually centres on the woman's imposture. What the reader is confronted with is not a (quasi-)medical example but rather a fraud case, conducted by a (poor) woman and uncovered by a 'rational' male surgeon. Half of this chapter lauds the surgeon for immediately suspecting the woman's body to be healthy, while he observes her body parts before he reports her to the magistrate:

> My brother [...] [observing] the areas around her ulcerated canker [to be] white and of good color and the rest of her body [to be in] very good condition, he thought to himself that this wench could not have canker, being so fat, plump, and full-cheeked, and he was sure that it was an imposture.
>
> (brackets in the original, Paré 1983, 75)

What remains of this 'monstrous' case is the impression that male surgeons cannot be fooled by deceptive (female) bodies. Furthermore, this chapter renders not only women's bodies but also their body parts, reproductive in particular, suspect. The only solution to exposing these deceptive or 'suspect' reproductive bodies seems to be rational male science.

There are more chapters in Paré's treatise that describe cases "about a hedge-whore beggar-woman pretending to be sick with saint fiacre's disease [haemorrhoids], and a long thick gut made by trickery [that] came out of her bum" or "about a fat wench from Normandy, who pretended to have a snake in her belly" by "setting [her] muscles in action" – all of them uncovered by rational male doctors, "learned [...] and very experienced" (chapter 24, Paré 1983, 81–82, chapter 25, 83–84). Paré describes these female "beggar-imposters" as "ugly," "full-bummed wench[es], chubby and shapely" who "put on a good show" (Paré 1983, 82–84). He ends chapter 25 by stressing that it is "necessary to uncover them [the women] whenever it is possible, and to accuse them before the Magistrate, to an end that punishment be meted out in proportion as the enormity of the case demands" (Paré 1983, 84).

Though Paré wrote in the sixteenth century, the maternal myths mentioned in his *Des Monstres et Prodiges* survived into the eighteenth century. This becomes especially clear by the example of the following very well-known birth narrative: the Mary Toft case (see e.g., Cody 2008; Harvey 2010; Williams 2012; Woods/Galley 2014; Buckley 2017). This odd event involved a young woman from the

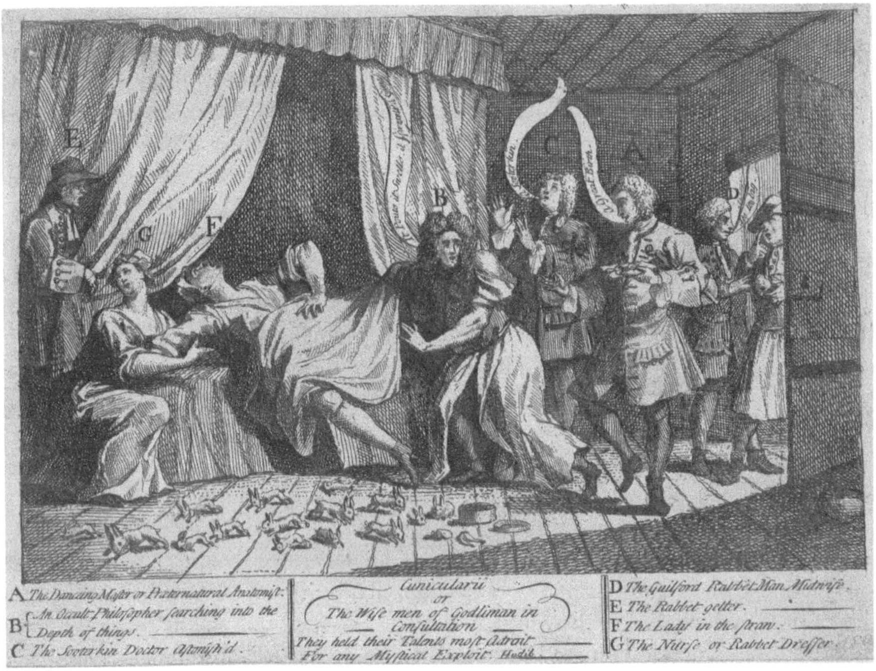
A The Dancing Master or Præternatural Anatomist.
B An Occult Philosopher searching into the Depth of things.
C The Sooterkin Doctor astonish'd.
Cunicularii or The Wise men of Godliman in Consultation
They held their Talents most Adroit For any Mystical Exploit. Hudib.
D The Guilford Rabbet Man Midwife.
E The Rabbet getter.
F The Lady in the straw.
G The Nurse or Rabbet Dresser.

Figure 4 William Hogarth's *Cunicularii, Or: The Wise Men of Godliman in Consultation* (1726). This graphic satire displays Mary Toft, supported by a female figure (left), in the centre after apparently having given birth to 17 rabbits and in labour with the eighteenth. She is surrounded by royal doctors or man-midwives (right), among them Sir Richard Manningham and Nathanael St. André as the captions imply (commons; see also the digital collection of the Metropolitan Museum of Art, The Royal Collection Trust or the Wellcome Collection, all open access).

small-town Godalming in South West Surrey, who in the year 1726 asserted to have given birth to as many as 17 rabbits and professed that she had done so as a result of severe craving for rabbit meat while pregnant – a classic example of the myth of maternal imagination that is very similar to the cases outlined in Paré's treatise. This wondrous case did not go unnoticed by the British medical establishment, and Toft was called to London by King George I. Under the observation of his royal doctors, Toft delivered the eighteenth rabbit (Figure 4).

Needless to say, this birth case is a myth. As it turned out, Toft had not given birth to actual rabbits but rather (dead) body parts thereof that she had apparently inserted into her vagina beforehand. After the fraud's exposure – as with the women mentioned in Paré – Toft was punished, in this case by imprisonment, though she was released a few months later. The more astonishing aspect, however, was how some of the seemingly rational medical men observing the case contributed to this myth themselves, as the historian Lisa Forman Cody emphasises (Cody [2005] 2008, 125). Cody outlines how King George's royal doctor Nathanael St. André, also trained in the field of (man-)midwifery, as well as the Scottish surgeon James Douglas and the elite physician Sir Richard Manningham among others, studied the case. While Douglas and Manningham had strong doubts about Mary Toft's claims, it was Nathanael St. André who believed his female patient and immediately published on this wondrous occurrence. Unsurprisingly, this caused severe damage to his reputation and St. André never fully recovered from rushing into print after the fraud was exposed (Cody 2008, 125–126, 132).

This "monstrous scandal" therefore does not trigger the question of what Mary Toft's body and mind were capable of, but rather draws attention towards the issue of whether (some) "medical men were able to recognize obvious truths" (Cody 2008, 127, 130, 133). This maternal myth thus mainly addresses the gullibility of medical men who had claimed to possess a more rational mind as opposed to the 'feeble' female body and soul. Cody further stresses that St. André had actually "followed the rules of best clinical practice" which in addition questions seemingly rational, objective medicine as opposed to apparent suspect female bodies and minds (Cody 2008, 127).

Most importantly, however, in spite of the obvious impossibility of Mary Toft's claims, "contemporary beliefs about the [...] dangers of pregnant women's minds" survived, especially among the common population (Cody 2008, 130, 145). The most remarkable aspect of the Mary Toft case is, in fact, that the belief in the myth of maternal imagination glossed over St. André's own medical scandal: Eventually, a woman had tricked others into believing her story and bodily performance. In line with Paré's reports, for instance, what remained was the take-home message that women's bodies – pregnant in particular (even those claiming to be) – were to be met with scepticism; only rational male medicine was able to recognise the 'truth,' despite St. André's own scandal, thus reinforcing the idea that pregnancy had to be monitored and controlled.

What is more, as Cody adds, this belief was equally transferred to the sphere of (female) midwifery: Thanks to their "delicate bodily frame" and "delicacy of mind," midwives were thought to be physically and emotionally too close to their birthing women – this supposed lack of distance thus also rendered them suspect from the outset (Cody 2008, 92, 95). Even more contradictory, as Sheena Sommers elaborates, at the same time men-midwives or obstetricians unsexed themselves by "transcend[ing] [their] own sexed bod[ies]", arguing to be able to combine medical objectivity and rationality with sympathy for their patients (Sommers 2012, 98, 100).[10] As Cody claims, in reality, however, man-midwives tended to treat their female patients more like "bodies or body parts," as "silent object[s], composed of dismembered parts [...] lacking subjectivity" (Cody 2008, 100). Current scholarship has attempted to rethink the myth of maternal imagination by acknowledging the potential of reproductive agency which will be revisited in the final parts of this book (see Buckley 2017). What follows first is a discussion of actual midwifery and obstetrical practices. The aim is to further carve out the (discursive) complexity surrounding the history of reproduction, childbirth and its (material) bodies of knowledge.

1.2.4 Midwifery & Obstetrical Practices

This chapter shifts the focus from maternal myths to actual documented practices of childbirth. Its goal is to highlight that pregnancy, birth and the assistance thereof are lived bodily experiences that cannot be grasped by centring on verbal or visual representations alone. Certainly, the research material used to reconstruct these practices also consists of words, representations and interpretations of these. The written material – or matter so to speak – on this subject continues to be important; this chapter's aim is rather to elevate the significance of the body as well as the material processes and practices that are involved in childbirth.

The following segment mainly deals with an introduction to the medical and cultural history of (man-)midwifery, the rise of obstetrics and a discussion of actual midwifery practices (Wilson 1995; Cody 2008; King 2007; Williams 2012; Woods/Galley 2014). Since it is impossible to recite all literary and cultural artefacts that address the female reproductive body, childbirth, midwifery, obstetrics and its agents, the subsequent chapters exemplarily discuss the practices of three well-known (man-)midwives: Sarah Stone (1701–1773), William Smellie (1697–1763) and his pupil William Hunter (1718–1783). It proceeds by concentrating on selected case notes, handbooks and obstetrical atlases and concludes that there is neither a single reason for the shift from midwifery to obstetrics nor were the practices and medical representations universal. It is safe to say, however, that both obstetric practices and representations contributed to an objectification of the female pregnant body by pathologising and also eroticising maternal corporeality. In this context, it is possible to draw a connection between the process of birth and the dissection table as will be shown after a concise reconstruction of the history of (man-)midwifery.

The medical historian Adrian Wilson devotes his research to the history of childbirth by treating it not only as a bodily but especially as a social event. In his pivotal study *The Making of Man-midwifery: Childbirth in England, 1660–1770* (1995), he emphasises that previous to the eighteenth century, the realm of childbirth had been a female-only space before the "man-midwife," later to be called 'obstetrician,' entered the scene (Wilson 1995, 1). Long before the advent of obstetrics, childbirth was viewed as a "social occasion for women," a "ritual" that involved the mother, the midwife and other women, so-called "gossips" in the birth process, thus creating an exclusive "culture of women" (Wilson 1995, 25). Births took place in a "distinct social place," the "*lying-in chamber*," in which the mother remained for another month after giving birth (emphasis in the original, Wilson 1995, 26).[11]

In her book *Giving Birth in Eighteenth-Century England* (2022), the historian Sarah Fox, however, relativises Wilson's claim and argues against birth as an exclusively female ceremony.[12] She reconceptualises birth as a process rather than an event that involved "rich networks of friends, family and neighbours" that "both shaped and maintained communities" (Fox 2022, 1–4). She thus asserts that the "'ceremony of childbirth' was of far-reaching importance beyond the collectivities of women that Wilson identified" and "therefore in the interest of both men and women" (Fox 2022, 4). Fox is less interested in the actual moment of birth and focusses more on the weeks before and after parturition and what they meant for the building of a community. In short, she investigates "what it was [like] to give birth in the eighteenth century" from the perspective of the pregnant women who described their experiences in "letters and diaries" (Fox 2022, 2). Although this socio-historical approach to (giving) birth is an equally insightful one, my book is rather concerned with the medicalisation of the material-discursive reproductive body that, also, took place in the birthing room.

Despite the birthing chamber's "central role in shaping eighteenth-century society" in terms of creating communities, as Fox claims, according to Wilson, access to this room was still restricted: Only women were allowed to visit the mother, while the husband took care of some of the household tasks (Wilson 1995, 27; Fox 2022, 3). Midwives attending the birth were usually married or widowed elderly women "of middle social status," although their rank and age could vary greatly (Wilson 1995, 30). They were generally known for their self-confidence, assertiveness and boldness, which, according to Wilson, was frequently interpreted as "stubbornness" by "frustrated medical m[e]n" (Wilson 1995, 30–31). For the duration of the month-long lying-in, the "wife's bodily energies and sexualities [...] belonged to her; what marriage had taken from her, the childbirth ritual temporarily restored" (Wilson 1995, 29). The birthing room thus lent the mother and her reproductive body a certain degree of agency as male access to both the room and her body was limited.

How, then, did the obstetrician enter the birth room? The answer is quite simple: Male practitioners were only called in case of difficult births (Wilson 1995, 12). These were instances in which potentially life-threatening complications occurred such as "fainting, vomiting, [...] tearing of the perineum, [...] haemorrhage [or] eclampsia", with puerperal fever as the "most dangerous [postpartum] condition of all" (Wilson 1995, 15).[13] In light of these exemplary complications, the question arises as to how often these difficult births occurred. Although Wilson admits the "impossibility of [...] precise rates" due to the few available sources that were published between 1730 and 1781, he concludes that, overall, only 1.5%–2.5% of all births "involved [...] major complications" (Wilson 1995, 18).

Particularly striking is the surprising rate of maternal mortality, which was as low as 1%–2%: As a result, the "vast majority of births [during this period] were normal" (Wilson 1995, 19). Wilson continues with what he calls the "problem of difficult births," reminding the reader that because 98% of births were normal, midwives hardly ever witnessed instances of complicated childbirth (Wilson 1995, 33). Paradoxically, this circumstance seemed to give observers – both male and female – reasons to argue that female midwives were not capable of delivering difficult births at all (Wilson 1995, 33). This assumption was especially expressed by male practitioners whose "work mainly consisted of delivering difficult births that midwives had been [apparently] unable to manage," thus further damaging their reputation (Wilson 1995, 33).

Another strategy to limit midwives' power was to criticise their skills: Male practitioners not only pointed at their "failures" but also were often not able to identify a skill like "stretching the mother's labiae" to increase the pain and hence accelerate the birth process (Wilson 1995, 36). Moreover, while male practitioners saw themselves as trained experts, midwives had gained their knowledge "from experience," and when their practices occasionally did not have the desired effect, it was the 'male midwife' who was then called (Wilson 1995, 36). In short, the male practitioner was only called in cases of emergency prior to the eighteenth century and was rather regarded "*as an adjunct to the midwife*" (emphasis in the original, Wilson 1995, 47, 59). He also sometimes practised techniques such as craniotomy, which involved destroying the child's skull with sharp instruments to remove it if it obstructed the birth canal (Wilson 1995, 49, 50). Ultimately, the "*surgeon was called to save the mother – not the child*" (emphasis in the original, Wilson 1995, 50).

This demonstrates that before the shift from midwifery to obstetrics, birthing women were generally reluctant to involve male practitioners. As Wilson emphasises, "mothers were not afraid of childbirth [...]: rather, they were afraid of *calling the male practitioner*" (emphasis in the original, Wilson 1995, 50, 51). The literary and cultural scholar Carolyn D. Williams confirms that while the man-midwife was only called in case of difficult births until about the end of the seventeenth century, practices changed in the eighteenth: "[I]nstead of being harbingers of doom rushed in at the latest minute, male practitioners became more closely integrated into the lives and birthing plans of the women wealthy enough to afford their services" (Williams 2012, 25). To call the male midwife, then, slowly became associated not only with the "safe delivery of a living baby" instead of a dead child but also with a certain level of class (Wilson 1995, 3; Williams 2012, 25;).

Wilson also emphasises how "mechanical descriptions" of the birth process by highly successful medical instructors and anatomists such as William Smellie and William Hunter led to the inclusion of childbirth into the field of medicine (Wilson 1995, 1, 3). Although the exact reasons for the shift from midwifery to obstetrics are unclear until today, Wilson proposes two possible explanations: fashion and forceps (Wilson 1995, 3). Not only did it become fashionable especially for upper-class pregnant women to hire a doctor or 'man-midwife,' but these practitioners also made use of fashionable instruments like forceps (Wilson 1995, 3). These new tools, although initially "disliked by mothers," were advertised as a 'safe' alternative to the delivery of babies by the hands of (female) midwives. Yet, this 'revolution' in the field of childbirth remains largely unexplained (Wilson 1995, 3).

In her 2005 pivotal study *Birthing the Nation – Sex, Science, and the Conception of Eighteenth-Century Britons*, Lisa Forman Cody asserts that although the shift from midwifery to obstetrics is still clearly "under-analysed," the "revolutionary nature" of this change should not be underestimated (Cody [2005] 2008, 3, 9). Cody's research is important not only because it stresses the phenomenon of man-midwifery as a distinctly British "domestic revolution", but also because it highlights the interconnection of the reproductive body, politics and national identity that "became bound together in eighteenth-century Britain", since children are usually regarded as the wealth of the nation (Cody 2008, 3–5, 11). Furthermore, despite the associated rationality pertaining to Enlightenment thought, "bizzare" myths of reproduction, maternity and birth continued to exist alongside new 'rational' insights in the emerging fields of science and (birth) medicine (Cody 2008, 7).

As opposed to previous historical scholarship that mainly centres on the "triumph of male science" and its aim to seize power over the (female) body, Cody argues that "eighteenth-century men's new-found authority over sex and birth occurred for specific sociological and political reasons" (Cody 2008, 9). Though my book refrains from discussing deliberate actions or concrete motivations for this power shift – as such suggestions are, I believe, highly speculative – it will nevertheless address the (political) effects of this change, namely the elevation of the (male) foetus at the expense of the maternal body and ultimately the female subject.

Regardless, as Cody outlines, male midwives or obstetricians succeeded in "conquering the reproductive body" and especially achieved this usurpation by "asserting [a] rational distance" (Cody 2008, 15). One of the possible reasons for the shift from midwifery to obstetrics might also involve the growing importance of population against the backdrop of Britain's colonial expansion: With a high population, the "English could swarm across and conquer the world" (Cody 2008, 20). It was after this shift, according to Cody, that the word "reproduction" was first used to describe "demographic expansion" instead of the previously applied term "generation" (Cody 2008, 21). Interestingly, Cody not only turns to written historical sources but also emphasises the relevance of (visual) images as essential to "communicat[ing] the [alleged] truths of [previously hidden] natural phenomena, [. . .] such as a dissected full-term foetus, and to define identities and social relationships" (Cody 2008, 24). Yet, her approach is predominantly a historical one.

In line with earlier scholarship such as Wilson's, Cody outlines how, until the end of the seventeenth century, pregnancy and childbirth had largely been regarded a "secret," a mysterious bodily process of which only mothers and midwives had knowledge (Cody 2008, 31). As a result, it was widely accepted that women had "natural authorities over birth" (Cody 2008, 31–32). As potential or actual mothers, midwives' practices, expertise and authority rested on experience, subjective "*feeling*" and "sympathetic attachment" to the women they assisted, while the male practitioner was only called in cases of emergency (emphasis in the original, Cody 2008, 35–36). C-sections, for instance, were not carried out until the early nineteenth century: Until then, "texts ordered male surgeons to puncture, crush, and decapitate the foetal head, and pull out the pieces of [the] dead baby with hooks" (Cody 2008, 40). Practitioners thus put the mother's life first. This would change throughout the course of the eighteenth century.[14]

Cody points to yet another reason for the shift from midwifery to obstetrics in addition to the need to call a male practitioner for difficult births – the rise of gynaecology (Cody 2008, 41). Men did not only "enter British birth rooms" in case of emergencies, but they also secured their "access to female clients" by disseminating gynaecological myths like hysteria, thus rendering the reproductive body (and its reproductive organs like the womb) feeble and in need of medical attention and supervision (Cody 2008, 41–43). As a result, "gynaecology and obstetrics began to meld" and hence contributed to the strengthening of the male midwife's authority (Cody 2008, 43).

Helen King, however, contradicts some of Cody's statements. In her book *Midwifery, Obstetrics and the Rise of Gynaecology* (2007), King radically disagrees with the common assumption that obstetrics and gynaecology originated in the eighteenth and nineteenth centuries (King 2007, 9). She argues that although Laqueur was right in saying that the 'one-sex model,' developed by Galen[15] during antiquity, dominated medical science until the eighteenth century, obstetricians like William Smellie continued to base their work on classical texts such as Hippocrates'[16] treatises (King 2007, 13–14). It is important to note that, according to King, Hippocrates "has always been invoked by those claiming radical difference from the male body and calling for a separate branch of medicine to treat women, on the grounds that there is not one sex, but two" (King 2007, 14). Therefore, King claims that eighteenth-century midwifery and obstetrics did not suddenly discard "ancient authority" – contradictory theories of sex, sexuality and reproduction "could exist alongside" one another (King 2007, 14, 17). She also questions Cody's statement that the eighteenth century saw the early beginnings of gynaecology and calls this claim "misleading" (King 2007, 19). On the contrary, King asserts that the field of gynaecology had rather always been "an area of male practice, theorizing, and indeed specialization, over many centuries" since classical antiquity and did not "meld" with obstetrics in the eighteenth century (King 2007, 19, 23).[17]

King thus strongly disagrees with Laqueur's and Cody's claim that the two-sex model originated in the eighteenth century and argues that in Hippocrates' treatises, especially in his *Diseases of Women*, "we find a woman, every part of whose body is gendered female" (King 2007, 26). She particularly opposes Cody's conclusion that man-midwives, by joining traditionally gendered characteristics like rationality with emotionality, transcended rigid gender relations: "Cody is going too far here; women's reproductive bodies had been available to men, and had been the object of their authoritative pronouncements, since ancient Greece" (King 2007, 27).

These somewhat contradicting studies therefore repeatedly confirm the historical complexity of pregnancy, childbirth and the reproductive body. While scholars consent that language, especially medical metaphors of the body as machine, contributed to the rise of man-midwifery, the exact circumstances of this shift remain unexplained. The same largely applies to the question of female agency during and after the shift from midwifery to obstetrics, an issue that I will seize upon in the final chapter of this book. What follows first are reconstructions of actual (man-) midwifery practices by the example of two major representatives of childbirth and their works, Sarah Stone and William Smellie, before I continue with Smellie's pupil, William Hunter.

In 2014, the demographer Chris Galley and the social geographer Robert Woods published an impressive and unique study on two of the best-known eighteenth-century (man-)midwives[18] – Sarah Stone and William Smellie – with the aim of providing both a female and male perspective on childbirth, whatever that may entail. Their extensive volume *Mrs Stone & Dr Smellie – Eighteenth-Century Midwives and Their Patients* (2014) distinguishes itself from other studies by including detailed case notes of both practitioners that illustrate the challenges (man-)midwives faced throughout the period, the techniques they used and the way they treated their female clients. Woods and Galley's main questions are how midwives actually assisted childbirth in the past, how they handled difficult births, how their knowledge was "established, communicated and received" and most importantly, what progress was made (Woods/Galley 2014, 1). As they claim, these questions have hitherto been neglected, which is why they shift their focus "towards the patients – pregnant women, the unborn and the new-born" (Woods/Galley 2014, 1). Admittedly, using the term 'patient' to describe the pregnant woman is rather unfortunate as it already pathologises female reproduction. Yet, Woods and Galley's contribution to the (social) history of midwifery and medicine represents a valuable addition to the medical humanities as it not only contextualises midwifery practices but also, and especially, emphasises childbirth and its assistance as a lived bodily experience.

Woods and Galley begin their investigation by outlining the birth process as such. In short, they describe it as a "natural" event that includes the necessity of the foetus to "undergo a corkscrewing motion" in the birth canal "in order to navigate its way out of the womb, through the first pelvis [...] and then the vagina" in several distinct phases from "contractions" to "corkscrewing" to the "expulsion of the placenta" (Woods/Galley 2014, 2). Although they acknowledge the birthing women's "considerable pain and effort – hence the term 'labour,'" it is surprising that they begin their study with such a strong focus on the foetus' struggle instead of the mother's, despite their claim to make the mother matter more (Woods/Galley 2014, 2–3). Nevertheless, one of the major strengths of this nearly 600-page-long volume is the confirmation that childbirth usually does not require any or just little intervention.[19]

The volume offers selected case notes produced by the (man-)midwives Sarah Stone and William Smellie in their entirety since Woods and Galley believe that only a "detailed and close reading" of these texts will enable to "enter the eighteenth-century birth chamber" and show "how practice developed and changed over the course of the eighteenth century" (Woods/Galley 2014, 4).[20] The subsequent sections concentrate on Sarah Stone's work *A Complete Practice of Midwifery* (1737) which she published after having already worked as a midwife for over three decades (Woods/Galley 2014, 67–68). Stone's case notes are unique not only because they were widely read by her contemporaries but they also offered a "selective, yet honest, account of her daily doings [and] the challenges she faced" (Woods/Galley 2014, 70). Such information is important as one aim of this book is to extend beyond mere representations of the reproductive body by exploring the actual (material) conditions of childbirth and (man-)midwifery.

To begin with, according to the available statistics Woods and Galley confirm what Wilson had already ascertained two decades earlier, namely that the maternal mortality rate was as low as 1%–2% on average (Woods/Galley 2014, 80). However, it has to be noted that, analogous to later obstetrical handbooks, most of Stone's recorded cases "ended badly" for the simple reason that she (also) mainly documented complicated births: Yet, her purpose was to "demonstrate to other [female] midwives how it was possible to tackle more difficult cases *without* calling in a man-midwife" and thus avoid their "business" being usurped by male practitioners (emphasis added, Woods/Galley 2014, 81, 87). For this reason, Stone elucidates her particular techniques that rely on the use of hands, fingers and a trust in experience instead of instruments. In fact, she emphasises that the "use of instruments" should be avoided *at all costs* to save her clients from "unwarranted interference and physical damage" (Woods/Galley 2014, 87). In Stone's view, there is "no substitute for *experience* and good judgement," particularly with regard to "timing of intervention" in the early stages of the birth process (emphasis added, Woods/Galley 2014, 87).[21]

The techniques Stone employs centre less on vision and more on touch; she promotes the use of her hands and fingers with the aim of "relieving [the] women of considerable suffering by shortening their labours and reducing risks to the unborn" (Woods/Galley 2014, 90). Her priority, however, is always to "save the mother" (Woods/Galley 2014, 93). Having been trained by her own mother for several years, Stone strongly believes in "[l]earning from experience" and also does not shy away from criticising other midwives "for [their] incompetence" (Woods/Galley 2014, 95). In general, Stone favours the use of "her fingers and hands as instruments," although she is also able to "perform craniotomies and post-mortem examinations when necessary" though these very rarely occur according to her notes (Woods/Galley 2014, 97).

Interestingly, as Woods and Galley outline, in her notes, Stone shows "every sign of cooperation" if the skills of "physicians, surgeons and men-midwives [...] were required" (Woods/Galley 2014, 97). She does not, however, reveal her "secret" of how to most effectively deal with flooding (the loss of blood), neither to her fellow midwives nor physicians and only passes on this information to her daughter who she also trained in midwifery (Woods/Galley 2014, 92). In general, Stone pays much attention to her clients' "pain, exhaustion and anxiety" and shows a great deal of sympathy and empathy towards them (Woods/Galley 2014, 98–99). On the basis of these historical notes, it is safe to say that Stone regarded birthing women as living and feeling subjects. It is only logical to assume that most midwives developed the ability to assist childbirth in a sympathetic manner, though this remains more or less speculative in view of this one exemplary case. Stone's use of language, however, further reveals how she viewed her clients.

Regarding her case notes' style, Stone employs a "simple, broadly non-technical language" with the aim of "enhancing accessibility" for all readers (Woods/Galley 2014, 98). Her notes contain a significant number of metaphors while lacking any kind of measurements; her focus is rather directed towards the question of how to reduce her female clients' pains as Woods and Galley further elaborate: "Stone demonstrates empathy with her patients because she has been pregnant herself. She tells her women's stories: *they are her subjects*, and she does not reduce them to physical objects needing to be manipulated" (emphasis added, Woods/Galley 2014, 98). Therefore, Stone's case notes are rather to be understood as a "scrapbook" instead of a "scientific treatise or a manual of midwifery practice" (Woods/Galley 2014, 99). Moreover, her subjective voice further "draw[s] the reader into Sarah Stone's own experienced world" (Woods/Galley 2014, 99). One has to consider, however, that the connection Woods and Galley draw between Stone's own experience of being pregnant and her abilities as a competent and sympathetic midwife risks a re-essentialisation of gender. This inevitably begs the question of how man-midwives and later obstetricians treated the female reproductive body.

As their volume title already suggests, Wood and Galley also investigate the midwifery practices of the famous eighteenth-century and Scottish-born male midwife William Smellie (1697–1763). Smellie is known as the "father of British midwifery" and substantially contributed to the field of childbirth and obstetrics through his four major publications.[22] In these books that all complement each other, Smellie "taught and demonstrated his skills as a midwife, as well as illustrating his work as a physician, surgeon, pathologist, apothecary and scientist" (Woods/Galley 2014, 159). Trained in medicine and midwifery in Lanark and Glasgow, he moved to London in 1739 to "seek better techniques for the safer delivery of mothers and their infants" and also started teaching midwifery from 1741 onwards (Woods/Galley 2014, 160–161).

Smellie's biography, however, shall not play a major role in this subchapter. Rather, the aim is to shed light on the little information available about his teaching methods and how he actually practised midwifery. *Mrs Stone & Dr Smellie* reconstructs Smellie's didactic methods from surviving syllabi and notes by his pupils. Based on these artefacts, his lectures covered the following:

> The theory and practice of that art [midwifery] are explained in the clearest manner. More particularly, the structure of the pelvis and uterus. Of the foetus in utero, and after parturition. The management of child-bearing women, during pregnancy, in time of labour, and after delivery. The manner of delivering women, in all variety of natural, difficult, and preternatural labours, performed on different *machines* made *in imitation* of *real women* and children.
>
> (emphasis added, Woods/Galley 2014, 161; see also Lieske 2008, 261)

Smellie lectured not only on the anatomy of the female reproductive body but especially on the "mechanics of childbirth": "While not the first to use 'machines' or 'phantoms' in his teaching, Smellie's mechanical genius ensured that his models were more lifelike, *accurately* imitating real women and foetuses" (emphasis added, Woods/Galley, 161). What strikes the eye in these passages is that although Woods and Galley, albeit very briefly, reference the established feminist scholar Pam Lieske as well as the historian Lisa F. Cody in a footnote, they do not critically reflect on the meaning of the presumably 'accurate' obstetrical machines; they leave the question open as to the effect of such machines on medical practices or the understanding of the female reproductive body.

Instead, Woods and Galley continue to describe how Smellie, in 1754 after realising the deficiency of some of his text book representations, assigned the Dutch artist Jan van Rymsdyk to produce detailed drawings of the female reproductive body that Smellie published in his *A Sett of Anatomical Tables* (1754).[23] Although some of these images are included in the original case notes Woods and Galley quote in their volume, they largely remain uncommented and seem to be taken for granted. The only evaluation of the images the authors undertake is to describe them as "beautifully engraved life-size figures" and "*accurate* representations of female anatomy, foetuses in utero and some of the problems associated with childbirth" (emphasis added, Woods/Galley 2014, 162). What these 'problems' are and to whom, is not further explained. Woods and Galley do not address the problem of 'accuracy' that shall be revisited later in this chapter.

Based on the transmitted notes regarding Smellie's midwifery practice, it has to be acknowledged that he, like Stone, equally focusses on difficult births, while the rate of maternal mortality is very similar to that of Stone's, close to 9%. In contrast to his female colleague, however, Smellie makes (more) use of instruments such as forceps in about 20% of the cases and calls them "artificial hands," maybe in an attempt to merge (human) touch with inert tools (Woods/Galley 2014, 173).[24] Woods and Galley continue to describe Smellie "employing due modesty by means of a bed quilt" when he proceeds with his examination and eventually "forms his judgement" (Woods/Galley 2014, 175). Like Stone, Smellie claims to use his fingers to give a "precise account of the changing position of the foetus' head" and "appears to be willing to let the birth take its course" before he "wraps the infant in cloths once born," cuts the umbilical cord and "ensures that the placenta is extracted by pulling gently on the cord" (Woods/Galley 2014, 175). Woods and Galley conclude that, in general, midwifery procedures apparently aimed at "minimum intervention"; Smellie therefore encouraged his pupils not to fatigue the mother, to "allow time, and be patient" (Woods/Galley 2014, 175, 178).

Smellie's successful handling of difficult births can be attributed to his "complete understanding of the mechanics of childbirth, in particular how the head of the foetus rotates in relation to the pelvis during childbirth" (Woods/Galley 2014, 178). Woods and Galley also point out that he was the "first to give a complete description of this process" and applaud that his "judicious use of forceps has saved lives" (Wood/Galley 2014, 178, 180). His books were also "written in a precise scientific style" and should be understood as "teaching vehicles [with the aim to] disseminate knowledge" towards his pupils (Woods/Galley 2014, 183). Woods and Galley do, however, identify a "certain lack of social grace" with regard to Smellie's practices and refer to a case where he immediately carried out a post-mortem after the mother's death; yet, they assign this behaviour to Smellie's "relentless pursuit of scientific knowledge and his overriding determination to save lives" (Woods/Galley 2014, 184).

Furthermore, the two authors claim that Smellie was "rarely critical of midwives," while they at the same time praise his "enlightened, paternalistic attitudes towards his midwives" (Woods/Galley 2014, 186).[25] According to the documented case notes, Smellie also kindly offered advice to his male colleagues on how to interact with attending midwives:

> This confidence [to call on male assistance] ought to be encouraged by the man, who, when called, instead of openly condemning her method of practice (even though it should be erroneous), ought to make allowance for the weakness of the sex, and rectify what is amiss, without exposing her mistakes.
> (Woods/Galley 2014, 186)

Woods and Galley indeed interpret this advice as possibly "patronizing" but at the same time remind the reader that Smellie's statements have to be read against the background of eighteenth-century attitudes towards sex and gender (Wood/Galley 2014, 186). While this might be correct, the question remains whether usually self-confident and experienced midwives like Sarah Stone, for instance, were actually in need of such infantilising treatment, generally speaking.[26]

Smellie's legacy is especially and "irrevocably linked" with the way he made use of his instruments, forceps in particular, that he continuously sought to improve (Woods/Galley 2014, 188). He was also apparently aware that his metal forceps, hooks and catheters "could cause unease among his patients" and therefore temporarily "experimented with wooden forceps" (Woods/Galley 2014, 188). Certainly, Smellie was not "without his critics" and was attacked by male colleagues and female midwives alike, especially by the midwife and polemicist Elizabeth Nihell; she was convinced that obstetricians had "no place in the birthing chamber" due to their gender, immodesty and use of instruments that "did more harm than good" (Woods/Galley 2014, 189–190, 266). As the historian Lyle Massey adds: "Nihell singled out Smellie to decry the brutality of the surgeon's forceps, advocating instead the softness of the [female] midwife's hands" (Massey 2005, 76). These attacks did not, however, reduce Smellie's fame and reputation, and Woods and Galley outline with reference to Pam Lieske, that by the mid-eighteenth century, man-midwifery had flooded London's medical marketplace (Woods/Galley 2014, 191).

One final aspect needs to be added though. Only in passing do Woods and Galley mention that the sheer number of Smellie's lectures "suggest that some may have been attended by curious gentlemen who were seeking some form of interesting diversion […] and had no intention of becoming midwives" (Woods/Galley 2014, 192). What these reasons for attending Smellie's courses might have been will be discussed in a later chapter. In any case, Woods and Galley are very laudatory of Smellie. In their view, the field of obstetrics significantly contributed to the development and improvement of childbirth. Though they might be right, Smellie's maternal mortality rate, for instance, is almost identical to that of Sarah Stone who hardly ever used instruments. This begs the question of how necessary instruments such as forceps, which could also cause severe damage to the mother's and infant's body, were (and still are) to ensure a safe birth. In general, what lies at the "heart of the debates about midwifery" are the "power relations within the birthing room" (Woods/Galley 2014, 265). What role medical illustrations played in this context will be discussed in the subsequent sections by the example of selected obstetrical atlases.

William Smellie educated a vast number of man-midwives. One of them was William Hunter (1718–1783), the eighteenth-century anatomist, medic and obstetrician who held several midwifery positions in London and published the well-known obstetrical atlas *The Anatomy of the Human Gravid Uterus Exhibited in Figures* (1774) (Woods/Galley 2014, 267).[27] What Woods and Galley mention briefly but emphatically, however, is that Hunter, in contrast to Smellie, "actively sought fame and fortune by building up a distinguished clientele" (Woods/Galley 2014, 269).[28] Yet, he did not publish much on midwifery throughout his lifetime and rather focussed on the anatomical details of the uterus and how to handle the placenta (Woods/Galley 2014, 269).[29]

Contrary to Smellie's understanding of the "uterus as machine," Hunter (apparently) aimed to increase scientific knowledge of the pregnant uterus in particular and, as Woods and Galley believe, "while this may not have had an immediate impact on the outcomes, their research did lay the foundations for subsequent advances during the nineteenth and especially the twentieth centuries" (Woods/Galley 2014, 271).[30] As Woods and Galley outline:

> By 1770 most male practitioners and increasing numbers of women had undertaken some form of training, the basic mechanics of childbirth were understood and, while there was still considerable debate as to what was considered to be best practice, it is likely that better techniques had brought about some improvement in outcomes. Interest in scientific midwifery blossomed, especially in London and increasingly in the provinces, but alongside these improvements many women still gave birth in similar circumstances to their ancestors, centuries earlier.
>
> (Woods/Galley 2014, 272)

To conclude: In general, eighteenth-century medicine witnessed an elaboration of dissection practices, in particular through "first-hand anatomical study" that especially Hunter demonstrated both in the scope of his "private anatomy classes" and his obstetrical atlases in which bodily layers were removed bit by bit (Jordanova 1989, 56). Yet, the practice of obstetrical representation was not without problems in terms of the pregnant female individual; in the scope of alleged medical advances, the maternal subject was simultaneously eroticised, violated and eventually erased with far-reaching consequences as the following subchapters discuss.

1.2.5 Representational Practices

This chapter already attempts to establish a first link between matter and meaning by taking a closer look at both (haptic) obstetrical practices and their representations. It argues, among other things, that practices of fragmentation, both haptic and visual, reduced the (maternal) woman's status as an individual while at the same time elevating that of the foetus. Considering representation alone, however, does not suffice. It is necessary to *entangle* it with the very real, material-medical practices that contributed to this phenomenon. The following sections thus turn to selected older and newer studies that deal with what we know about the history of science, medicine and gender while focussing on dissected reproductive bodies.

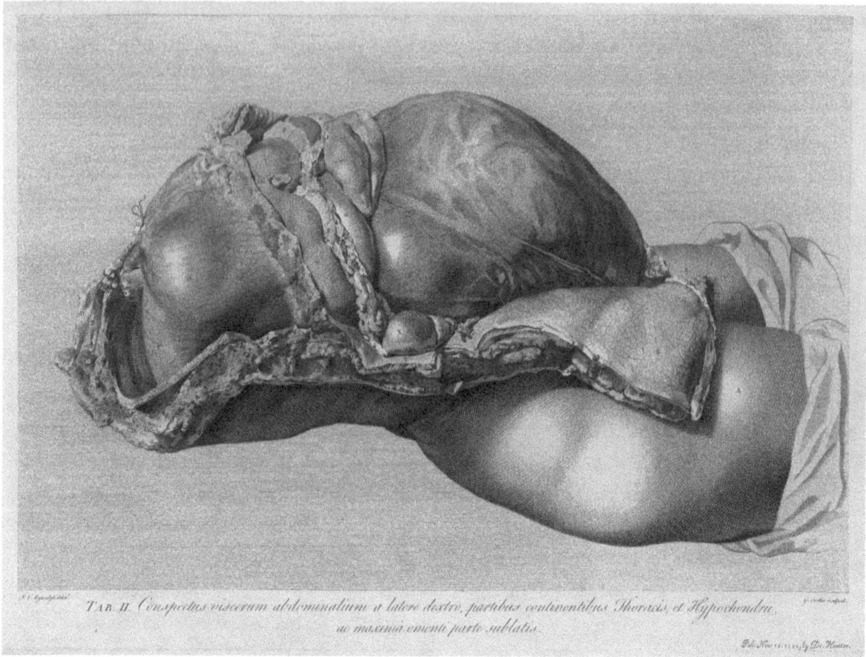

Figure 5 Excerpt from William Hunter's *Gravid Uterus* (*Anatomia uteri humani gravidi tabulis illustrate*) (1774) with illustrations by Jan van Rymsdyk. Plate 2 shows a female torso or cadaver whose abdomen has been opened, displaying a uterus in an advanced state of pregnancy (commons; Wellcome Trust; see also the digital collection of the National Library of Medicine).

In the classic and ground-breaking study *Sexual Visions – Images of Gender in Science and Medicine between the Eighteenth and Twentieth Centuries* (1989), the historian Ludmilla Jordanova refers to one of the plates William Hunter included in his obstetrical atlas *Gravid Uterus* (1774). Plate 2 in Hunter's atlas displays a severely fragmented pregnant female torso, partly covered by drapes, which leaves no doubt that what the viewer is dealing with here is an image of a dissected cadaver. In the description Hunter added to this plate, he claims that it shows "the whole mass of the abdominal visera [sic] … in its *natural* situation" (emphasis added, Jordanova 1989, 47) (Figure 5).

Hunter's addition to this image raises the question of whether a depiction of a carefully draped or artfully arranged female abdomen can actually be understood as 'natural.' In order to discuss this issue, it is necessary to turn to the very real, *material* dissection practices that resulted in this representation. Most importantly, what are the effects of these practices on both the birthing subject and the foetus?

Jordanova stresses that Hunter's illustrations are "[d]rawn from actual dissections […] in such a way that the three-dimensional quality of maternal and foetal tissue is foregrounded," just like a topographer would proceed, hence the geographical metaphor of the 'atlas' for his obstetrical book *Gravid Uterus*

(Jordanova 1989, 48). Hunter thus seems to aim at anatomical 'accuracy,' but since no representation is unmediated, this claim needs to be scrutinised. Jordanova argues that this particular mode of visualisation is connected with pathology, "disease and death, the monstrous and the morbid" (Jordanova 1989, 48–49). What is more, Hunter's illustrations also demonstrate the "multiple intertwinings" not just "between body image and sex roles," as Jordanova claims, but also between eroticism and violence. She distinguishes between three kinds of violence: (1) *epistemological* (or metaphorical by associating femininity with nature in need of being conquered by science), (2) *actual* (or material) and (3) *representational* violence (Jordanova 1989, 60). What follows is a concentration on the last two categories of violence that further underscore the entanglement of matter and meaning.

The second form of violence Jordanova mentions is "quite literal" and refers to both the "actual dissection of female corpses" and the "performance of experiments or surgery upon women" (Jordanova 1989, 60). Though dissection as such was understood as a "massive violation" by many of his contemporaries, Hunter dissected several women who had died in the midst of parturition (Jordanova 1989, 60). What is more, medical violence was particularly directed towards female genitals; though not required to access and expose the gravid uterus during Hunter's anatomical performances, he also "sectioned the clitoris" (Jordanova 1989, 61). Generally, eighteenth-century medical texts shifted their focus from reproductive body parts to more "explicit illustrations of female genitals," as opposed to those depictions of earlier centuries that were "represented in directly erotic terms" (Jordanova 1989, 61). As Jordanova emphasises: "The more 'accurate' representations of the Enlightenment are not indicative of a matter-of-fact acceptance of 'private' parts, but of increasing scrutiny and voyeurism" (Jordanova 1989, 61).

By turning to the plates in Hunter's *Gravid Uterus*, Jordanova calls attention to the viewer's position in relation to the woman's cadaver; it results in the viewer's eye being drawn into the vulva and vagina while the "cut-off thighs, [and] the sectioned clitoris may all be seen as implicitly violent" (Jordanova 1989, 62). The same holds true for Smellie's atlas: In plate 3, the image's "unfamiliar angle" of the female genitals, the child's head and the use of forceps to pull it from the mother's (dead) body create a "shocking and violent effect" (Jordanova 1989, 62) (Figure 6).

Jordanova goes one step further and calls such depictions pornographic, which makes sense if one considers the common feature of pornography and these medical illustrations: violence. However, as she stresses, these representations should not be understood as a way to "sanction [...] men's sadism towards women"; rather, violence and idealisation go hand in hand (Jordanova 1989, 62). She concludes that in "both idealizing and the violating modes, body image and sex roles remain welded together" (Jordanova 1989, 63).

The literary scholar Karen Newman builds on Jordanova's work among others and shifts the focus from violence and pornography to the question of how the proliferation of these obstetrical representations added to the concept of individualism during the Enlightenment in the eighteenth century (Newman 1996, 44). She refers to the impressive and "first and only" collection in the obstetrical museum in Bologna that displays the "entire range of obstetrical knowledge and practice"

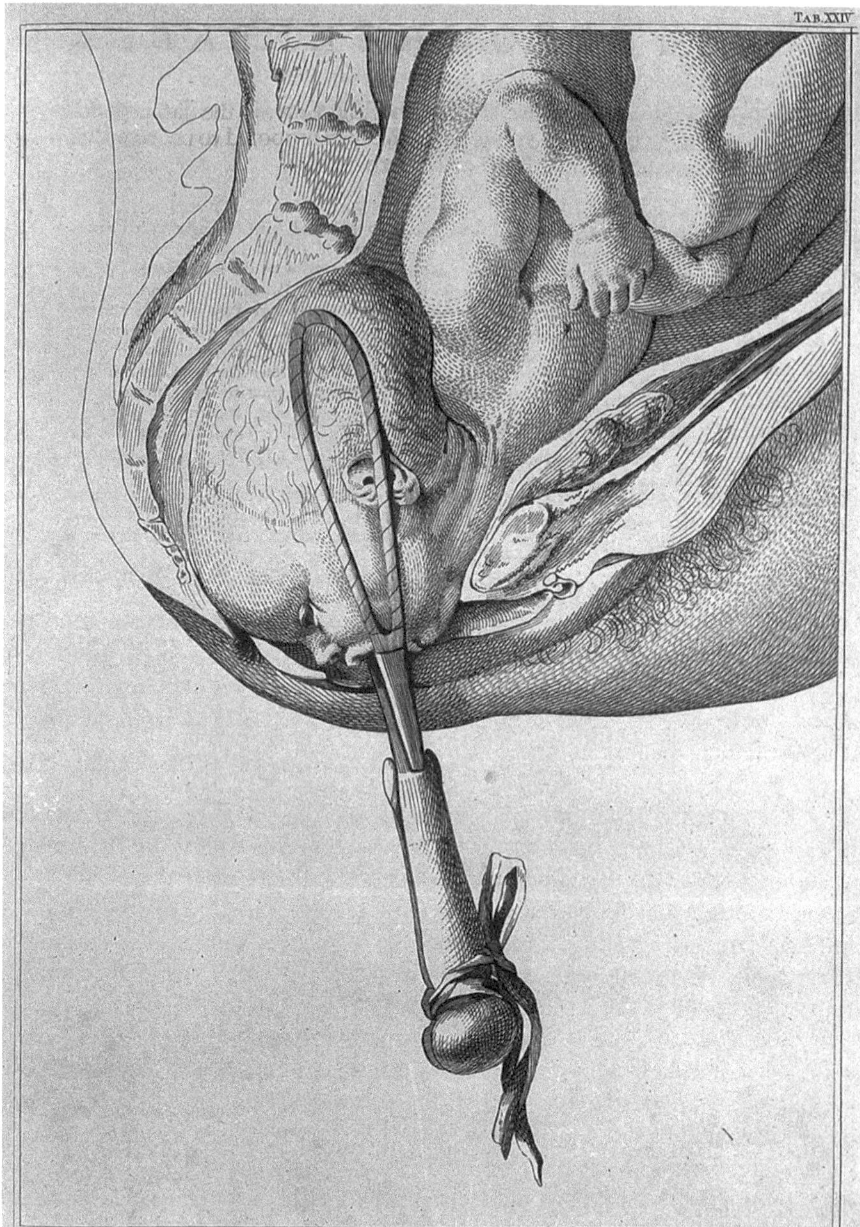

Figure 6 Excerpt from William Smellie's *A Sett of Anatomical Tables* (1754). Plate 24 displays a similar image as described by Jordanova – an unfamiliar angle of a child being extracted from a fragmented female body with dissected genitals (commons; Wellcome Trust; see also the digital collection of the National Library of Medicine).

(Newman 1996, 45). Although the collection was initially meant to educate female midwives, it quickly became the domain of male obstetricians who included the use of instruments. As Newman outlines, this transition from midwifery to obstetrics is particularly exemplified in the frontispiece of *Man-Midwifery Dissected; Or, the Obstetric Family-Instructor* (ca. 1793/1795), published by the English illustrator and caricaturist Samuel William Fores' (1761–1838) and titled "A Man-mid-wife" (Newman 1996, 48) (Figure 7).

The regulation of reproduction through obstetrics started to gain relevance from the late seventeenth century onwards as population or "demographic growth" was strongly linked to the power of the state (Newman 1996, 49). In contrast to female-dominated midwifery which built its knowledge on experience and close interaction with the birthing women, trained doctors were usually "sharply separated from the bodies of the sick, particularly those of women" (Newman 1996, 51). Newman illustrates how the female reproductive body was increasingly constructed as a "series of parts to be manipulated" by the introduction of instruments such as forceps, pelvimeters and specula that mostly medical men had access to (Newman 1996, 51). This fragmentation of the female form led to the repression of the body as a whole that manifested itself not only in obstetrical illustrations but also in wax models; these represented an "abdomen [that is] split open, the layer of skin and muscles folded back, [...] and the thighs mere stubs" (Newman 1996, 51–54). I would like to emphasise that, of course, fragmentation is often a necessary mode of depiction. At the same time, most of the current haptic and visual representations displayed difficult births, thus contributing to the pathologisation of pregnancy and parturition.

The Bologna collection also includes models of "monstrous births" – wax models of new-born infants with missing or deformed limbs displayed in a seated position on little tableaus that were believed to be the product of the myth of maternal imagination (Newman 1996, 57–59, see also Buckley 2017). Instruments to remove these babies from the maternal body are shown in the "mode of photographic representation" that "detaches them from their utilitarian purpose, lighting them dramatically so as to aestheticize and thereby suppress the frequently horrific damage that these instruments could inflict on fetus and mother alike" (Newman 1996, 58–61).[31] As earlier chapters of this book have already hinted at, many of these "startingly naturalistic" and highly detailed representations of the gravid uterus move the foetus to the fore and represent it as a seemingly autonomous "living infant," often resembling an individual person (Newman 1996, 62). The "emotive effect" of this mode is powerful, as Newman continues; it not only reinforces identification with the foetus but also evokes a "'narrative' of developing 'life'" that lends reproduction a dramatic character (Newman 1996, 62, 64).

Such material practices and their representations, therefore, were entangled with political discourses still dominant in the eighteenth century. Newman mentions John Locke's *Second Treatise of Government* (1689), especially the chapter "Of Paternal Power" in which he stresses the right of all "children of men" to individual autonomy; however, as Newman emphasises, Locke refers to sons in particular,

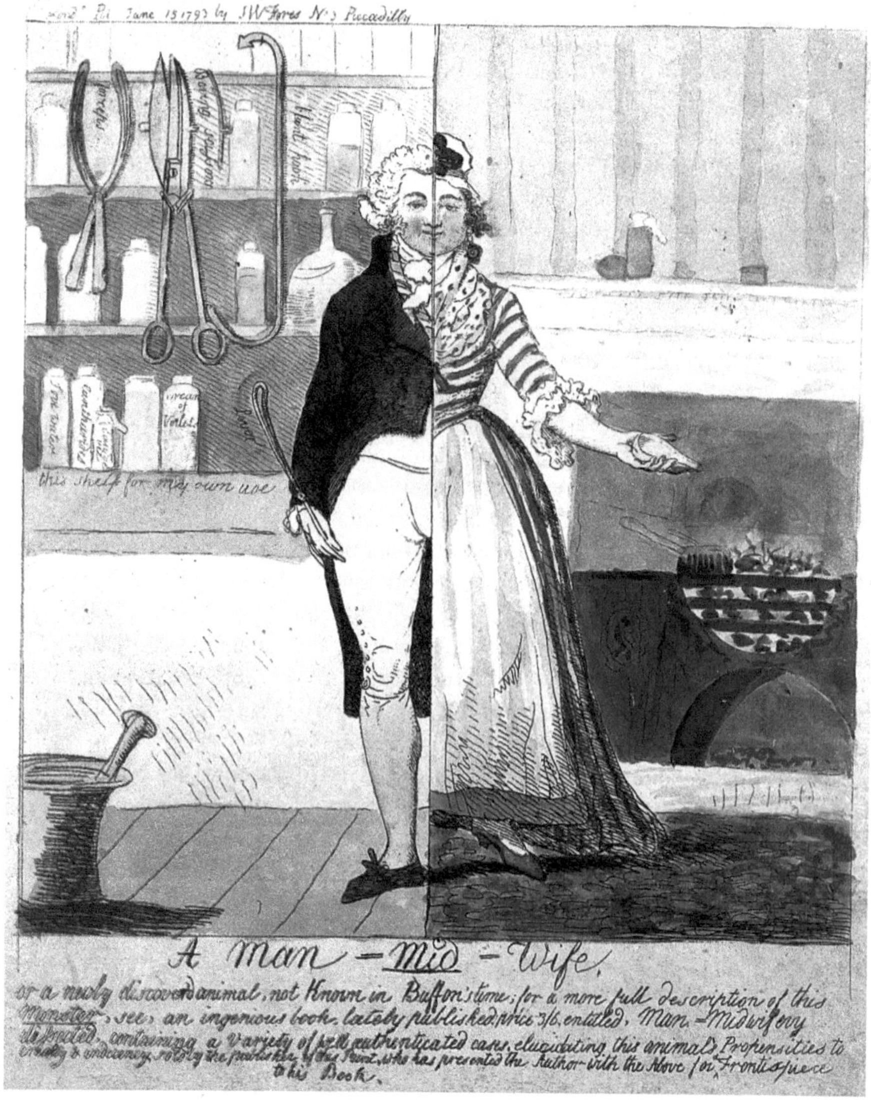

Figure 7 Isaac Cruikshank's satirical etching *A Man-Mid-Wife* (1793). It displays two human figures joined together in the middle, one a male doctor set in an overtly medicalised environment and holding obstetric forceps in one hand, the other a female midwife holding a shell in hers in front of a fireplace and set in what seems to be a parlour (commons; see also the digital Wellcome Collection, open access).

which enables him to discuss individualism "without evoking the woman's body" (Newman 1996, 65). Newman also cites Donna Haraway's study on primates, *Primate Visions* ([1989] 1990), that argues along similar lines by underscoring that "female bodies violate western women's liberal singularity [...] and compromise their full claims to citizenship"; by always being "potentially pregnant," a woman's body "betrays [her] individuality" and is reduced to "men's fantastic self-reproductive projects" (Haraway 1990, 353; Newman 1996, 65–66).

Newman explains that the effects of this impossibility to be regarded as an individual were far-reaching: "Woman's failed singularity – her reproductive body – justified the refusal to extend to women the rights claimed for universal 'Man' and thereby helped to deflect the threat to gender hierarchies posed by Enlightenment liberalism" (Newman 1996, 66). What is more, as Newman continues, parallel to the woman's downgrade in medical representations the foetus was not only elevated to a human individual but also assigned with a gender – male:

> The autonomous human child represented in midwifery manuals, obstetrical atlases, anatomical sculpture, modern medical dictionaries, and new medical specialities is independent of the woman's body, whole and undivided, always male,[32] and virtually never dissected, opened, wounded, or permeable; it is the image *par excellence* of rights-bearing Enlightenment Man ferociously rendered in the fabled state of nature.
>
> (Newman 1996, 67)

As a result, obstetric discourses and practices rendered the (male) foetus superior – a little man with legal rights – but at the cost of the maternal subject. Needless to say, this form of "fetal imagery" does in no way represent 'reality' or 'hard' obstetric facts as it lacks the depiction of fluids or the mother's uterine muscles (Newman 1996, 67). Moreover, the strong focus on the foetus as a "fully formed child" evokes sympathy for the unborn while at the same time preventing identification with the mother who is only visible as a chunk of flesh (Newman 1996, 67). These representations therefore stress "fetal personhood" while simultaneously erasing the mother, mainly through dismemberment, a problem that the following subchapters will address (Newman 1996, 68).[33]

Certainly, the fragmentation of the human body was not just reserved for females; yet, the female body is particularly gendered as it is not almost always pregnant, but poses a threat to the "identificatory process" by enabling identification with the foetus, not the mother (Newman 1996, 88, 97). Newman refers to Hunter's often-cited illustration in his atlas *Gravid Uterus* which displays a pregnant torso and conventional whole foetus (Figure 8).

However, the image of the opened, fragmented and violated female body also shows unnecessarily mutilated genitals that contrast the opaque foetal body in staggering detail (Newman 1996, 98). Interestingly, as Newman continues, "the French word *detaillier* means 'to cut in pieces'"; she thus argues that Hunter's engravings are to be understood as a "madness for the particular, a naturalism beyond denotative instrumentality in which the lavish format […] and excessive detail collapse the conventional schema of obstetrical representation" (Newman 1996, 98–99). As opposed to the foetus' "inviolate intact body," the maternal body is a chunk of flesh into which the unborn is "wedged" (Newman 1996, 101). According to Newman, this "anatomy butchery […] threatens any logic of individualism" by not only functioning as a *memento mori* for the viewer but also reminding them "of the fragility of the separation of inside and outside, self and other" (Newman 1996,

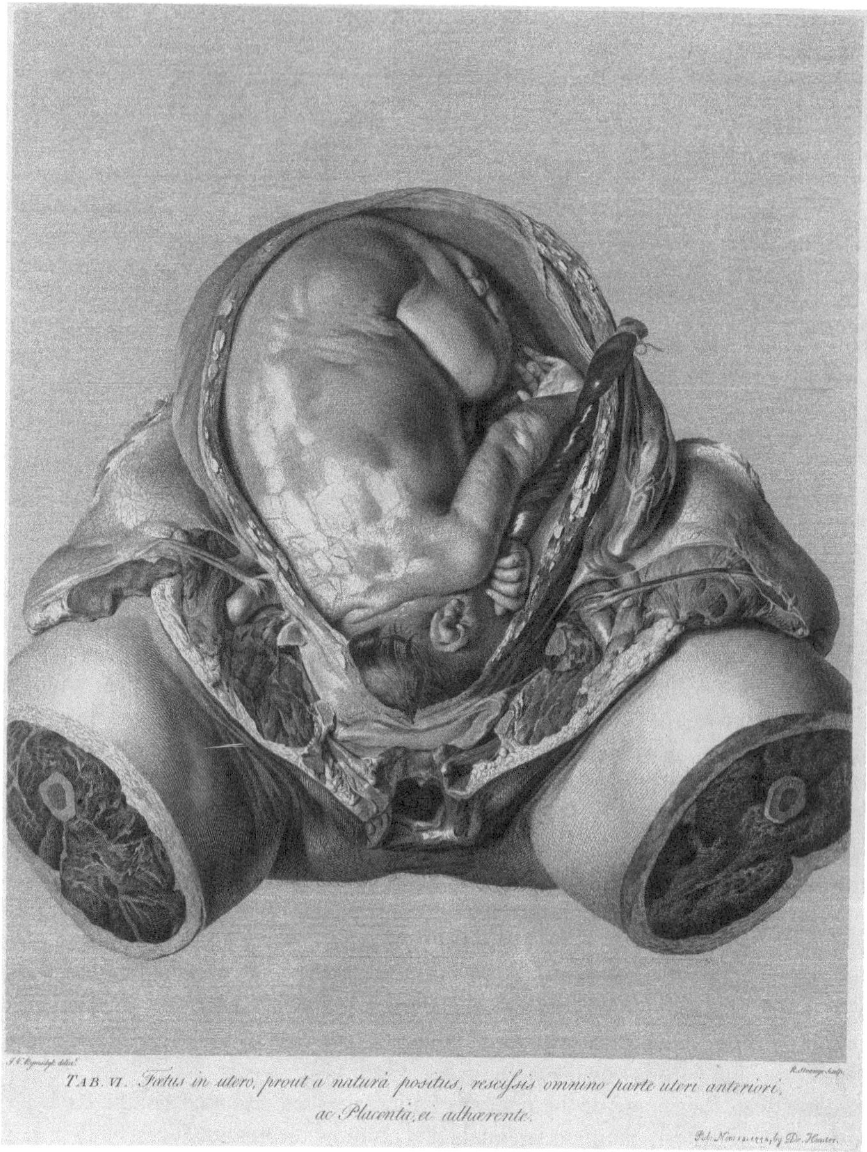

Figure 8 Excerpt from William Hunter's *Gravid Uterus* (1774). This iconographic and often-cited plate shows a severely butchered female torso. The legs are amputated, revealing the bones and flesh, and the genitals including the labia and clitoris are dissected. A fully developed child, curled up in a ball, with dark hair is wedged into the cadaver's centre, drawing the viewer's attention towards it (commons; Wellcome Trust; see also the digital collection of the National Library of Medicine).

101–102). What is more, I argue, these representations are directly connected to or entangled with their very real material practices of dissection.

The art historian Lyle Massey emphasises that both Smellie's and Hunter's obstetrical atlases mostly build on plates instead of (written) text and are thus visually linked to the dissection table or theatre to investigate childbirth's complexity (Massey 2005, 73). Along the lines of Jordanova and Newman, Massey describes these images as "[s]tark, brutal, and fetishistically naturalistic"; they lead to a new form of pathologisation of the female reproductive body (Massey 2005, 73). For Massey, these obstetrical atlases underscore the formation of what Michel Foucault called the 'clinical' or 'medical gaze' in his work *The Birth of the Clinic* (1963) (Massey 2005, 73). Massey also outlines how obstetricians sought legitimacy for their emerging profession by combining midwifery and "anatomical dissection" (Massey 2005, 74–75).

This is exactly where the obstetrical illustrations come into play. Earlier representations of the female reproductive body such as those to be found in *Historia de la Composicion del Cuerpo Humano* (ca. 1560), published by the Spanish anatomist Juan Valverde de Amusco, or in *De Conceptu et Generatione Hominis* (1580), by the Swiss surgeon and man-midwife Jakob Rüff, displayed the gravid female body not only in standing or sitting positions but also in a more holistic manner, "whole and apparently alive" (Massey 2005, 75, 77) (Figure 9).

Smellie and Hunter, however, "break with the conventions" of showing the pregnant woman as a living subject and instead concentrate on the genitals or "pelvic region [...] as it might appear either in delivery or on the dissection table [...] partitioned rather than whole, and, in some instances, dead rather than alive" (Massey 2005, 76). As a result, Smellie and Hunter create a "visual link between [material] anatomical dissection and the process of birth," thus legitimising their ('new') profession as man-midwives or obstetricians (Massey 2005, 77). This demonstrates that obstetrical representations are not only inextricably linked to but rather entangled with material-medical practices.

As Massey continues with reference to Wilson, Hunter, however, centred on 'normal' births and their processes; yet, by doing this, he managed to "usurp her [the midwife's] role" (Massey 2005, 78). What is more, he claimed his illustrations to be rational, scientific and especially 'universal' as he states in his own preface to the atlas *Gravid Uterus*:

> The art of engraving supplies us [...] with what has been the great desideratum of the lovers of science, an *universal language*. Nay, it conveys clearer ideas of most *natural objects*, than words can express; makes stronger upon the mind; [...] an immediate comprehension of what it represents.
>
> (emphasis added, Hunter in Massey 2005, 80)

Hunter elevates the image as a "universal language" that allows for more 'accurate' access to "most natural objects," in this case, reproductive bodies, thereby promoting "visual tools of archempiricism" (Massey 2005, 80). He also refers to the Dutch anatomist, physician and writer Govard Bidloo whose plates in the atlas *Anatomia*

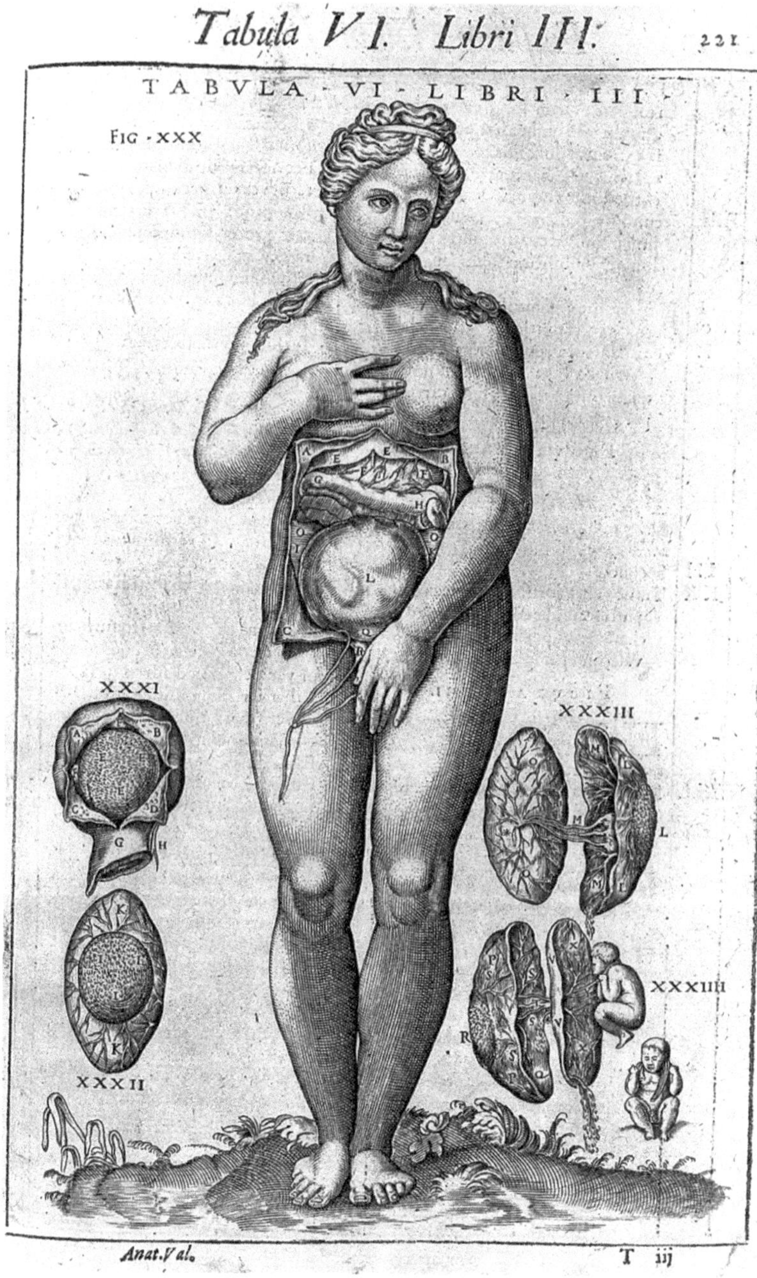

Figure 9 Excerpt from Juan Valverde de Amusco's *Historia de la Composicion del Cuerpo Humano* (ca. 1560). Page 101 contains a holistic representation of a female pregnant body that evokes the idea of subjectivity. At the same time, the lower right corner shows an extracted uterus or placenta and next to it an unrealistic image of a foetus resembling a fully developed little person (commons; Wellcome Trust; see also the digital collection of the National Library of Medicine).

Humani Corporis (1685) are to be understood as a "watershed moment" in anatomy's history as they make use of "new representational strategies" (Massey 2005, 80). What strikes the eye is that Bidloo's plates show not only the fragmented female reproductive body but especially the "actual tools and arrangements of the dissection table" (Massey 2005, 80). For example, Bidloo's illustrations include the "pins and strings" with which the tendons of the material body were separated to uncover the cadaver's musculature (Massey 2005, 80). Massey asserts that this particular representation "transport[s] the viewer into the laboratory itself" (Massey 2005, 80). In other well-known plates, Bidloo and his illustrator Gérard Lairesse also chose to display details like a fly sitting on "anatomical preparations"; these additions make unambiguously clear to the viewer that the represented bodies are "actual cadavers" and not "figments of the artist's imagination" (Massey 2005, 80, 83).

Like Hunter's atlas, Bidloo's work also contains images of dissected female pregnant bodies. Here, too, the reproductive body is represented "as though on the dissection table" with its "truncated [...] head, arms and legs" (Massey 2005, 80, 85). The abdominal wall is peeled off, exposing the foetus curled up in a ball and looking as if asleep, a representational strategy Hunter later adopted. As Massey emphasises, Bidloo insists that his "engravings directly reflect actual dissections," stressing in the texts accompanying his plates that he had changed nothing (Massey 2005, 81) (Figure 10).

Massey draws particular attention to another well-known and often-cited table VI in Smellie's atlas that shows an arm representation during birth. The image is violent: What the viewers see is a severely fragmented female torso, the legs cut off above the knees, exposing bones and raw meat, the abdomen slit open, and in it, a child with dark hair whose arm is stuck in the birth canal while its fingers on the outside of the woman's body clutch a tip of the cloth that is partially covering the 'mother's' thighs. As Massey continues, Smellie "claimed that even though the fetus seems to flex its fingers coyly, the detail was recorded as perceived, not added for art's sake. He implied that nothing had come between the representation and the objectivity of observation" (Massey 2005, 81). Smellie thus insisted on the "unadulterated reality" of his illustrations, thereby making "claims to scientific authority" and "unmediated" representation (Massey 2005, 81–82). This statement is, of course, highly questionable as scholars such as Stuart Hall, for instance, have demonstrated that representations of events or even objects are, *per se*, never unmediated (Hall 1997, 5) (Figure 11).

Massey returns to *Gravid Uterus* and outlines how Hunter alleges to represent a "normative picture of human gestation, reducing the plural to the singular"; more importantly, 'his' bodies are supposed to be "read not as individual cases [or individuals?] [...] but as standard icons of various stages in gestation morphology" (Massey 2005, 82). The removal of symbols and landscapes that dominated earlier illustrations is further meant to denote Hunter's "notion of pure objectivity" that enabled him to claim professional authority over childbirth (Massey 2005, 83). Death is a recurring motif in Hunter's images which becomes especially clear in his plate 6 (VI) – the "dissected edges and cuts seemingly available in *tactile* as well as visual terms" underscore that the viewer is "*participating* in an anatomical dissection" (emphases added, Massey 2005, 84). Massey's considerations allow for two inferences: (1) the impossibility of unmediated 'things' and thus purely objective representations, and (2) the *entanglement* of the dissected body with both the viewer and the representation; they are all simultaneously participating or 'acting.'

Massey concludes her publication with a critique of Michel Foucault's research. She wonders why, given his "concern with how the clinical gaze re-*visualized* both medical practice and the body," Foucault almost completely ignores the proliferation of "late-eighteenth-century visual material concerned with pathological and anatomical dissection" (emphasis in the original, Massey 2005, 85). Hunter's obstetrical atlases, however, are crucial as they link the aesthetics of anatomical dissection with its "ontological" implications: "Hunter's pictorial approach was indelibly tied to the [material] *act of dissection* – the opening of the body to postmortem scrutiny – and the adequate representation of dissection as proof of medical knowledge," thus elevating the obstetrician's status (emphasis added, Massey 2005, 85).

On a final note, Massey makes a slight distinction between Smellie's and Hunter's illustrations. She argues that Smellie's work, in contrast to Hunter's, is "oriented more toward midwifery and dissection" and treats the issue of death "more delicately" by pointing not only to the danger of difficult births but also towards the "*living, embodied* presence of both infant and mother. Neither is shown dead, even though each is featured through the lens of dissection" (emphasis added, Massey 2005, 88). Massey sums up the main difference between Smellie's and Hunter's representational practices as follows:

> Whereas Hunter employs anatomy to deanimate birth and to pacify and deaden the female body in pursuit of a normative account of gestation, Smellie's atlas invokes dissection in order to underscore the relation between the body's interior and exterior during the *active, living* process of childbirth. The two atlases ultimately make divergent visual statements about the relation between the female body, illness, and childbirth, and in the process they also make different epistemological claims about the relation between *representation, practice*, and anatomical *knowledge*.
>
> (emphasis added, Massey 2005, 89)[34]

Along similar lines, the cultural historian Karen Harvey argues that Hunter, by alienating body parts, vests "authority on the medical expert" (Harvey 2010, 47). Most importantly, however, the effect of this representational mode is especially the increasing erasure of the maternal subject (Harvey 2010, 48). Although Smellie's and Hunter's obstetrical atlases differ in their diverging foci in terms of dead bodies and living processes as Massey argues, according to Harvey they have one particular thing in common with regard to the representation of the foetus:

> [both] visualize foetuses almost alive (yet now lost) in an attempt to save the unborn [...]. These are dead babies in a book about saving babies. One powerful response to these illustrations is to want to lift these babies off the page and deliver them safely. Such a response is conditioned by the deployment of artistic techniques of realism.
>
> (Harvey 2010, 48)

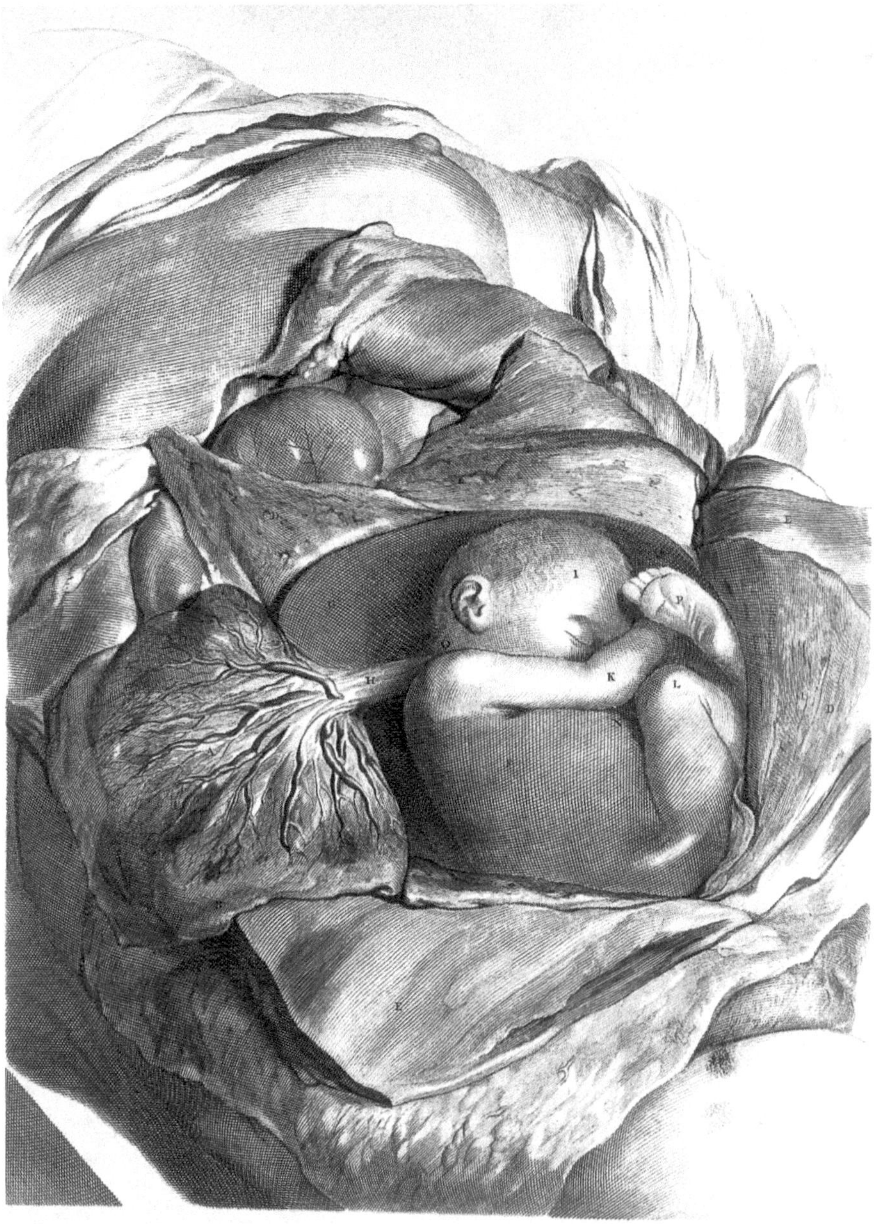

Figure 10 Excerpt from G. Bidloo's *Anatomia Humani Corporis* (1685). Plate 56 displays a dissected pregnant female torso, the layers of flesh peeled off, revealing what seems to be an almost fully developed 'sleeping' child still attached to the placenta. The mother's breast and nipple are exposed, but her head is covered with drapes, thus contributing to the maternal subject's objectification and erasure (commons; Wellcome Trust; see also the digital collection of the National Library of Medicine).

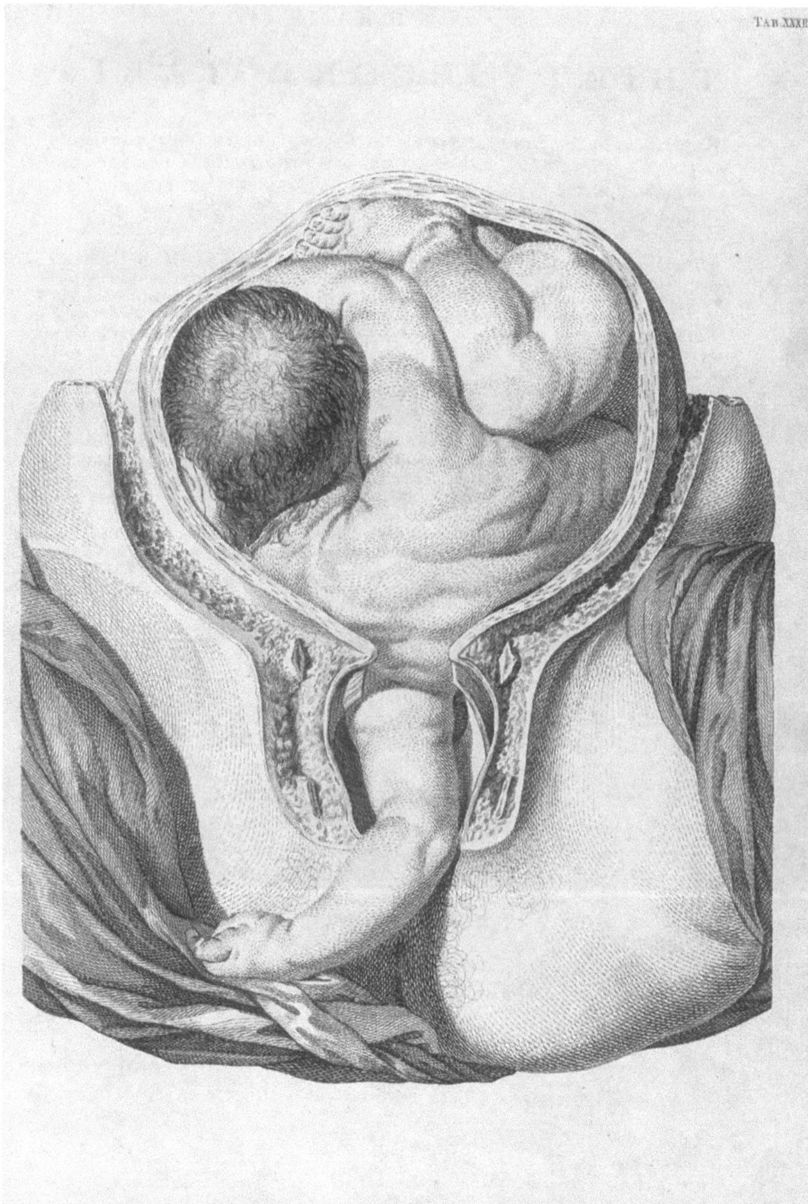

Figure 11 Excerpt from William Smellie's *A Sett of Anatomical Tables* (1754). Plate 32 strongly resembles Hunter's well-known and often-cited plate 6 (VI): It shows an equally butchered pregnant female torso with a child stuck in the mother's birth canal. The image of the child's arm exiting the dissected vagina and vulva and grabbing the cloth wrapped around its mother's thighs evokes the impression that it is still alive and needs to be saved from the female corpse, though both mother *and* child are, in fact, dead (commons; digital collection of the National Library of Medicine).

As Rebecca Whiteley adds in her impressive book *Birth Figures – Early Modern Prints and the Pregnant Body* (2023), these and other early-modern images offer a "peek into the still-living interior" and often even represent the foetus "as a cherubic toddler, with curly hair, big eyes, chubby cheeks, and a self-conscious expression" (Whiteley 2023, 2). Sarah Schäfer-Althaus further adds that the unborn babies in both Smellie's and Hunter's atlases are "perfect aesthetic visualizations of life-in-death," reducing the female reproductive "transcient body [...] to a [mere] carcass holding the foetus" (Schäfer-Althaus 2020, 37). Most importantly, as Whiteley concludes, such "[b]irth figures still form a part of the visual culture of pregnancy and midwifery for professionals and laypeople today" (Whiteley 2023, 3).

So far, this subchapter mostly dealt with visual representations of the female reproductive body. But there is more to the practice of obstetrics and the transmission of 'knowledge.' The following sections introduce a particular representational practice that (further) merges matter and meaning: the obstetrical wax model. In order to fully grasp the meaning of the (material) reproductive body's entanglement with its representations, it is necessary to revisit Jordanova's *Sexual Visions* (1989). In her pivotal work, Jordanova criticises not only Foucault's abstract discourse theory but especially his contribution to the pathologisation of the female reproductive body that began in the eighteenth century. Interestingly, Jordanova already addresses the material conditions of obstetric practice that are interlinked with representations of reproduction. However, she does not yet have the appropriate language to talk about the entanglement of matter and meaning, a gap this book attempts to fill in Chapter 1.3 after elaborating on Jordanova's ground-breaking work in more detail.

Jordanova asks how eighteenth-century medical practices were interconnected with body images and calls for merging the "imaginative realm" with the "accounts of [the] anatomical, physiological and pathological" (Jordanova 1989, 44). Her study offers valuable insight into the actual material practices involved in the production of representations of the female reproductive body, both visual and haptic. Jordanova investigates anatomical models made from wax that were produced and "dispersed all over Europe" in the eighteenth century (Jordanova 1989, 44).[35]

These "Venuses" were not, as one might assume, life-sized skeleton-like replicas of the female body but highly sexualised and overtly passive 'imitations' of women lying on "silk or velvet cushions" with "[e]yebrows, lashes, [...] pubic hair" and facial expressions recalling "sexual and religious ecstasy"; these models also had removable body parts such as torsos and layers of artificial flesh that could be peeled back like the skin of an orange and hence enabled the viewer to look deep into the female reproductive body, leading to a "coupling of seeing and knowing" (Jordanova 1989, 44–45, 47).[36] Needless to say, these fragmented artificial 'female' bodies further contributed to the objectification of the maternal subject. What is more, they added another dimension to visual representation: matter.[37]

According to Jordanova, the "representational logic" of these 'hyper-realistic,' female wax models is that their "meticulous detail" not only led to a "sense of the uncanny" but especially highlighted how (biological) sex and gender were *entangled* with eighteenth-century medical discourses; as she points out, science and medicine's main goal was to affirm the "material intricacy of the physical world" by "exploring and representing human anatomy and physiology" (Jordanova 1989, 45, 47). The mode of 'realism,' therefore, was utilised in science and medicine to demonstrate 'accuracy' which in turn assumed the "supposedly unmediated eye of the camera," a conviction that is highly problematic as outlined earlier:

> Representation accordingly consists of recording or transcribing an objective natural world. This approach is as seductive as it is fallacious. It is [therefore] possible to challenge every one of the foregoing assumptions; that the eye simply records the real world, that the camera does the same, that unmediated perception of any kind is possible, that historically we move ever closer to clear vision and hence to accurate representation and so on.
>
> (Jordanova 1989, 46)

Jordanova further complicates the notion of 'accurate' representations that are, simply speaking, a matter of impossibility and stresses the *entanglement* of matter and meaning when she points out that "[i]n effect, those who offer representations are always selecting and choosing [...] rather than merely reflecting a pre-given world" (Jordanova 1989, 46). She thus calls for critically thinking about seemingly 'realistic' representations of the material female reproductive body. For Jordanova, there is neither a "referent beyond" the viewer nor a "supposedly objective world" that is reflected in a one-way, linear or causal manner of object first and representation second (Jordanova 1989, 47). On the contrary, in terms of the female wax models, the excessive bodily details "add nothing" to the anatomical 'accuracy' of these material representations; "they even form a bizarre and striking contrast to the exposed internal organs and muscles that look like [fragmented] chunks of meat" (Jordanova 1989, 47).

For Jordanova, especially the wax models resemble eroticised "sleeping beaut[ies]" that invite the viewer to gaze into the female body's interior that links "abstract femininity" and 'seeing and knowing' with the "*material reproductive processes* associated with women" (emphasis added, Jordanova 1989, 50).[38] As a result, "[n]ot only were these [...] aspects bound together as an ensemble, but they were also political in a quite direct way" in that they "express relations of [male] power and authority" (Jordanova 1989, 50). In particular, female sexual body parts – including breasts, the uterus and ovaries, for instance – became the main markers of both anatomical and social differences (Jordanova 1989, 58).

In a more recent publication, the feminist and medical historian Marica D. Nichols builds on Jordanova's work and redirects her focus from Venuses made of wax to those found in obstetrical atlases. In her contribution to Jolene Zigarovich's volume *Sex and Death in Eighteenth-Century Literature* (2013), she deals with medical handbooks and focusses on the anatomical Venus, more precisely on the two representational modes of *Venus divinitas* and *Venus vulgaris* (Nichols 2013, 103). She starts by referring to Titian's sixteenth-century oil painting *Sacred and Profane Love* (1512) that displays two female figures "on either side of a well before an Arcadian landscape," one naked and one fully clothed (Nichols 2013, 103). When, as a student, asked by a professor which one was which, she was surprised to learn that the naked Venus in Titian's painting represents "sacred love [...] purity and otherworldliness," whereas the dressed Venus is associated with "[p]rofane love [...] mercenary wordliness [...] greed and lust" (Nichols 2013, 103) (Figure 12).

Sixteenth-century societal order relied on "proper sexual conduct"; as Nichols explains, the "dual figures of *Venus divinitas* and *Venus vulgaris* were an ideological representation of the need to contain and control the sexual nature of women" (Nichols 2013, 103). Needless to say, the dual trope of whore versus saint has a long tradition in myth and (fictional) literature alike; however, Nichols stresses that this concept of femininity also influenced "medico-scientific literature" (Nichols 2013, 104–105). Her aim is thus to uncover the way especially the *Venus vulgaris* manifests itself in eighteenth-century depictions of the female reproductive body (Nichols 2013, 105). An examination of how these bodies were represented in medical texts is essential, as "[i]mages in atlases were not merely an ideal, but the medico-scientific *norm* for how the female body should be" (emphasis in the original, Nichols 2013, 105).

In line with Jordanova, Nichols outlines how the rise of "new realism" in medical texts rendered the female reproductive body an erotic or pornographic object; the medical atlases, she argues, achieved this shift by borrowing the trope of the *Venus vulgaris* as opposed to the *Venus divinitas* that proliferated in most of the earlier anatomical depictions of the female reproductive body (Nichols 2013, 104). Along the lines of Newman, Nichols reminds her readers that the female nude body in medical texts, however, does not just evoke (sexual) desire, but also "fear and loathing" as it functions as a "constant reminder of the inevitability of death and decay – [...] a *memento mori*" (Nichols 2013, 105; see also Newman 1996, 101–102).

Furthermore, Nichols focuses on female hair – pubic hair in particular – that fulfils several cultural functions. Since female sexuality had to be controlled as it potentially threatened the "family, the state, and the soul itself," earlier depictions of the female reproductive body in the mode of the *Venus divinitas* displayed a shaved *mons veneris* (mound of Venus) in order to contain the "leaky female body" (Nichols 2013, 105). As Nichols explains, the shaved female body functioned as a "visual declaration of its subordination to male artists and viewers"; as a result, the "unshorn pubis" represented the *Venus vulgaris* (Nichols 2013, 105). It is thus not surprising that pubic hair is often featured in erotic literature where it was meticulously described as an "important indicator" of female sexuality and maturity (Nichols 2013, 105).

It is fascinating to acknowledge that although the "taboo against revealing female genitalia was deeply engrained in eighteenth-century society and [apparently] extended to medical practitioners," those very "medical men" who sought "professional respectability" simultaneously included such images in their anatomical works (Nichols 2013, 108). Despite accusations towards men-midwives potentially

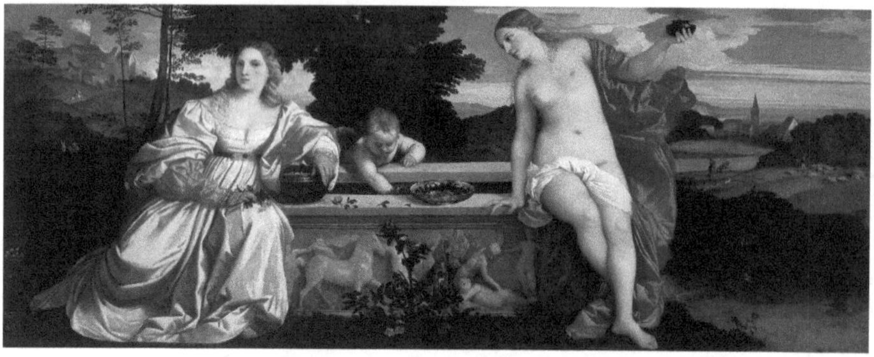

Figure 12 Titian's oil painting *Sacred and Profane Love* (1514). The clothed Venus on the left represents profane love or the *Venus vulgaris*, whereas the naked figure on the right, lacking any signs of pubic hair, stands in for sacred love or the *Venus divinitas*. According to Nichols, these modes dictate how the female reproductive body should be (commons; see also Nichols 2013, 103–105).

acting as sexual predators, obstetricians added pubic hair to their illustrations with the effect that their obstetrical atlases "reduced women to their sex and sexual functions at the very time new ideals of sexual continence for middling and elite women were emerging" (Nichols 2013, 108). In fact, as Nichols argues, this new mode of representing the female reproductive body rendered the Venuses "profane – not divine – goddesses" (Nichols 2013, 109).

Nichols compares images from Bidloo's and Smellie's obstetrical atlases. She points out that the former's exemplary depiction only hints at the woman's pubic hair and also "draws attention away from the woman's genitals" towards the unborn, while the latter's illustration "is straight on," focussing on the vulva "[n]early at eye level" and a detailed drawing of "each pubic hair" (Nichols 2013, 112). What is more, "[i]f the perspective is that of a man-midwife, then the female body is doubly exposed"; Smellie's image shows removed cloth that should have covered the naked body, thus revealing "uterine mysteries" (Nichols 2013, 112). Nichols argues that the woman's "sexual functions" are the focus of Smellie's images rather than the foetus which "blurs the line between the medical and the erotic dead female" (Nichols 2013, 112).[39]

In a final step, Nichols focuses on Smellie's anatomical table IV[40] to demonstrate in more detail how medicine and pornography are linked in these texts. Interestingly, she mentions the medical-material practices involved in the production of this illustration: "most of the images are compositions that Smellie and his artists arranged with prepared female body parts and preserved fetal corpses" and were also used to teach midwifery in his lectures: "In these 'experiments,' the female corpse had become quite literally an obstetrics phantom, giving birth strictly through the efforts of the male accoucheur" (Nichols 2013, 114). Unsurprisingly, the foetus was depicted as a little individual and the 'mother' as a "composite of several dissected bodies possessed by the anatomist" (Nichols 2013, 114).

Nichols argues that Smellie's table IV displays the female genital "opened as if in arousal, the labia and clitoris seemingly engorged, the vaginal opening slightly dilated" (Nichols 2013, 114–115). Again, she refers to the material conditions involved in this eroticised depiction: "This image is clearly the work of artistic imagination – what in reality must have been a desiccated, bloodless hunk of flesh is presented as vital, plump, even aroused" (Nichols 2013, 115). The "presence and amount of [pubic] hair" further aligns the image with the trope of the *Venus vulgaris*, "eager for coitus" (Nichols 2013, 115). Nichols concludes that although eighteenth-century obstetrical atlases claimed to be rational, objective and disinterested, quite the opposite is the case. Details such as cloth and pubic hair – a signifier for profane female sexuality – operate as a visual "frame, drawing the eye into the sexual organs," thus aligning medical texts with erotic literature (Nichols 2013, 115). In table IV, the vulva is the "center point" and thus "complicates claims of the scientific detachment of the image by bringing it into the realm of art" and blurring the lines between medicine and pornography (Nichols 2013, 116).

This subchapter's final section revisits the female anatomical wax models. Though claimed to be produced for educational purposes only, they also served as a "main attraction" for non-medical viewers (Nichols 2013, 117). In fact, the art scholar Roberta McGrath describes these models as an "antecedent for pornography" as they allow a violent view into the female body (McGrath 2002, 16). As McGrath explains, the life-sized Venuses were "exhibited in every major European city in the late eighteenth and early nineteenth centuries" and distinguished themselves from earlier material representations as follows:

> Unlike earlier ivory miniature models which were often dressed, and which adopt a religious pose with hands clasped in prayer and eyes and legs closed, these animated, almost life-like mannequins resemble closely what would become the standardised pose of the pornographic model. These early suggest a sexualised female body that the observer, presumed male, might penetrate. The dolls, undressed and skinned, revealed at their core the 'truth' of femininity: a womb containing a tiny, removable foetus.
>
> (McGrath 2002, 16)

Although, as Nichols suggests, "we have no evidence that any usable sex dolls actually existed, clearly someone looked at the wax Venuses and envisioned the possibility" (Nichols 2013, 117). Nichols concludes that these "quasi-medical displays" merged the medical with the erotic or pornographic, "conflating the 'dead,' exposed, and opened female body with medical inquiry" (Nichols 2013, 117). As a result, the dissected *Venus vulgaris* "promised the male viewer absolute possession and knowledge of the female body" through its "fragmentation and dissolution" (Nichols 2013, 118).[41] What both visual and haptic representations especially did, however, was entangle meaning with matter. This acknowledgement is not new as established scholars like Jordanova, Harvey, McGrath, Massey or Nichols have discussed. Yet, their studies lack an appropriate language to talk about the problem of representation, that is its entanglement with materiality.

1.2.6 Problematising Representation

The previous subchapters that dealt with different representational practices of reproduction – from Smellie's and Hunter's (textual) atlases to (haptic) wax models to representational modes of the *Venus vulgaris* – raise the following questions: What role do *material* practices play in medical representations of reproduction? How are (bodily) matter and (visual) meaning entangled with each other? In order to discuss these questions, it is first necessary to problematise anatomical representations as such before turning to the role of materiality. As the following sections demonstrate, changing representational modes were (and are) not simply the result of an increase in realism or scientific advancements. What is more, they can have very real (gender-)political implications.

As early as the late 1980s, the feminist science historian Londa Schiebinger critically reflects on representations of the female body in her contribution to Laqueur and Gallagher's volume *The Making of the Modern Body* (1987) and offers an impressive historical survey on the female skeleton. Schiebinger outlines how, up until the first half of the eighteenth century, the male skeleton was considered the norm; in this context, she especially stresses how anatomical representations – such as significantly smaller female skulls or larger pelvises – were "laden with cultural values" (Schiebinger 1987, ix).[42] She argues that female body parts illustrated by men in their medical texts "were to become politically significant" against the background of the gradually changing position of women in Europe who were relegated to different spheres based on their anatomy (Schiebinger 1987, 42).[43] Schiebinger contends that such modes of representing female body parts were in no way "simply the product of the growth of realism in anatomy" (Schiebinger 1987, 43). On the contrary, they had very real, material consequences.

In terms of reproduction, Karen Newman argues along similar lines. In her extended and ground-breaking essay *Fetal Positions – Individualism, Science, Visuality* (1996), she contends that "certain modes of visualizing science have profoundly determined 'fetal politics'" that in turn (still) affect "contemporary abortion debates" (Newman 1996, 1–2). Newman especially highlights that, although "obstetrical and embryological images" are never identical, they "share a core schema" – the elevation of the foetus and simultaneous erasure of the mother (Newman 1996, 2). She examines the extent to which the meanings of these visualisations vary historically (Newman 1996, 2). As mentioned earlier, Newman adds to the discourse of sexuality by historicising reproduction's "relation to individualism" that arose in the scope of the Enlightenment (Newman 1996, 3). She argues that it was this era in which the foetus's status as an autonomous subject was cemented. In her view, not only verbal but especially visual representations of the reproductive body significantly contributed to this paradigm shift. Furthermore, the discursive elevation of the foetus's status to personhood survived and still affects current political debates on issues such as abortion.

Newman turns to verbal and visual artefacts alike. For her case studies, she prefers Bruno Latour's[44] term "inscription" as opposed to "visualization", since she believes all "*visualizations* of science" to be laden with "symbolic value" (emphasis in the original, Newman 1996, 8). Also, instead of being fixed, practices of inscriptions are "mobile; their symbolic value or social meaning can be marshalled on behalf of particular interests" (Newman 1996, 8). Newman sides with prominent feminist studies that have described how "fetal imagery effaces women's reproductive bodies" by representing "a solitary fetus" while simultaneously evoking an "erasure of the woman's body" (Newman 1996, 8). In particular, she points to images produced in the second half of the twentieth century that "through extreme enlargement and cropping [show] only [the foetus'] head and hands" to the degree that "the fetal image is manipulated to appear like a sleeping human baby" (Newman 1996, 10). These images thus lend the foetus a sense of personhood while the mother is rendered invisible.

Interestingly, Newman stresses that the "presentation of the fetus as autonomous has a much longer history" than one might assume (Newman 1996, 26). In fact, these practices of inscription had been "remarkably constant" until the dawn of the Enlightenment (Newman 1996, 26). From about the second until the seventeenth century, fetal images were displayed as "likewise wholly stylized, conventional, and unrealistic homunculi [...] represented in fantastic gymnastic postures" and almost always "illustrate[d] a core schema [...]: a uterus separated from the female body and a seemingly autonomous fetal figure" (Newman 1996, 27) (Figure 13).

Moreover, these "quasi-objective" and very detailed depictions were often published in midwifery and obstetrical manuals in the eighteenth century and showed "no indication of dependence on the maternal body" whatsoever (Newman 1996, 28–29, 42–43). Such illustrations depict an increased focus on the foetus that is portrayed as a "'lifelike' [little] 'human,' an autonomous individual" and the simultaneous "suppression [...] of the female gestating body" (Newman 1996, 44). Newman emphasises how these images belong to the "many discursive modes that contributed to Enlightenment conceptions of individualism" (Newman 1996, 44). In this case, however, the foetus's status is elevated at the cost of the mother's; her body and thus her status as an individual is eradicated.

Such practices of inscriptions also play a key role in Roberta McGrath's *Seeing Her Sex: Medical Archives and the Female Body* (2002). Here, she deals with "visual inscriptions of the reproductive female body" from the mid-eighteenth to the early twentieth century (McGrath 2002, 1). McGrath investigates "how the modern medical gaze" rendered the female body "as spectacle, as sexual object"; women thus became "*the* object of male speculation" (emphasis in the original, Newman 1996, 1). "[S]exual difference," Newman argues, "lies at the heart of [the] Enlightenment"; it was the (long) eighteenth century in which the reproductive body was understood as a "new terrain, a final frontier of carnal knowledge" (Newman 2002, 1). McGrath confirms Newman's conclusion that in today's reproductive medicine, the "female body has disappeared" and asks "how and why a living, breathing subject became [...] a thing, an object dismembered and taken apart [...] and finally dissolved" (Newman 2002, 1).[45]

McGrath places special focus on the "new discipline of obstetrics" and analyses the "most widely discussed" atlases by obstetricians such as William Smellie and William Hunter (McGrath 2002, 64). She stresses the "profound effect" these medical books had on subsequent practices of inscriptions and also emphasises how "[f]rom the eighteenth century onwards, there was no question of distinguishing between bodies and their representation; bodies were seen in the terms set out by the atlases" (McGrath 2002, 64). In other words, medical men "learned the craft of anatomy [mainly] from atlases rather than from [haptic] bodies" (McGrath 2002, 64). In line with Schiebinger and Newman, McGrath thus equally problematises these representations to be found in new obstetrical manuals as a means to access the 'real,' material reproductive body.[46]

It cannot be overstated, as Schiebinger and Newman already implied, that medical illustrations, including these obstetrical handbooks and their bodily images, "never were, or are, straightforward, unmediated representations"; they were (and are) rather products of "how men understood women" (McGrath 2002, 65). More precisely, these visual inscriptions represented the anatomist's "view of women's bodies": As McGrath points out, "[n]othing was accidental" – the obstetrician made careful choices about how the reproductive body "should be seen" (McGrath 2002, 65). Many of these atlases represented the reproductive body "as merely a germinator" and ignored the mother both "as an independent being" and as the essential precondition for life (McGrath 2002, 66). Hence, the woman and her body were made invisible as if they played no role at all in the creation of life. Instead, anatomists centred solely on specific reproductive body *parts* and thus rendered the woman "symbolically dead" and "already in pieces," and those who passed away "near to term" were regarded "valuable objects" (McGrath 2002, 66).

Reproductive subjects were thus reduced to inert "[birth-]machines" or "dead object[s] [...] divided [...] into [...] productive parts which could be isolated or extracted"; obstetricians even "cut off and discarded those parts [...] – head, arms, legs – which they perceived as unnecessary components" (McGrath 2002, 66). McGrath concludes that this "violent activity joined engraving to anatomy" as both practices of dissecting and engraving were "material acts" (McGrath 2002, 66). As a result, these atlases demonstrated a "complete separation of mother and foetus," rendering both the "anatomist and the foetus [...] active while woman was inactive" or "inert" (McGrath 2002, 67). This leads to the question of how material or matter is intertwined with representation.

The literary scholar Pam Lieske takes up the notion of materiality and offers a specific and innovate approach to the history of the reproductive body by investigating the "*material* representation of maternity and childbirth" (emphasis added, Lieske 2012, 70). Lieske draws attention to so-called "obstetrical machines" that have a lot in common with the previously mentioned wax models; these machine-like artificial corpora were produced by male midwives for training and demonstrate "the Enlightenment's fascination with the pregnant female body" (Lieske 2012, 71). Obstetrical machines were full-sized replicas of pregnant bodies and usually comprised a "torso with the legs amputated above the knees" (Lieske 2012, 71). What distinguishes them from other anatomy models is that they were

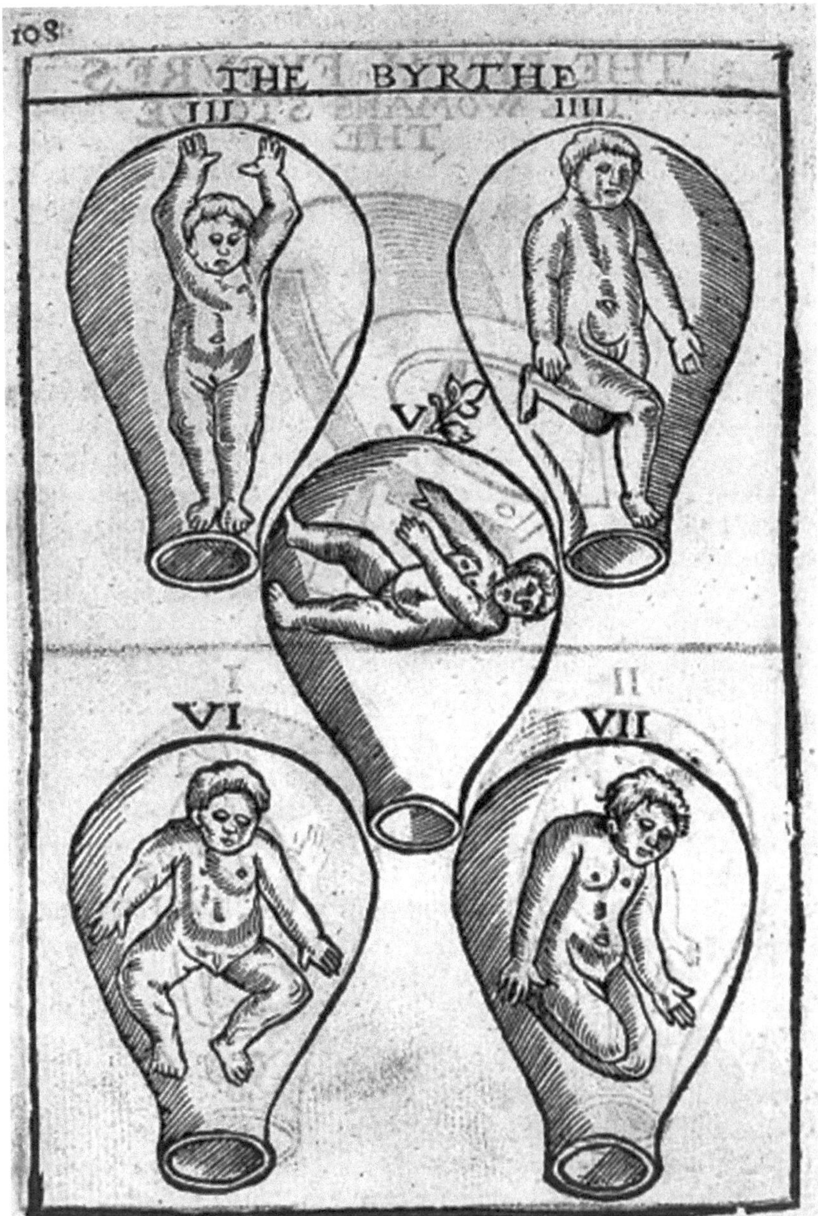

Figure 13 Excerpts from Eucharius Rösslin's *The Birth of Man-kinde; Otherwise Named the Woman's Book*, first published in 1540, reprinted and quoted in midwifery manuals numerous times until the second half of the seventeenth century. The selected image consists of unrealistic representations of foetuses that rather resemble fully developed little 'people' with full hair and adult-looking limbs, "jumping, dancing, diving, tumbling in unfettered freedom" (Wellcome Collection; see also Newman 1996, 28–29).

normally "mechanized, with a frame of human bone" and, as Lieske continues, these "obstetrical machines were to be seen and, above all, to be used" (Lieske 2012, 71). Lieske outlines their material characteristics as follows:

> While a foetus and pelvic cavity were common features in all machines, depending upon the credentials of the medical men who owned them and the ways in which they were used, the contents and technical sophistication of devices varied widely. Some machines may have been little more than a female pelvis with a canvas bag inside, while others were extravagantly built, with contracting uteri, shifting fluid, and orifices that opened and closed [...].
> (Lieske 2012, 71)

Although obstetrical machines as well as all other forms and depictions of the pregnant body could differ widely from one another, they all had one thing in common: They not only represented the way male physicians saw the reproductive body but also – literally – embodied the *material* manifestation of dominant medical metaphors that reduced the mother to a fragmented birth machine, deprived of personhood. In fact, these machines had the same effect as the obstetrical images in Smellie's and Hunter's atlases: They divided the reproductive body into parts and thus rendered the womb an apparatus for the efficient production of infants. One has to consider, however, that these devices were used to train both obstetricians and midwives alike, although the male doctor continued to function as the instructor and thus maintained discursive power.[47]

Other scholars have equally taken up the question of how material practices are entangled with anatomical representations. In her essay "Visualizing Reproduction: A Cultural History of Early-Modern and Modern Medical Illustrations," Karen Harvey formulates a response to a 2007 interdisciplinary conference exhibition displaying anatomical illustrations of the female reproductive body. In this paper, she explicitly calls for recognising the "material medical practices" involved in these phenomena (Harvey 2010, 37). Harvey particularly asks how the interdisciplinary medical humanities can benefit from a cultural analysis of such representations; she argues that "[h]istorians gain a tremendous dividend from acknowledging that medical images are linked to [material] *practices*, those of recording and dissection, for example" (emphasis added, Harvey 2010, 37). Harvey here already mingles matter (the dissected bodies) with representation (the medical illustrations). She emphasises the "choices made in the creation, manipulation and use of images" by medical practitioners and artists; these help to understand not only early-modern (medical) culture but also "current [medical] practices" (Harvey 2010, 37).

It is important to stress at this point that the following considerations are *not* to be understood as a farewell from the concept of representationalism – on the contrary, representations of the reproductive body continue to be relevant. The point this book wants to make is that representationalism alone does not suffice to fully grasp the relevance of certain practices. It is thus necessary to consider not only representational but also *material* practices that were (and still are) involved in the production of the reproductive body's meaning *and* matter. Harvey's essay contains many relevant sections that hint at the problem of representationalism as the *only* tool of analysis. She states that, in the field of cultural history,

> [a] representation is [regarded] not the thing itself but a depiction, a re-presentation [...]. Representations are acts of human creation [...], and as such are made intentionally and with intent. Indeed, representations are constructed to *do* something, and historians are interested in the cultural work they do. Defining culture as a *text* to be read is another important statement of intent. 'Text' does not refer simply to a document; instead, 'text' refers to something that is woven, has texture, and levels of meanings that are not always self-evident.
>
> (emphasis in the original, Harvey 2010, 38)

As Harvey outlines, cultural historians mainly remain on the level of language, while agency is only ascribed to representations; the "levels of meanings" therefore mainly reside on the traditional plain of representationalism (Harvey 2010, 38). The following references to Foucault's discourse theory in Harvey's paper confirm this reading: "a discourse is the framework of thoughts and ideas and practices within which those objects are created" (Harvey 2010, 38). However, in this respect, bodies are repeatedly rendered passive objects awaiting inscription.

Although Harvey is interested in "different 'modes' of visual representation," she recalls that "changing representations are not in any straightforward way the result of improvements in scientific or medical knowledge" and thus argues along the lines of Schiebinger (Harvey 2010, 39). While cultural historians focus on the question of how these representations "reflect and reinforce current ideas about women [...] or even the content of medical knowledge," their goal is also to highlight "how these images worked to shape expertise as a precise *kind* of knowledge" (emphasis in the original, Harvey 2010, 39). After referencing McGrath's, Fissell's and Cody's studies that trace the power shift from midwifery to obstetrics and criticise the erasure of the mother's body in medical representations, Harvey, however, concedes the following:

> Historians are reminded of the rootedness of these 'texts' in *lived experience*: they are *not simply representations* but bound up closely with *practice*. Indeed, we must also consider the *realities* of producing these illustrations from dissected cadavers, which had to be kept fresh while artists sketched each stage of the dissection and also maneuvered them around to reveal different angles. Limbs, not necessary for a depiction of the centre of the mother's body, were likely to have been removed so that less body mass had to be kept fresh and the body could be moved around more easily.
>
> (emphasis added, Harvey 2010, 43)

Harvey, though generally focussing on representational modes throughout her essay, also implies that representationalism alone does not suffice to fully grasp medical illustrations of material bodies. What needs to be considered *in addition* are the material practices involved in this knowledge production. As she continues: "In viewing these illustrations *not simply as distinct representations* or texts to be read, but in a number of specific contexts – the context of *medical practice* [...] – our interpretation of these engravings is necessarily revised" (emphasis added, Harvey 2010, 43). As a result, it does not suffice to consider the "choices made in the creation, manipulation and use of *images*" but also the manipulation of *matter*, i.e., the body (emphasis added, Harvey 2010, 43). Only by making the body's materiality 'matter' more, it will be possible to fully understand how the body's 'reality' and its medical representations are entangled.

As an interim conclusion, it is safe to say that anatomical representations of the reproductive body are not simply representations that reside on the level of language. These 'texts' are also deeply rooted in material practices. It is not just the images that 'act'; the dissected cadavers, the manipulation of both body parts and modes of visualisation, the physician's and artist's intervention and also the viewers all interact and thus lend both sides of the coin – matter and meaning – agency. Harvey already recognises this but does not yet have the appropriate language at hand. As the previous sections have demonstrated, the history of reproduction has been investigated by historians, feminists and literary and cultural scholars alike. While the majority of these studies agree that the power shift from midwifery to obstetrics was rather gradual than abrupt and, most importantly, far more complex than generally assumed, there seems to remain one significant gap regarding the discursive formation of the reproductive body: *matter*.

It is important to recognise that the only available access to eighteenth-century knowledge consists of both verbal and visual texts, in other words: *language*. Since physical matter – bodily materiality in particular – is ephemeral due to decay, what is left for analysis are 'only' *(re)presentations* of that matter. Medical, literary and cultural artefacts thus form the sole gateway to the history of the reproductive body. This realisation is by no means new. Yet, it seems as if not only the body's *materiality* plays a key role in the shaping and reshaping of discourses around pregnancy and childbirth – the material practices of representation tend to have hitherto been largely neglected in the historiography of the reproductive body.

Foucault's work on the history of the clinic in the 1960s and of sexuality in the 1970s is path-breaking in that he identifies a heightened interest in sex and sexuality during the eighteenth and nineteenth centuries due to new scientific and medical insights. Foucault, however, exclusively remains on the level of discourse. Moreover, he ignores the history of the reproductive body in particular and the medical-material practices involved in its representation. The same gap can be identified in Laqueur's studies, published in the 1980s. Although he traces the history of the male and female reproductive body, he equally evades a discussion of the relationship between representation and matter. In the same decade, Martin, Schiebinger and Jordanova extend beyond a mere history of reproduction and offer valuable contributions to the field of medical historiography from a feminist viewpoint. Despite their recognition of language's power to shape the discursive reproductive body, their acknowledgement that representations are not just products of realism and their critique of Foucault's profusely abstract discourse theory, all three fail to offer a way out of representationalism's dead end. Nonetheless, their studies can be understood as a fruitful problematisation of purely discursive analyses of reproduction that seem to ignore the body's material dimension.

The 1990s are characterised by extended thoughts on reproductive models during the Enlightenment (Laqueur) and a concise history of childbirth in Britain (Wilson). Newman's work on reproduction is pivotal in that it particularly emphasises the body's erasure in medical manuals and especially questions the inadequateness of models of representation and reality, while McGrath criticises women's lack or loss of agency during birth due to disempowering obstetrical discourses. In the 2000s, scholars like Cody identified a link between power shifts in childbirth and historico-cultural developments of the British nation, whereas King contradicted previous theories expressed by historians such as Laqueur who had claimed that the eighteenth century witnessed a relatively abrupt discursive change regarding the understanding of sex and sexuality. Yet, despite these diverse discussions, the role matter or materiality played for these presumed shifts still remains a blind spot.

It is only in the 2010s that scholars seem to unanimously underscore the complexity of eighteenth- and nineteenth-century reproductive discourses and demonstrate unequivocally that the shift from midwifery to obstetrics was not medically necessary (Waddington, Williams, Buckley). However, none of them explicitly address the importance of matter in their studies and continue to remain on the level of discourse. Only Lieske is one of the few scholars who deals with (the power of) materiality and childbirth by the example of the obstetrical machine. How the problem of representation can be solved, though, continues to be unclear.

What follows is a proposal of how to find a way out of representationalism's impasse by including matter or materiality in discourse analysis. The aim is by no means to dismiss representation or discourse altogether. The goal is rather to demonstrate why the *material* body is good to think with – or rather *through* – in terms of reproduction, medicine, literature and culture. In short, I argue that a historiography of reproduction by means of a purely (Foucauldian) discursive analysis that is predominantly concerned with one side of the coin – representation – falls short as it ignores the role *matter* and *material practice* played (and continues to play) for the understanding of pregnancy and childbirth. The challenge is thus to find a way to merge the discursive with the material reproductive body.

Notes

1 The Restoration of Charles II in 1660 enabled not only the advent of a longer period of peace and prosperity after many years of war and political upheaval due to the British Civil Wars and the Interregnum, but it also made possible the continuation of key developments in the field of science, technology, anatomy and medicine.

2 Many eighteenth- and early nineteenth-century thinkers and writers such as Samuel Johnson, Laurence Sterne and Samuel Taylor Coleridge believed in the "supremacy of [...] reason [and] were deeply threatened by the fragility of the flesh" (Schama 2004, x). This 'fear of the flesh' is partially rooted in the ideas of René Descartes whose name coined the term Cartesian dualism.

3 In 1543, Vesalius, who is often referred to as the 'father' of human anatomy, published a series of books titled *De Humani Corporis Fabrica Libri Septem* (*On the Fabric of the Human Body*) that also contained detailed illustrations of dissected human bodies.

4 Anatomical representations of dead bodies, however, demanded the involvement of skilled artists to spread this 'carnal knowledge.' Hence, what had already begun during the Renaissance continued during the eighteenth century – the arts and sciences merged and led to the "resurrect[ion of] the body in a more secular guise" (Porter 2004, xiii).

5 Sarah Fox confirms in *Giving Birth* (2022) that, although the body was "in transition" during this period, "holistic ideas of health and management remained an important framework," not only "for understanding the body" as such, but also for "managing childbirth" (Fox 2022, 5).

6 As Evelyn Fox Keller emphasised in *Reflections on Gender and Science* ([1985] 1995), the Cartesian dualism renders the flesh – traditionally associated with femininity – inferior as opposed to the masculine connoted mind (Keller 1995, 61–64). These associations have very real consequences, such as the exclusion from certain work places or the lower rate of women choosing STEM-related study courses.

7 In *Geschichte unter der Haut* (*The Women beneath the Skin: A Doctor's Patients in Eighteenth-Century Germany*) ([1987] 1988), the medical historian and feminist Barbara Duden equally conceives the reproductive body as a discursive construct. Duden's work is only referenced in passing here as her focus rests on the German physician Johannes Pelargius Storch and his female patients and thus belongs to the German history of science and medicine.

8 Martin builds on Laqueur's earlier work and pursues the question how new liberal ideas expressed by political philosophers like Thomas Hobbes and John Locke in combination with the events of the French Revolution defied the "natural order" of things including religion, the monarchy and (gender) politics during the Age of Enlightenment (Martin 1987, 32). Martin exposes how steadily growing uncertainties with regards to social systems were 'healed' by science in the eighteenth century, in particular by the claim that women's and men's "social roles [...] were grounded in nature, by virtue of the dictates of their bodies" (Martin 1993, 32).

9 Pallister published an English translation of Paré's *De Monstres* titled *On Monsters and Marvels* that is in turn based on the Malgaigne edition of 1840 (Pallister 1983, xxix).

10 See Isaac Cruikshank's satirical print *A Man-Mid-Wife* (1793) that is equipped with the subheading "'or a newly discover'd animal, [...]; for a more full description of this Monster, see, an ingenious book, [...] entitled, Man-Midwifery dissected [sic], [...] elucidating this animal's Propensities to cruelty & indecency [...]."

11 See also my book chapters on midwifery and obstetrics (Henke 2022, 2023, 2025) in which I equally quote these and other numbers.

12 See also Wilson's more recent book *Ritual and Conflict: The Social Relations of Childbirth in Early Modern England* (2013), where he repeats this claim.

13 Wilson further describes 'monstrous' operations such as craniotomy that involved crushing the infant's skull inside the birthing subject's body to extract the foetus if it became stuck in the birth canal, cutting off infants' arms or C-sections, the latter a rather uncommon practice in eighteenth-century Britain as the mother seldomly survived (Wilson 1995, 20–22).

14 In line with Wilson, Cody also stresses that although "[i]nfant mortality rates could be quite high," statistics suggest that "[m]aternal mortality rates" were as low as "1 to 2 percent," which leads to the conclusion that "most mothers survived" childbirth (Cody 2008, 41).

15 Aelius Galenus, Claudius Galenus, Galen or Galen or Pergamon (AD 129–216) was a Greek philosopher but also surgeon whose work significantly influenced the development of anatomy among many others.

16 Hippocrates of Kos (460–370 BC) was a Greek physician and known as the 'father of medicine' (see also King 2008).

17 For more information on the 'culture' of gynecological science and its development from the early nineteenth century onwards, see Ornella Moscucci's *The Science of Woman. Gynaecology and Gender in England, 1800–1929* (1993).
18 The term "(man-)midwives" or "(man-)midwife" is used here and elsewhere for readability when addressing both female and male midwives.
19 However, the repeated use of the term 'normal' and 'natural' birth processes is also not entirely unproblematic from a feminist viewpoint as it equally runs danger of pathologising or 'othering' certain kinds of birth.
20 They remind their readers, however, that "[m]edical case notes represent a particular and highly specialised genre" that needs to be critically read as they are never "simple, neutral or objective," let alone universal, an insight that goes without saying in the field of literary and cultural studies (Woods/Galley 2014, 43, 51). Yet the current midwifery case notes share some common characteristics. They usually include the woman's circumstances (age, health condition, social status etc.), the reason why the midwife was called, the procedures, the outcomes and reflections, other simple information such as "date, time, place" as well as further attendants present (Woods/Galley 2014, 53).
21 Her clients are described as "not the poorest of the poor," although Stone seems very "aware that midwives and medicines could be costly" (Woods/Galley 2014, 88). Moreover, Stone's notes make clear she is mainly called for emergency cases in the areas of Somerset to which she usually has to ride on horseback for miles, so most of her cases describe the "gruelling nature of a rural midwifery practice" (Woods/Galley 2014, 88–89).
22 These consist of 1) the midwifery textbook *A Treatise on the Theory and Practice of Midwifery* (1751, dated 1752, reprinted 1752, third edition 1754); 2) the two case notes volumes *A Collection of Cases and Observations in Midwifery. By William Smellie, MD, To Illustrate His Former Treatise, or First Volume, on That Subject* (1754) as well as 3) *A Collection of Prenatural Cases and Observations in Midwifery. By William Smellie, MD, Completing the Design of Illustrating his First Volume on that Subject* (1764) and, most importantly, the obstetrical atlas 4) *A Sett of Anatomical Tables, With Explanations, and an Abridgement of the Practice of Midwifery; with a view to illustrate a Treatise on that Subject, and Collection of Cases* (first edition 1754, second edition 1761). According to Woods and Galley, the latter book also comprises the "original engravings" from the later published *Anatomical Tables with Explanations, and an Abridgement of the Practice of Midwifery, with a View to Illustrate a Treatise on the Subject, and Collection of Cases. By William Smellie, MD. A New Edition, Carefully Corrected and Revised, with Notes and Illustrations, Adapted to the present Improved Method of Practice* [...] (1787) (see Woods/Galley 2014, 158).
23 See also Massey (2005, 77).
24 Woods and Galley describe Smellie's "general procedure" as follows: On arrival in the birthing room, he first takes his patient's pulse, then talks to the attendant midwife or nurse, "but not apparently to the woman on whom he conducts a physical examination" (Woods/Galley 2014, 175).
25 Woods and Galley quote case 180 in which the obstetrician Smellie lectures (female) midwives as follows: "[the midwife] ought to be perfectly mistress of the art of examination in time of labour, together with all different kinds of labour, whether natural or preternatural, and the methods of delivering the placenta; she ought to live in friendship with other women of the same profession, contending with them in nothing but knowledge, sobriety, diligence, and patience; she ought to avoid all reflections upon men-practitioners; and when she finds herself at a loss, candidly have recourse to their assistance" (Woods/Galley 2014, 186).
26 In Woods and Galley's volume, Smellie ends his advice with a sentence that also points to the fear of obstetricians regarding possible retributions by midwives and writes: "These gentle methods will prevent that mutual calumny and abuse which too often

prevail among the male and female practitioners; [...] and on such occasions he must expect to meet with retaliation from those midwives whom he may have roughly used" (Woods/Galley 2014, 186).

27 Woods and Galley describe this book as his "greatest publication" and a "work of remarkable beauty" that "combined science with art" by displaying "foetal development together with the structure of the uterus and placenta" (Woods/Galley 2014, 267). Although they reference Lyle Massey's important contribution "Pregnancy and Pathology" (2005) in a footnote that deals with the effect of Hunter's obstetrical illustrations, they here too do not critically evaluate the meaning and implication of these literally 'graphic' depictions of the female reproductive body.

28 Hunter also worked for King George III's wife, Queen Charlotte of Mecklenburg-Strelitz, whose birth process he documented in detail (Woods/Galley 2014, 269; see also Massey 2005, 77).

29 Interestingly, Hunter seemed to have advised against the unnecessary use of forceps and "famously [...] suggested" the following to midwives: "When a woman's pains grow less and less, and the head is properly presented, the labour may well be finished by the forceps [...]; but this should be done very cautiously, and gently. For one woman and child that the forceps have saved, it has destroyed ten" (Woods/Galley 2014, 269).

30 See also Cunningham's *The Anatomist Anatomis'd. An Experimental Discipline in Enlightenment Europe* (Cunningham 2010, 165–185).

31 Newman further identifies the instrument's "phallic shape"; hooks, speculum, head pullers and forceps hence demonstrate a "male-dominated technology linked to the growing status of obstetrics" (Newman 1996, 61).

32 Certainly, the representation of the foetus as "always male" also has to do with the still prevalent idea that the male body was considered the norm and the female body merely an inferior version of it (see Aristotle's and Galen's one-sex model).

33 The strategy behind this kind of bodily fragmentation is that it "discipline[s] the cultural threat posed by [the] reproductive body and assure[s] the self-evidence of sexual difference" as Newman infers: "The woman-as-reproductive body [...] cannot be allowed to encroach upon or trouble the identificatory relay between observing subject and fetal body. The privilege of disembodiment that defines the individual paradoxically requires the profoundly embodied and coded bodies of women, but those bodies must always be represented at some remove from the fetus and the process of birth" (Newman 1996, 82).

34 In addition, Hunter's focus, as opposed to Smellie's, is on texture which becomes clear when considering the representation of the foetuses' skin and hair. In Hunter, the foetus' "skin has something of that quality of newborn skin – soft, milky, almost translucent" (Harvey 2010, 46). Furthermore, "[w]hereas as the unborn's hair in Smellie is indicated with just a few lines, in Hunter the hair is thick, built up with line after line until it becomes a solid mass beneath which you can see nothing" (Harvey 2010, 46). In Harvey's view, Smellie's images "display little of the texture of the Hunter atlas" and are therefore to be understood as "pure instruction" (Harvey 2010, 46). What is more, while Smellie focuses on the birth process, Hunter is rather interested in the "nature of the gravid uterus" (Harvey 2010, 47).

35 See Joanna Ebenstein's very impressive *The Anatomical Venus* (2016) containing powerful photographs of eighteenth-century life-sized obstetrical wax models displayed in a science museum in Florence. Examples can be found in Zoe Williams' *The Guardian* article titled "Cadavers in pearls: meet the Anatomical Venus" (2016): https://www.theguardian.com/artanddesign/2016/may/17/anatomical-venus-anatomy-human-biology-joanna-ebenstein-books. Last access: November 2024.

36 A further noteworthy representational practice or trope that ties in with the fragmentation of the female reproductive body is the so-called 'anatomical Venus' that, contrary to the term 'Venus' that evokes "mythological, biblical, [and] anthropological" images,

summons "erotic plots of romance, types of the seductress" often featured in eighteenth-and early nineteenth-century novels (Newman 1996, 86–88). Their sexual power, however, is warded off by rendering them "objects to be exposed and manipulated" (Newman 1996, 88). What is more, they are "always pregnant" and thus signal their "sexual specificity" (Newman 1996, 88).

37 Since scholars also commonly ask about the way male bodies were represented, it is important to note that masculine models existed as well but with one major difference: flesh, or rather the lack thereof. Jordanova writes: "Others represent men, either the whole body or sizeable parts of it. Yet, I know of no male models which show the complete body either covered with flesh or recumbent" (Jordanova 1998, 44–45). Therefore, only female wax models were covered in a flesh-like texture while some were also embellished with "flowing hair, pearl necklaces, removable parts and small foetuses" (Jordanova 1998, 45).

38 Jordanova emphasises that we also need to investigate the actual *uses* of such (material) representations that "were not restricted to a narrowly medical context but enjoyed wide circulation" (Jordanova 1989, 49). Jordanova assumes that the (haptic) wax models "make certain reactions very likely" and argues that they "invited sexual thoughts" by evoking the desire of "mentally unclothing a woman" (Jordanova 1989, 49–50, 55). Of course, the wax models were "already naked"; however, their "removable layers" contributed to the model's eroticism as these could be peeled off, allowing "ever deeper looking into the chest and abdomen" and thus enabling "shared metaphors" like "penetration and unveiling" (Jordanova 1989, 55). This "interest in depth" was immensely relevant for how people understood gender and sex; the "actual unveiling of women's bodies" made "visible the emblematic core of their [women's] sex" – reproduction (Jordanova 1989, 57–58).

39 As Nichols adds, the cloth in these obstetrical images serves yet another function: It contributes not only to the age-old (masculine) trope of unveiling 'nature's secrets,' but also recalls a form of (eroticised) striptease (Nichols 2013, 112). In this respect, she refers to the anatomical atlas *Anatomie Generale des Viscères* (1752) by the French anatomist and artist Jacques Fabien Gautier d'Agoty that includes several images of dissected pregnant women. The particular feature of these illustrations is that, contrary to the male figures that are both completely shorn and dissected, the female forms are only partially dissected except for their faces that seem to flirt with the viewer, "inviting him to examine the secrets of her half-dissected body" including her "thick bush of [pubic] hair": As Nichols infers, this is a "depiction of a striptease continued beyond mere nudity" (Nichols 2013, 112).

40 This deliberately omitted graphic image can be found here on page 19/168 (page 7): https://wellcomecollection.org/works/wzrtz7z5/items?canvas=19 (last access: March 2025).

41 In this context and with regards to Smellie's and Hunter's atlases, Sarah Schäfer-Althaus adds that "[i]n death, the anatomist has the ultimate control over the female reproductive body [...]. He becomes the director of the narrative, spectacle and gaze, which through its visual documentation can now be enjoyed repeatedly – in public and private – by the dissector and [...] by everyone willing to pay for [these images]" (Schäfer-Althaus 2020, 34).

42 See also Schiebinger's *Nature's Body – Gender in the Making of Modern Science* (1993) for a more general history of science, sex and sexuality.

43 According to Schiebinger, anatomists depicted female skulls "as smaller" to demonstrate the superiority of men's intellectual capabilities (Schiebinger 1987, 43). The same holds true for the female pelvis, which was depicted markedly larger in order to find ('scientific') arguments against "women's participation in the public sphere" by restricting them to the realm of housework and childcare (Schiebinger 1987, 43).

44 See Latour's "How to Talk About the Body? The Normative Dimension of Science Studies" (2004).
45 McGrath traces the history of anatomy and outlines how until the 1750s, dissected bodies consisted only of criminals who were publicly "gibbeted in chains" as a "post-mortem punishment" (McGrath 2002, 63). After the Murder Act of 1751 that allowed the substitution of criminals' corpses to anatomy schools, the "supply of bodies" significantly increased leading to the "spectacle['s]" return to the private sphere (McGrath 2002, 63). As a result of the "increased demand for corpses" in the field of anatomy, a "market for bodies" emerged; since the majority of "murderers were male," however, female reproductive bodies were treated as commercial goods: "pregnant female cadavers were doubly rare" (McGrath 2002, 63) After the Anatomy Act (1832) in the nineteenth century, "dead bodies [...] became ordinary articles of medical trade [...] cadavers were sold like meat in bits and pieces: half of whole, limbs or trunks, a head or a foot" (McGrath 2002, 63).
46 McGrath further explains that eighteenth-century obstetrical atlases were "multi-authored works" and involved anatomists and artists alike (McGrath 2002, 64). The images used in these books displayed "moments in pregnancy" that were "so impossibly dramatized as to be untrue to life" (McGrath 2002, 64). The procedure was as follows: The surgeon first dissected the bodies and then commissioned an artist to create drawings "from the dead woman and her foetus as they lay on the anatomist's slab" (McGrath 2002, 64). Interestingly, as McGrath points out, William Smellie and William Hunter both hired the Dutch engraver and painter Jan Van Rymsdyk (McGrath 2002, 64). Despite employing the same artist, however, their atlases were "very different" both with regards to their form and content (McGrath 2002, 64).
47 Lieske criticizes previous historical studies for largely neglecting the wide use of these obstetrical machines that hence "fall into a hazy void where their role in midwifery training is acknowledged, but details on what machines may have looked like and how they were used remain hidden" (Lieske 2012, 72). Yet, she also questions the "well-intended but misplaced feminist sensibilities" of some studies as they "view obstetrical machines as a combination of misogynistic popular entertainment and bad science [and] ride the coat-tails of eighteenth-century, anti-male midwifery critics" (Lieske 2012, 72). Naturally, the current thesis also seeks to avoid a one-sided perspective; it rather aims at a more balanced historical re- or deconstruction of reproduction by acknowledging its material-discursive complexity.

References

Buckley, Jenifer. 2017. *Gender, Pregnancy and Power in Eighteenth-Century Literature: The Maternal Imagination*. Basingstoke: Palgrave Macmillan.

Browner, Stephanie. 1992. "Review of Thomas Laqueur, *Making Sex*." *Victorian Studies* 35: 221–222.

Cody, Lisa Forman. [2005] 2008. *Birthing the Nation: Sex, Science, and the Conception of Eighteenth-Century Britons*. Oxford: Oxford University Press.

Cunningham, Andrew. 2010. *The Anatomist Anatomis'd: An Experimental Discipline in Enlightenment Europe*. Farnham: Ashgate.

Deutscher, Penelope. 2017. *Foucault's Futures: A Critique of Reproductive Reason*. New York: Columbia University Press.

Duden, Barbara. 1988. *The Women beneath the Skin: A Doctor's Patients in Eighteenth-Century Germany*. Cambridge, MA: Harvard University Press.

Ebenstein, Joanna. 2016. *The Anatomical Venus*. London: Thames & Hudson.

Foucault, Michel. [1976] 1978. *The History of Sexuality*. New York: Pantheon.

Foucault, Michel. 1994. *The Birth of the Clinic: An Archaeology of Medical Perception.* New York: Vintage Books.

Fox, Sarah. 2022. *Giving Birth in Eighteenth-Century England.* London: University of London Press.

Gowing, Laura. 2003. *Common Bodies: Women, Touch, and Power in Seventeenth-Century England.* New Haven, CT: Yale University Press.

Greenfield, Susan C., and Carol Barash. 1999. *Inventing Maternity: Politics, Science, and Literature, 1650–1865.* Lexington: University Press of Kentucky.

Hall, Stuart. 1997. "Introduction." In *Representation: Cultural Representations and Signifying Practices*, edited by Stuart Hall, 1–13. Thousand Oaks, CA: SAGE.

Haraway, Donna. 1990. *Primate Visions: Gender, Race, and Nature in the World of Modern Science.* Abingdon: Routledge.

Harvey, Karen. 2010. "Visualizing Reproduction: A Cultural History of Early-Modern and Modern Medical Illustrations." *The Journal of Medical Humanities* 31 (1): 37–51.

Henke, Jennifer S. 2022. "Mary Wollstonecraft, *Maria: or, The Wrongs of Woman* (1798)." In *Handbook of the British Novel in the Long Eighteenth Century,* edited by Katrin Berndt and Alessa Johns, 449–466. Berlin; Boston, MA: De Gruyter.

Henke, Jennifer S. 2023. "Contesting Spaces of Knowledge: Reproduction, Medicine and Literature." In *Contradiction Studies: Mapping the Field/Inaugural Conference on Concepts of Contradiction in the Humanities,* edited by Kerstin Knopf, Gisela Febel, and Martin Nonhoff, 233–256. Heidelberg: Springer.

Henke, Jennifer S. 2025. "Matters of Interest: Entangling the Maternal Body." In Undue Burdens: Reproductive Rights and Bodily Autonomy in the Long Eighteenth Century, edited by Fiona Brideoake, Ula Lukszo Klein, and Nicole Garret. University of Virginia Press.

Hunter, William. 1774. *The Anatomy of the Human Gravid Uterus Exhibited in Figures.* London: D. Wilson.

Jordanova, Ludmilla J. 1989. *Sexual Visions: Images of Gender in Science and Medicine between the Eighteenth and Twentieth Centuries.* Madison: University of Wisconsin Press.

King, Helen. 2007. *Midwifery, Obstetrics and the Rise of Gynaecology: The Uses of a Sixteenth-Century Compendium.* London: Routledge.

King, Helen. 2013. *The One-Sex Body on Trial: The Classical and Early Modern Evidence.* London; New York: Routledge.

Laqueur, Thomas, and Catherine Gallagher, eds. 1987. *The Making of the Modern Body: Sexuality and Society in the Nineteenth Century.* Berkeley: University of California Press.

Laqueur, Thomas. [1990] 1992. *Making Sex: Body and Gender from the Greeks to Freud.* Cambridge, MA, London: Harvard University Press.

Latour, Bruno. 2004. "How to Talk About the Body? The Normative Dimension of Science Studies." *Body & Society*, 10(2–3): 205–229.

Lieske, Pam. 2012. "'Made in Imitation of Real Women and Children': Obstetrical Machines in Eighteenth-Century Britain." In *The Female Body in Medicine and Literature*, edited by Andrew Mangham and Greta Depledge, 69–88. Liverpool: Liverpool University Press.

Lieske, Pam, ed. 2008. *Eighteenth-Century British Midwifery, Volume 5: The State of Midwifery Considered, William Smellie and His Critics.* London: Pickering and Chatto.

Martin, Emily. [1987] 1993. *The Woman in the Body: A Cultural Analysis of Reproduction.* Buckingham: Open University Press.

Massey, Lyle. 2005. "Pregnancy and Pathology: Picturing Childbirth in Eighteenth-Century Obstetrical Atlases." *The Art Bulletin* 87 (1): 73–91.

McGrath, Roberta. 2002. *Seeing Her Sex: Medical Archives and the Female Body*. Manchester: Manchester University Press.

Newman, Karen. 1996. *Fetal Positions: Individualism, Science, Visuality*. Stanford, CA: Stanford University Press.

Nichols, Marcia D. 2013. "Venus Dissected: The Visual Blazon of Mid-Eighteenth-Century Medical Atlases." In *Sex and Death in Eighteenth-Century Literature*, edited by Jolene Zigarovich, 119–138. New York; London: Routledge.

Paré, Ambroise. 1983. *On Monsters and Marvels*. Translated by Janis L. Pallister. Chicago, IL: University of Chicago Press.

Pallister, Janis L. 1983. "Introduction." In *On Monsters and Marvels*, by Ambroise Paré, xi–xxii. Chicago, IL: University of Chicago Press.

Park, Katharine, and Robert A. Nye. 1991. "Destiny Is Anatomy." *New Republic*: 53–57.

Porter, Roy. 2004. *Flesh in the Age of Reason*. London: Penguin.

Saunders, J. B., and Charles O'Malley. 1973. *The Illustrations from the Works of Andreas Vesalius of Brussels*. New York: Dover Publications.

Schäfer-Althaus, Sarah. 2020. "Dissecting Birth: Obstetrics, Bodily Transience, and the Anatomist's Gaze in Eighteenth-Century Medical Atlases." In *Transient Bodies in Anglophone Literature and Culture*, edited by Sarah Schäfer-Althaus and Sara Strauß, 15–36. Vol. 91 of *Anglistik und Englischunterricht*. Heidelberg: Winter.

Schama, Simon. 2004. "Foreword." In *Flesh in the Age of Reason*, by Roy Porter, vii–xiii. London: Penguin.

Schiebinger, Londa. 1987. "Skeletons in the Closet: The First Illustrations of the Female Skeleton in Eighteenth-Century Anatomy." In *The Making of the Modern Body: Sexuality and Society in the Nineteenth Century*, edited by Thomas Laqueur and Catherine Gallagher, 42–82. Berkeley: University of California Press.

Smellie, William. 1754. *A Set of Anatomical Tables, with Explanation and an Abridgement of the Practice of Midwifery, with a view to illustrate a treatise on that subject, and collection of cases*. London: D. Wilson.

Sommers, Sheena. 2012. "Transcending the Sexed Body: Reason, Sympathy, and 'Thinking Machines' in the Debates over Male Midwifery." In *The Female Body in Medicine and Literature*, edited by Andrew Mangham and Greta Depledge, 89–106. Liverpool: Liverpool University Press.

Stone, Sarah. 1737. *A Complete Practice of Midwifery: Consisting of Upwards of Forty Cases or Observations in that valuable Art, […]. Recommended to All Female Practitioners in an Art so important to the Lives and Well-Being of the Sex*. London: printed for T. Cooper, at the Globe, Paternoster Row.

Waddington, Keir. 2011. *An Introduction to the Social History of Medicine: Europe since 1500*. London: Red Globe Press.

Wahrman, Dror. 2008. "Change and the Corporeal in Seventeenth- and Eighteenth-Century Gender History: Or, Can Cultural History Be Rigorous?" *Gender and History* 20: 584–602.

Whiteley, Rebecca. 2023. *Birth Figures: Early Modern Prints and the Pregnant Body*. Chicago, IL; London: University of Chicago Press.

Wertz, Richard W., and Dorothy C. Wertz. 1977. *Lying-In: A History of Childbirth in America*. New York: Free Press.

Williams, Carolyn. 2012. "Difficulties, at Present in No Degree Clear'd Up: The Controversial Mother, 1600–1800." In *The Female Body in Medicine and Literature*, edited by Andrew Mangham and Greta Depledge, 16–33. Liverpool: Liverpool University Press.

Wilson, Adrian. 1995. *The Making of Man-Midwifery: Childbirth in England, 1660–1770.* Cambridge, MA: Harvard University Press.

Woods, Robert, and Chris Galley. 2014. *Mrs Stone & Dr Smellie: Eighteenth-Century Midwives and Their Patients*. Liverpool: Liverpool University Press.

Zigarovich, Jolene, ed. 2013. *Sex and Death in Eighteenth-Century Literature*. New York; London: Routledge.

1.3 Framework

Beyond Representationalism

1.3.1 The Future of Feminist Eighteenth-Century Studies

Before turning to the problem of representationalism as the only tool for a historiography of the female reproductive body during the Enlightenment, it is first necessary to briefly address the future of feminist eighteenth-century scholarship in general. In her eponymous volume (2018), the editor Robin Runia ascertains an "uncomfortable undercurrent" in eighteenth-century research that feminism "has done its work" (Runia 2018, 1). Runia laments the increasing neglect of 'female' issues and the consequential "loss of [feminist] scholarship" in this field (Runia 2018, 1). Her aim is thus to reaffirm the "relevance of feminist recovery within contemporary scholarship" and especially to "move *beyond*" a focus on the eighteenth-century novel and include other forms of literature as well (emphasis added, Runia 2018, 1–2). She does not understand the term 'beyond' as a claim that feminist eighteenth-century scholarship has already been completed, but rather uses it to "encourage us to step back," to take on new perspectives regarding the representation of women, and especially to embrace the fruitful "inconsistency [of] scholarly approaches" to eighteenth-century literary and cultural artefacts (Runia 2018, 3, 5). It is precisely this goal that this book equally aims at: It seeks to revisit and reframe representations of the (material) female reproductive body in eighteenth-century literature and culture by, to use the now common catchphrase, 'making matter matter' again.

In terms of embodiment, the feminist English scholar Cynthia Richards adopts Runia's critique in her chapter on history and trauma and adds one crucial aspect to the above-mentioned considerations that, as Richards claims, is still under-researched in eighteenth-century scholarship: the *body*. Richards stresses how "deconstruction and new historicism operate within closed systems" that draw a clear distinction between texts and bodies (Richards 2018, 13). Furthermore, while new historicism allegedly amended "deconstruction's failure to examine the *material* conditions of the text's production, [it] added yet another layer between those represented bodies and our own" by strictly distinguishing historical bodies from our own (present) bodies and bodily experiences (emphasis added, Richards 2018, 13): "Bodies of the past were not identical with bodies of the present, but took shape and form in

DOI: 10.4324/9781003467977-4

a historical context and a rhetorical framework that necessarily divided them from our current understanding of materiality" (Richards 2018, 13).

Richards criticises this "closed system of representation" and the "limits of historicism" by acknowledging eighteenth-century literature's impact on today's readers and their lives because scholars tend to ignore the significance of the body "(or lack thereof)" in their studies (Richards 2018, 13, 15). She hence calls for making bodies (more) relevant again and advocates the necessity to merge the physical or material with the historical (Richards 2018, 15). History, as Richards continues, cannot be separated from the (material) body and "our lived [bodily] experiences"; above all, history is never "fixed in time" but rather a "porous, not a closed, structure" that has different meanings for different people at different times (Richards 2018, 17).[1]

Although Richards' focus lies on trauma and bodily loss through the example of rape in eighteenth-century novels like Samuel Richardson's *Clarissa* (1748) among others, her reflections regarding the body prove to be particularly useful for this book's objective, namely to raise awareness for the (historical) discursive body's entanglement with its materiality. This becomes even clearer when considering the field of disability studies that "focuses on the lived experience – and the particularities of bodies" (Richards 2018, 24). More importantly, studies of this kind deal with the ways "environments can frame bodies" in terms of their normativity and "what it means" to deviate from socio-culturally constructed norms (Richards 2018, 24). For Richards, disability and trauma studies "provide a [...] language" to talk about (wounded) bodies and help comprehend how our reaction to these bodies "frames our understanding of the human" (Richards 2018, 24–25). She insists on the possibility to "make newly visible the body" in literature and culture of the eighteenth century (Richards 2018, 25). Ultimately, Richards urges us to *rethink* and take seriously bodily images not only to help acknowledge the "provisional nature of our own" but also to allow these "embodied readings" to resonate with our own lives (Richards 2018, 27). In sum, the future of feminist eighteenth century lies in a *(re)thinking of the female body* in order to make it (more) visible again. One way to achieve this is to bring the body's materiality to the fore and reread it from a materialist viewpoint.

1.3.2 (Re)Thinking (with) the Body

What is the body anyway? Is it "universal, decontextualized," a "*tabula rasa*, simply awaiting inscription by culture" (DeMello 2014, 5)? The anthrozoologist Margo DeMello answers this question with an unequivocal 'no' in her 2014 introduction to body studies (DeMello 2014, 5). Bodies are rather to be understood as social constructs that are "always changing" and subject to "power relations," which determine what it means to have or 'be' a female, male, abled, disabled, black, white or other kind of body (DeMello 2014, 5). DeMello stresses that "bodies are never 'blank' or unmarked" – they are always already laden with cultural meaning (DeMello 2014, 7).

Traditionally, the body has been regarded as separate from the mind. Only relatively recently, scholars have begun to dissolve this mind/body problem that reaches back to classical antiquity. This division was finally cemented in the seventeenth century when the French philosopher and scientist René Descartes famously coined the Cartesian dualism of mind and/over body. From a feminist perspective, prioritising the mind over the body poses a particular problem as Evelyn Fox Keller points out in her criticism of the natural sciences. According to her, these disciplines are "deeply rooted [in] popular mythology that casts objectivity, reason, and mind as male, and subjectivity, feeling, and nature as female" with all its common consequences including the debarment of women from the practical realm of science or the (gendered) split between the public and private sphere (Fox Keller 1995, 7). Fox Keller explains how such a "feminist perspective on science confronts us with the task of examining the roots, dynamics, and consequences of this *interacting network* of associations and disjunctions – together constituting what might be called the 'science-gender system'" (emphasis added, Fox Keller 1995, 8).

Fox Keller thus clearly demonstrates how (material-)discursive constructions or "interactive networks" of representing the (material) body have significantly influenced – or are rather inextricably entangled with – most rational and 'objective' fields such as the natural sciences. What is more, as DeMello adds, to classify bodies as either female or male, inferior or superior, normal or abnormal, enables social control (DeMello 2014, 11). With reference to the anthropologist Terence Turner, DeMello emphasises how the body "becomes the symbolic stage on which the dramas of society are enacted" (DeMello 2014, 11). In other words, the body becomes a performative power arena in which agents struggle for discursive authority.

Of course, this fight for power also holds true for medical bodies that, to use Michel Foucault's term, are equally 'disciplined' by both society and medicine. Foucault's major contribution to the field of body studies is indisputable and has triggered a significant number of scholarly responses. Yet, older and newer research on the body's discursivity continues to understand it merely as a "canvas on which patterns of significance are inscribed and counter-inscribed" (DeMello 2014, 13). They simply assume the body to lack any form of agency and understand it as a passive object, a container to be 'filled' with meaning, thus reaffirming the problematic body/mind dualism. It was only in the late 1980s and early 1990s that scholars like Emily Martin recognised the importance of medical practices that not only (literally) "fragmented [women's bodies] into parts" but also reduced them to their ability to reproduce (DeMello 2014, 16–17). In fact, the issue of reproduction is "perhaps the best example of a biological concept that is deeply culturally constructed" (DeMello 2014, 58). As the biologist Lynda Birke stresses in *Feminism and the Biological Body* (1999), "women are defined primarily as 'wombs on legs'" (Birke 1999, 12; see also DeMello 2014, 59).

Along similar lines, the philosopher and gender theorist Judith Butler explains in *Bodies that Matter: On the Discursive Limits of "Sex"* (1993) that femininity has been associated with materiality since classical antiquity due to a "set of etymologies which link matter with [the Latin] *mater* and *matrix* (or the womb) and, hence, with a problematic of reproduction" (Butler 1993, 31; see also DeMello 2014, 59). Butler, however, equally remains on the levels of discourse in her predominantly Foucauldian approach to body and matter, thus potentially reaffirming the hierarchical binary between mind over materiality. How, then, can the female reproductive body be freed from the limits of representationalism? How can scholars make the body's 'matter matter' again?

1.3.3 Material Cultures & The Problem of Representation

Despite the persistence of the mind/body division, twentieth- and twenty-first-century scholars have aimed at an "alternative way of understanding the body" (Hillman/Maude 2015, 1). As the literary critics David Hillman and Ulrika Maude point out in their 2015 volume on the body in literature, scholarship has shifted towards recognising the constitutive entanglement of body and mind or soul that, at the same time, is still not unproblematic: "although many recent philosophers, scientists and writers seem to suggest that the body *is* the self, [this recognition] also poses a serious challenge to received notions of identity and subjectivity" (emphasis in the original, Hillman/Maude 2015, 1). Yet, the editors agree that everyday life is always an "embodied experience" and give examples such as "sex and childbirth, eating and defecation, pleasure and pain, desire and repulsion," thus making the concept of embodiment central to their collection (Hillman/Maude 2015, 1).

With their volume, Hillman and Maude address the question of bodily representations in literature. They draw heavily on Foucault's discourse theory while simultaneously acknowledging an "eclectic theoretical pluralism" of current approaches to the question of how bodies are represented in literary and cultural texts (Hillman/Maude 2015, 2). Simultaneously, they concede that there are, in fact, "no [material] bodies in literature":

> Not only there is no obvious way for the concrete materiality of the body to be fully present in or on the written page; even more profoundly, there would seem on the face of it to be an apparent *mutual exclusivity* of the body and language – the one all brute facticity, the other presupposing precisely the *absence of matter*. And yet, over the last three or four decades, critics and theorists have found myriad ways of addressing the representation of the body and embodied experience in literature. […] *literature* may after all be the *body's closest companion*.
>
> (emphasis added, Hillman/Maude 2015, 3)

Here, Hillman and Maude point to the problem of representing the body in literary artefacts. For them, the body is "always already mediated through representation" (Hillman/Maude 2015, 3). Yet, as they continue, "it may be the object that is given to discourse […] so that literature might in fact be understood as *the* place par excellence for the body to express itself" (emphasis in the original, Hillman/Maude 2015, 3). Although it seems as if the two scholars are tapping into the trap of approaching the body via representationalism only, they admit both the body's "illusory absence" as well as its "illusory presence," leading to an "endless aporia of presence and absence" or a kind of feedback loop (Hillman/Maude 2015, 4). In fact, literature confronts the reader with the "legible materiality of the body" and hence opens up opportunities for resistance or agency or, as they call it, "forms of [bodily] unruliness" (Hillman/Maude 2015, 4–5). Hillman and Maude thus already point to the limits of a purely Foucauldian discourse analysis and recognise the possibility of bodily agency: "For the body is never simply a passive depository of cultural fantasy or the workings of power; it resists all reification and fixity" (Hillman/Maude 2015, 5). How this problem is to be solved, however, remains largely unanswered in their volume, especially with regard to the question of how meaning and matter are entangled with one another.

The English scholar Stacey Alaimo and the postmodern feminist and political scientist Susan Hekman offer a way out of the "impasse" of representationalism that, as they claim, has been "caused by the contemporary linguistic turn in feminist thought" (Alaimo/Hekman 2008, 1). In their ground-breaking volume *Material Feminisms* (2007), they begin by criticising feminist scholarship's previous aversion to the body's materiality and their excessive focus on language and "social constructionist models" (Alaimo/Hekman 2008, 1). Although Alaimo and Hekman recognise poststructuralism and deconstruction's productivity for feminist issues, they regret that "postmodernism has not fulfilled its promise as a theoretical grounding for feminism" (Alaimo/Hekman 2008, 2). While postmodern studies have revealed the social construction of binaries such as female/male, they seem to have continuously accepted one dominant dichotomy nearly "without question: *language/reality*" (emphasis added, Alaimo/Hekman 2008, 2).

In short, Alaimo and Hekman criticise postmodernist studies for focussing almost entirely on discourse while dismissing the body's materiality, which has led to a distorted discussion of such issues (Alaimo/Hekman 2008, 3). As the current and the previous chapters demonstrate, numerous studies have been published on the body since the second half of the twentieth century. Yet, as Alaimo and Hekman confirm, "nearly all of the work [...] has been confined to the analysis of discourses *about* the body" (emphasis in the original, Alaimo/Hekman 2008, 3). Alaimo and Hekman thus call for a material-oriented discourse analysis from which fields such as feminist science studies in particular could profit:

> We need a way to talk about these bodies and the materiality they inhabit. Focussing exclusively on representation, ideology, and discourse excludes lived experience, corporeal practice, and biological substance from consideration. It makes it nearly impossible for feminism to engage with medicine or science in innovative, productive, or affirmative ways – the only path available is the well-worn path of critique.
>
> (Alaimo/Hekman 2008, 4)

Alaimo and Hekman identify recent studies that offer alternative ways to talk about the body in or through literary and cultural artefacts. These approaches "bring the material back into science without losing the insights of social constructionism" (Alaimo/Hekman 2008, 5). They refer to theorists such as the sociologist and philosopher Bruno Latour who attempted to merge materiality with ontology and ascribed matter with a kind of agency in the scope of the 'actor-network-theory' (short: ANT).[2] This book, in contrast, shall rather utilise theories developed by *feminist* science scholars like Donna Haraway, N. Katherine Hayles and Karen Barad who explicitly criticise those forms of (gendered) essentialisms that "continue [...] to haunt feminism" (Alaimo/Hekman 2008, 17).

Similar to Robin Runia, who wants to move 'beyond' established feminist scholarship by going a step back and taking on new perspectives regarding the representation of women and their bodies, Alaimo and Hekman aim to "move *beyond* discursive constructions and [...] radically *rethink materiality*" without abandoning the achievements of postmodernism (emphasis added, Alaimo/Hekman 2008, 6). What all of these proposed approaches by scholars such as Haraway, Hayles, Barad as well as Alaimo and Hekman seem to have in common in this context is not only the conviction of an *entanglement* of matter and discourse but also the belief that materiality and thus bodies equally share one aspect in particular: *agency* (Alaimo/Hekman 2008, 7). Put simply, matter and meaning cannot be separated; both are inextricably interwoven with one another. This insight has a number of consequences, especially for the way we understand the medical body.

The sociologist Chris Shilling further confirms the impossibility of a disentanglement of the social from the biological and refers to the example of plastic surgery among others: "If [...] medical forces make it possible to extort increasing control over bodies, undermining the idea that they are unalterable biological organisms, this raises questions [...] about *how* we should manage and control our bodily being" (emphasis in the original, Shilling 2016, 4). As a result, when using the word 'bodies,' Shilling refers to the "embodied human *as a whole*" that underlines the "academically neglected physical and organic dimension of existence" (emphasis in the original, Shilling 2016, 6). Moreover, for Shilling, bodies interact with each other; he describes these interactions as "*inter*-corporeal," as "mutual corporealit[ies]" that are also entangled with (social) metaphors, thus creating a complex network of relations "*within*" and "*between*" biological organisms and society (emphasis in the original, Shilling 2016, 17, 19).

Shilling explains that debates surrounding the questions of whether humans *have* or *are* bodies are still ongoing (Shilling 2016, 23). The most controversial discussions, however, have always taken place in one particular field – *reproduction* (Shilling 2016, 24). By insisting on the fundamental difference between "sexed bodies" in the eighteenth century, science and medicine contributed to the "social subordination" of women due to their seemingly inferior bodies (Shilling 2016, 26–27). It cannot be overemphasised that it was especially the shift from the one- to the two-sex model that enabled the denial of basic human rights to women during the Enlightenment as they were (again) regarded as bodily (and thus mentally) inferior to men (Shilling 2016, 28).[3]

"What the sexed body means" evokes controversial debates to this very day (Shilling 2016, 36). It was not until the 1990s that scholars like Judith Butler argued that the sexed body's social (and material) significance rests in its performance or "performativity" (Shilling 2016, 36, 38). Yet, Butler has been criticised by feminist scholars for largely ignoring the body's materiality both in *Gender Trouble* (1990) and *Bodies that Matter* (1993) (Alaimo/Hekman 2008, 3). Despite some of the critical responses to Butler's theories, her concept of gender performativity has nevertheless proven useful for making the body matter, as Shilling emphasises: "We do not have to 'do away' with the material body to acknowledge the importance of performance: irrespective of what sexed bodies are, they become *visible*" (emphasis added, Shilling 2016, 40). One way to make the body and its materiality visible again is to utilise the image of the cyborg, a powerful myth that contributes to the dissolution of the dichotomy between meaning and matter, representation and 'reality' as well as feminism and materiality.

1.3.4 Cyborg Imagery & The Importance of Embodiment

In her pioneering essay "A Cyborg Manifesto – Science, Technology and Socialist-Feminism in the Late Twentieth Century" (1985), the feminist biologist and philosopher Donna Haraway proposes an "ironic political myth" that merges feminism with materialism (Haraway [1985] 2000, 291). She employs the image of the cyborg as a "way out of the maze of dualism" and embraces the confusion it causes (Haraway 2000, 292, 316). Haraway's cyborg imagery proves useful for a first approach to the body as it dissolves the boundaries or, as she puts it, "troubling dualisms" or "self/other, mind/body, culture/nature, male/female [and] reality/appearance" (Haraway 2000, 313). For Haraway, the division between reality and fiction is an illusion since the cyborg, a "hybrid of machine and organism," is the very product of both "imagination and material reality" (Haraway 2000, 291–292). What is more, Haraway understands the early cyborg-as-machine as a "caricature of [the] masculinist reproductive dream," an important aspect that will be revisited later in this book (Haraway 2000, 293).

Haraway's cyborg myth describes "transgressed boundaries, potent fusions and dangerous possibilities" for "progressive people" to investigate in the scope of politically motivated projects (Haraway 2000, 295). This is also one of this book's aims – to create a *productive confusion* as to how the reproductive body can be (re)thought against the backdrop of a feminist agenda. In this context, Haraway mentions that the "cyborg world" is not just about (masculine) control of the planet or warfare, but also or especially about the "final appropriation of women's bodies" (Haraway 2000, 295). In any case, Haraway perceives these "monstrous [...] unities" as "potent myths for resistance" (Haraway 2000, 295). It is therefore possible to utilise her cyborg imagery to both highlight the fragmentation of female identity as the 'other,' and to expose the effect of the divisions between body/mind, reality/fiction or matter/meaning that especially entail the following: sexual objectification (Haraway 2000, 299). In Haraway's view, a woman "does not exist as a subject, or even potential subject, since she owes her existence as a woman to sexual appropriation" (Haraway 2000, 299). The cyborg therefore sheds light on this form of fragmented identity: "[It] is a kind of disassembled and reassembled, postmodern collective and personal self. This is the self [that] feminists must code" (Haraway 2000, 302).

At one point, Haraway criticises the way "new technologies" in the field of reproductive medicine have intensified the perspective of the body as a "utility-maximizing machine" and explains: "Among the many transformations of reproductive situations is the medical one, where women's bodies have boundaries newly permeable to both '*visualization*' and '*intervention*'" (emphasis added, Haraway 2000, 306). The power struggles involved in the reading of such representations are obvious: "Of course, who controls the interpretation of bodily boundaries in medical hermeneutics is a major feminist issue" (Haraway 2000, 306). The current investigation thus seeks to rethink the reproductive body by emphasising the blurry or rather entangled boundaries between body and mind, reality and fiction or matter and representation.

The pregnant body itself can be conceptualised as a cyborg body: It transforms during pregnancy and amalgamates with obstetric science and technology: Here, the material body merges with technical instruments that dissect, dissemble and fragment the female form, thus rendering it a hybrid cyborg body. Along similar lines, the English scholar Clare Hanson addresses the maternal body's "conceptual indeterminacy" (Hanson 2004, 87). For her, the pregnant body clearly intersects between the material and cultural:

> Its most striking characteristics is its mutability, as it expands, dilates, contracts and expels. It is also leaky and permeable, losing mucous, blood and milk [...]. [...] Its borders, then, are indeterminate. Additionally, it has the property of divisibility, beginning as one and becoming two and for this reason, it calls into question the idea of the indivisible subject which underpins the Western philosophical tradition.
>
> (Hanson 2004, 87)

The pregnant body therefore challenges the notion of individuality due to its indeterminate or hybrid state. Being neither one nor two, it poses a potential threat to the self that can only be warded off through (social or medical) control. For the philosopher and feminist psychoanalyst, Julia Kristeva, the pregnant body is equally "located at the intersection of biology and culture" (Hanson 2004, 95; see also Kristeva 1982). Kristeva's concept of the "abject maternal body," as Hanson outlines, aligns the reproductive body with repulsion: Individuation requires a "moment of abjection" by which the self is established (Hanson 2004, 95). In other words, the reproductive body needs to be rendered 'monstrous' or 'othered' in order for the subject to constitute itself.

It is this form of hybrid 'monstrosity' that Haraway celebrates by the example of the cyborg as it not only unsheathes the "limits of language" but also challenges seemingly stable distinctions between body and mind, nature and culture or materiality and representation (Haraway 2000, 315). Hence, for Haraway, the cyborg is the "most promising monster" (Haraway 2000, 292). She thus calls for taking cyborg imagery seriously, not by engaging in an "anti-science metaphysics," but by acknowledging that science, culture and materiality are inextricably linked (Haraway 2000, 316). This realisation should be embraced, as "[t]he machine is us, our processes, an aspect of our embodiment. We can be responsible for machines; *they* do not dominate or threaten us. We are responsible for boundaries; we are they" (emphasis in the original, Haraway 2000, 315). Haraway introduces this theory at the zenith of postmodernism in 1980, a philosophical movement that challenges objectivity, universality and the understanding of matter.

At the turn of the millennium, the literature and science scholar N. Katherine Hayles draws a similar connection between representation and reality in *How We Became Posthuman – Virtual Bodies in Cybernetics, Literature and Informatics* (1999). In particular, she laments the "erasure of embodiment" in the field of information technology and cybernetics or rather the, in her view, false concept of disembodied information (Hayles 1999, 4). It is especially the "materiality/information separation" and the resulting "information/materiality hierarchy" that Hayles wishes to challenge (Hayles 1999, 12). She criticises the current conviction that "information can circulate unchanged among different material substrates" and tackles the question of "how *information lost its body*" (emphasis in the original, Hayles 1999, 1–2, 4).

According to Hayles, embodiment is central to what it means to be human; she is highly critical of the humanist assumption that the liberal subject "*possess[es]*" a body rather than "*being* a body" and thus attempts to dissolve the distinction between mind and materiality (emphasis in the original, Hayles 1999, 4):

> I see the deconstruction of the liberal humanist subject as an opportunity to *put back into the picture the flesh* that continues to be erased in contemporary [posthumanist] discussions about cybernetic subjects. [...] my dream is a version of the posthuman [...] that understands *human life is embedded in a material world* of great complexity, one on which we depend for our continued survival.
>
> (emphasis added, Hayles 1999, 5)

For Hayles, both the human and posthuman "coexist in shifting configurations that vary with historically specific contexts" and, similar to Haraway, she celebrates the "pleasurable shock" this claim causes (Hayles 1999, 6). In this context, Hayles critically evaluates cybernetics' "powerful dream" of reaching immortality by disembodying ourselves and "becom[ing] the information we have constructed" (Hayles 1999, 13).

However, she reminds us that "for information to exist, it must *always* be instantiated in a medium" (emphasis in the original, Hayles 1999, 13). It is the, in her view, false understanding of information as "separate from the medium" that creates a distinction between information and matter (Hayles 1999, 13). Hayles argues that "*feedback loops* run between technologies and perceptions, artifacts and ideas" (emphasis added, Hayles 1999, 15) and explains this statement by the simple example of the message:

> In information theoretic terms, no message is ever sent. What is sent is a signal. Only when the message is encoded in a signal for transmission through a medium – for example, when ink is printed on paper or when electrical pulses are sent racing along telegraph wires – does it assume material form. The very definition of "information", then, encodes the distinction between materiality and information [...].
>
> (Hayles 1999, 18)

As a result, maintaining a distinction between information and matter creates a hierarchy between the two. This leads to the (unfortunate) conclusion that information is "more mobile, more important, more *essential* than material forms" (emphasis added, Hayles 1999, 19). Hayles' aim is thus to reunite information with matter by "putting back together parts" and moving towards a more complex understanding of information and matter's mutual entanglement (Hayles 1999, 13). In order to achieve this, she calls for a historiography of the body's erasure: "Once we understand the complex interplays that went into creating the condition of virtuality, we can [...] see it as the result of historically specific negotiations" and "fully recognize the importance of the embodied processes constituting the lifeworld of human being" (Hayles 1999, 20). In short, Hayles wants to re-establish the link between matter and information by stressing that there is no information without embodiment. In line with Haraway's cyborg imagery that does not want to dissolve the individual but rather calls for its responsibility, she reminds her readers: "You are the cyborg, and the cyborg is you" (Hayles 1999, xiii). Having said this, how can such posthumanist approaches be harnessed for an analysis of the female reproductive body in literature and culture?

The English scholar Paul Sheehan builds on Haraway's and Hayles' work and states that the cyborg myth is "analogous" to the "monstrous or grotesque body [...] made legible through somatic disfiguration" (Sheehan 2015, 245–246). Sheehan adds that the cyborg and/as monstrous body is not only to be understood as posthuman but more precisely as "*other than human*, where otherness is defined by the principle of transformation" (emphasis in the original, Sheehan 2015, 246). Sheehan turns to "myth, rather than science" and names Mary Shelley's *Frankenstein, Or: The Modern Prometheus* (1818) as the "richest source for mythological posthumanism" (Sheehan 2015, 246).[4]

The point Sheehan wants to make is that from the very beginning, "god and man are affiliated" before the "counter-Promethean turn" occurs when Victor sees his 'monstrous' creation, made out of a conglomerate of dead (human) body parts, for the first time and turns away from it in horror (Sheehan 2015, 247). As Sheehan outlines: "The 'horror' here is the horror of posthuman non-integrity, of an assemblage that refuses to cohere into a totality" (Sheehan 2015, 247). In his view, the "monstrous, mythic body" has one main function: to criticise science, "or at least [...] scientific naturalism," if not even, I would add, fantasies of scientific omnipotence (Sheehan 2015, 248). The following sections build on the notion of 'god' and (wo)man's affiliation or 'entanglement' of meaning and matter that helps to extend beyond representationalism as the only tool of analysis.

Considering the materiality of the female reproductive body as the 'equal' side of the coin by conceptualising it as an interactive entanglement with its representations opens up a number of possibilities. As Meghan L. Burke points out in her 2009 essay on absent mothers and the male usurpation of maternity in eighteenth-century fiction, it is especially the maternal body that functioned as the main threat to man-midwives during the shift from midwifery to obstetrics: "Rather than viewing their pregnant patients as women with whom they worked, many men viewed them as no more than potentially dangerous, *oppositional objects*" (emphasis added, Burke 2009, 368).

The mechanisms of control and "rational intervention" were in turn entangled with a number of other objects, "often in the form of [...] prized surgical instruments" (Burke 2009, 368). These, as Burke continues, "could be viewed as veritable weapons against the seemingly malevolent 'secrecy' of the female body" (Burke 2009, 368). Burke concedes that, by rendering the female reproductive body passive by the late eighteenth century, obstetricians made mothers' active participation and thus agency during birth obsolete. This power shift is literally visible in medical illustrations of the time that, in contrast to earlier depictions produced in seventeenth-century midwifery manuals, showed "virtually no part of the mother except graphically severed torsos and thighs of obviously 'dead' (and therefore obsolete) women" (Burke 2009, 372).

The literary and cultural studies scholar Mihaela Ursa equally criticises the "disappearance of the mother" from cultural as well as medical representations (Ursa 2014, 132). By the example of twenty-first-century in vitro fertilisation, she further identifies an increased "empathy towards the idea of technologized bodies and technologized means of body generation" (Ursa 2014, 132). At the same time, Ursa contends that the erasure of the reproductive body and thus mother "does not necessarily prove matrophobic intent, but accentuates the antinaturalistic trend in body technologies while disempowering the female body, especially in its gestating and birthing form" (Ursa 2014, 132). The disappearance of the reproductive body, as she argues, can be grasped by certain posthumanist strands that criticise the phenomenon of disembodiment in/and technology, expressed by scholars such as Hayles, as we have seen (Ursa 2014, 132). The following subchapter proposes a particular posthumanist approach to reproduction that merges the material with the discursive and offers a way out of the maze of dualism and representationalism.

1.3.5 A Material-Discursive Approach

The first and daring paragraph of Karen Barad's contribution "Posthumanist Performativity: Toward an Understanding of How Matter Comes to Matter" (2008)[5] sums up the problem the previous and extensive chapters have been leading up to – the neglect or rather mistreatment of matter and materiality in current humanities studies:

> Language has been granted too much power. The linguistic turn, the semiotic turn, the interpretative turn, the cultural turn: it seems that at every turn lately every 'thing' – even materiality – is turned into a matter of language or some other form of cultural representation. [...] Language matters. Discourse matters. Culture matters. There is an important sense in which the only thing that does not seem to matter anymore is matter.
>
> (Barad 2007, 132; Barad [2003] 2008, 120)

To be precise, the feminist philosopher and quantum physicist Barad does not criticise the total absence of matter (as a topic) from discourse analyses, but rather laments its continued replacement with 'matters of language' that continues to uphold the hierarchy between representation and 'reality' and thus renders matter "passive and immutable" (Barad 2008, 120). In line with scholars like Haraway and Hayles, Barad equally scrutinises representationalism's and social constructivism's "belief in the power of words to mirror preexisting phenomena" (Barad 2008, 121). How, then, can we escape the dilemma of words over matter and extend *beyond representationalism*? There is consensus among new materialists that discursive practices cannot be excluded from analysis. However, in order to challenge the attempt to "turn everything (including material bodies) into words" Barad suggests "*performative* alternatives to representationalism," which will be outlined later (emphasis added, Barad 2008, 121).

In general, Barad shifts the focus away from the question of how (accurately) language 'mirrors' reality to "matters of *practices/doing/actions*" as well as issues of "ontology, materiality, and *agency*" (emphasis added, Barad 2008, 122). Barad uses physical optics[6] as a metaphor to underscore how representationalism becomes "caught up" in reflection (Barad 2008, 122). In the extensive study *Meeting the Universe Halfway – Quantum Physics and the Entanglement of Matter and Meaning* (2007), they build on Haraway's critique of reflection or reflexivity (as part of representationalism) that reaffirms the boundary between "copy and original and the search for the authentic and really real" (Haraway in Barad 2007, 71). Instead of being content with reflection, Barad calls for paying closer attention to *diffraction*[7] that they utilise as a trope throughout their work (Barad 2007, 71). Diffraction, as opposed to reflection, is marked not by "themes of mirroring and sameness," but by "patterns of difference" (Barad 2007, 71).

Barad's explicit aim is *not* to use the diffraction metaphor analogous to the actual "physical phenomenon" of the patterns produced by the dispersal of light or particles – they rather want to "disrupt the widespread reliance on an existing optical metaphor – [...] reflection" that centres on similarities and differences between seemingly stable and preformed entities: "diffraction, as I argue, does not concern homologies but attends to specific *material entanglements*" (emphasis added, Barad 2007, 88). Barad's diffraction metaphor is useful for an analysis of the body as it helps to dissolve the boundaries between language and 'reality.' On the basis of this theory, it is possible to claim that representations – verbal, visual or even haptic – of the body are not mere reflections of that matter; they rather (re)create one another due to their continuous and inextricable *entanglement*. The relationship between language and the body is therefore not static but, according to Barad, an ongoing "*doing* – [an] *enactment* of boundaries" (emphasis added, Barad 2008, 122).

In addition to diffraction, Barad thus introduces the term 'performativity' that they, in contrast to Butler who regards the body as passive, use to attribute agency to matter. Barad's goal is to rethink performativity from a "materialist, naturalist, and posthumanist" standpoint and thus demonstrate that matter is anything but passive and rather an "active participant in the world's becoming"; they term this process "intra-activity" as opposed to int*er*-activity that implies an int*ra*-action between two seemingly stable and preformed entities (Barad 2008, 122). Barad's concept of posthumanist performativity offers an impressive way out of the maze of representationalism by radically rethinking matter and/as discourse.[8] By building on the work of Judith Butler, Andrew Pickering,[9] Bruno Latour, Joseph Rouse and Donna Haraway, Barad suggests a posthumanist performativity that allows for an understanding of matter, discourse, science, society, human and nonhuman as *entangled* (Barad 2008, 126).

Although Barad admits that Foucault's discourse theory, heavily relying on power structures, already "links discursive practices to the materiality of the body," it nevertheless falls short as his approach fails to analyse "*how* [exactly] discursive practices produce material bodies" in the first place (emphasis in the original, Barad 2008, 127). In other words; despite Foucault acknowledging the body's historicity in his first volume of *The History of Sexuality* (1976), he does not address how history and matter are intertwined without creating an order between the two.

Barad rather asks about biology's and history's *simultaneousness* and in what way "historical forces are always already biological" (Barad 2008, 127). What they criticise in particular is Foucault's failure to recognise matter's "*active* role" in shaping its own historicity: Barad thus ascribes materiality its own power and agency (emphasis in the original, Barad 2008, 128). In order to grasp the materiality of "*all* bodies – 'human' and 'nonhuman,'" Barad proposes a "material-discursive" approach to cultural, material and/or scientific practices that both focus on and dissolve the *relation* between discourse, matter and agency, which they term "agential realism" (emphasis in the original, Barad 2008, 128–129). Just as it is impossible for Barad to "fully explicate" Butler's, Foucault's, Haraway's and Rouse's ideas in their work, the following sections equally aim at a condensed rendition of Barad's performative metaphysics (Barad 2008, 129).

In short, Barad chooses another point of departure, namely that of metaphysics in order to highlight the "intertwined practices of knowing and becoming" (Barad 2008, 130). They draw on the physicist Niels Bohr's "philosophy-physics" that opposes the assumption of "'things' as ontologically basic entities" (Barad 2008, 131). As Barad outlines, Bohr thus questions the Cartesian dualism of mind over body to the degree that he even objects to language's function as a medium, since the "triadic structure of words, knowers and things" are inseparable (Barad 2008, 131). Instead of talking about the "position" of a seemingly independent object with clear boundaries, both Bohr and Barad prefer to think the 'act' of observation as a "property of the *phenomenon* [or episteme]," because object and observation 'happen' simultaneously: "*phenomena are the ontological inseparability of agentially intra-acting 'components*'" (emphasis in the original, Barad 2008, 132–133).[10]

Put simply, matter and representation are always already inseparable. Put even simpler: Everything – humans, nonhumans, bodies, words, representations, reality, subjects, objects, relations, relata etc. – are *entangled* in what could be called a 'cosmic soup'. A 'split' between them is only temporarily achieved by the int*ra*-action that 'enacts' boundaries within a certain phenomenon. But what exactly are 'phenomena' and how do they work? Barad suggests the term 'apparatus' that they use synonymously with phenomena. Apparatuses, however, are not to be confused with mere instruments or (mediating) machines. Rather, they are "themselves phenomena" or, as Barad puts it, performative practices: "*apparatuses are dynamic (re)configurations* of *the world, specific agential practices/intra-actions/performances through which specific exclusionary boundaries are enacted*" (emphasis in the original, Barad 2008, 134):

> In summary, the universe is agential intra-activity in its becoming. The primary ontological units are not "things" but phenomena – dynamic topological reconfigurations/*entanglements*/ relationalities/(re)articulations. And the primary semantic units are not "words" but *material-discursive practices* through which boundaries are constituted. This dynamism is *agency*. Agency is not an attribute but the ongoing reconfigurings of the world.
>
> (emphasis added, Barad 2008, 135)

As a result, neither things nor meanings are (pre)determined. Boundaries between matter and matter but also between matter and meaning are produced through material-discursive practices. The same holds true for (human) bodies, which is why Barad merges posthumanism with a material-discourse analysis: "'Human bodies' and 'human subjects' do not preexist as such; nor are they mere end products. 'Humans' are neither pure cause nor pure effect, but part of the world in its open-ended becoming" (Barad 2008, 139).

Furthermore, as Barad repeatedly emphasises, matter is never passive or a "blank slate […] passively awaiting signification; […] *matter is substance in its intra-active becoming – not a thing, but a doing, a congealing agency*" (emphasis in the original, Barad 2008, 139). Matter, according to Barad, is thus an "*active* 'agent' in its ongoing materialization. […] Bodies are not objects with inherent boundaries and properties, they are material-discursive phenomena" (emphasis in the original, Barad 2008, 140–141). As a result, in Barad's approach, "no priority is given to either materiality or discursivity" (Barad 2008, 143). It is essential to note that when Barad assigns matter (or the body) with agency, they do not mean "human intentionality or subjectivity"; rather, Barad refers to "'cyborgian' forms of agency" as a "matter of intra-acting; it is an enactment, not something that someone or something has. [...] Agency is not an attribute whatsoever – it is 'doing'/'being' in its intra-activity" (Barad 2008, 144).

Barad stresses that such a "posthumanist materialist account of performativity" questions materiality's pre-existence or its (assumed) status as an "effect of human agency" (Barad 2008, 145). As they continue: "Nature is neither a passive surface awaiting the mark of culture nor the end product of cultural performances" (Barad 2008, 145). Barad outlines how especially feminist science studies have already pointed to the problem of the Cartesian or nature/culture dualism, which thwarts an understanding of how "*matter comes to matter*" (emphasis in the original, Barad 2008, 140, 145). In accordance with Bohr, they emphasise that the

> "knower" does not stand in a relation of absolute externality to the natural world being investigated – there is no such exterior observational point. [...] "We" are not outside observers of the world. [...] rather, we are part *of* the world in its ongoing intra-activity. [...] "Humans" are part of the world-body space in its dynamic structuration. [...] we know because "we" are *of* the world. [...] *Onto-epistem-ology* – the study of practices of knowing in being – is probably a better way to think about the kind of understandings that are needed to come to terms with how specific intra-actions matter.
>
> (emphasis in the original, Barad 2008, 146–147)

The recognition that representations cannot be analysed on the basis of accuracy alone is not new as mentioned earlier with reference to Stuart Hall. However, Barad's rethinking of matter and meaning helps "mainstream science studies" to include constructs such as gender or sexuality that have too often been regarded as "preformed categories of the social" (Barad 2007, 87). In Barad's view, these studies "fail to attend to 'gender-in-the-making' – the production of gender and other social variables as constituted through technoscientific practices" (Barad 2007, 87). In line with feminist science studies, Barad calls for investigations of "gender-and-science-in-the-making" and invites mainstream science studies to question the culture/nature binary, and especially to recognise "*that* it [the dichotomy] matters" and to ask "*how* it matters and *for whom*" (emphasis in the original, Barad 2007, 87).

Representationalism or the 'reflection' metaphor hence does not suffice in order to achieve this goal: "reflexivity is based on the belief that practices of representing have no effect on the objects of investigation" (Barad 2007, 87). The diffraction metaphor, however, can be utilised as a tool for (re)thinking matter and meaning in the scope of (feminist) science studies:

> Diffractively reading the insights of feminist and queer theory and science studies approaches *through* one another entails thinking the "social" and the "scientific" together in an illuminating way. What often appears as separate entities [...] does not actually entail a relatio of absolute exteriority at all.

> Like the diffraction patterns illuminating the indefinite nature of boundaries [...] the relation of the social and scientific is a relation of "*exteriority within*."
>
> (emphasis added, Barad 2008, 122)

In chapter four of *Meeting the Universe Halfway*, Barad includes a table that summarises their approach by contrasting 'diffraction' with 'reflection.' What follows is a condensed quote of this juxtaposition to demonstrate that aspects of mimesis are insufficient when talking about representation and reality, language and matter or literature and the body (See Figure 14).

The point Barad wishes to make with their concept of agential realism is that it helps to understand that "knowledge-making practices" cannot be investigated by turning to representationalism alone:

> knowing, thinking, measuring, theorizing, and observing are material practices of intra-acting within and as part of the world. [...] We do not uncover preexisting facts about independently existing things as they exist frozen in time like little statues positioned in the world. [...] The point is not simply to put the observer or knower back *in* the world (as if the world were a container and we needed merely to acknowledge our situatedness in it) but to understand and take account of the fact that we too are part of the world's differential becoming.
>
> (emphasis in the original, Barad 2007, 90–91)

Reflection	*Diffraction*
mirror image (division between entities)	**diffraction pattern** (differences from within, *entanglement*)
mimesis (reflections, 'objectivity', homology)	**differences materialised** (differences that matter)
representationalism (preformed boundaries, subject/object	**performativity** (no pre-existence of subject/object, *intra-actions*)
ontology/epistemology (knower/known binary)	**onto-epistem-ology** (knowing as material practice, *entanglement*)
reading against (fixed)	**reading *through*** (transdisciplinary)
→ reflecting on representations	**→ how practices matter**

Figure 14 A condensed rendition of Karen Barad's main differences between reflection and diffraction (see Barad 2007, 89–90).

What is more, as Barad stresses by referring to physical optics again, the "details of diffraction patterns [strongly] depend on the details of the apparatus [...]. If any of these parameters is changed, the pattern can be significantly different" (Barad 2007, 91). They emphasise that "[a]ttention to fine details is a crucial element of this methodology" (Barad 2007, 92). Barad thus advocates thinking the material and discursive "*through* one another" instead of against one another (emphasis added, Barad 2007, 92–93). The methodology they suggest hence "enables a *critical rethinking* of science and the social in their relationality. [...] Like the diffraction patterns illuminating the indefinite nature of boundaries [...] – the relation of the social and the scientific is a relation of '*exterior within*'" (emphasis added, Barad 2007, 93).

Barad's approach is relatively abstract and has received significant critical attention. The subchapter's final section is therefore devoted to a brief discussion of some (alleged) conceptual ambiguities and problems the German sociologists Katharina Hoppe and Thomas Lemke address in their article "Die Macht der Materie: Grundlagen und Grenzen des agentiellen Realismus von Karen Barad" (2015). Hoppe and Lemke correctly outline Barad's main premisses and emphasise the latter's claim that because causality is only implemented by in*tra*-action, there cannot exist a prior 'direction' of power relations [Translation: Then the question arises as to what 'plenitude' and 'capacity' [of matter] refer to here – if not to the idea of a unified, stable substance and an original force inherently present in matter.] (Hoppe/Lemke 2015, 264). They also acknowledge that with 'agency,' Barad does *not* mean properties of subjects or objects but the enactment of changes through in*tra*-activity (Hoppe/Lemke 2015, 264).

However, Hoppe and Lemke question Barad's ambivalent use of the term 'matter' and argue that Barad risks upholding the division between matter and meaning by ascribing materiality a dynamic agency: "dann ist zu fragen, worauf sich 'Fülle' und 'Vermögen' [der Materie] hier beziehen – wenn nicht auf die Idee einer einheitlichen, stabilen Substanz und einer ursprünglichen Kraft, die Materie immer schon innewohnt" [Translation: Then the question arises as to what 'plenitude' and 'capacity' [of matter] refer to here – if not to the idea of a unified, stable substance and an original force inherently present in matter.] (Hoppe/Lemke 2015, 270). Hoppe and Lemke's question is understandable. Yet, they immediately recognise this conceptual ambivalence as an important strategy: "Die gleichzeitige Betonung radikaler Relationalität und die Hervorhebung eines quasi-fundamentalen Stellenwerts von Materie verleiht Barads Kritik am Sozialkonstruktivismus und Poststrukturalismus ihre besondere Schärfe" [Translation: The simultaneous emphasis on radical relationality and the assertion of a quasi-fundamental status of matter lends Barad's critique of social constructivism and poststructuralism its particular sharpness.] (Hoppe/Lemke 2015, 270–271).[11]

Ironically, Hoppe and Lemke themselves give a concrete example earlier in their publication for the entanglement of matter and discourse when they address a topic that can be linked to that of this book: prenatal risk assessment. With reference to Nete Schwennesen and Lene Koch's article "Visualizing and Calculating Life: Matters of Fact in the Context of Prenatal Risk Assessment" (2009), they demonstrate the applicability of Barad's agential realism (Hoppe/Lemke 2015, 268).

Schwennesen and Koch's empirical study that is based on observations of prenatal diagnostic examinations highlights the entanglement of matter and discourse, of meaning and the reproductive body, in a vivid manner:

> [...] so werde der Fötus in verschiedenen Materialitäten in den Praktiken der Wissensproduktion erst hervorgebracht [...]. Im Kontext der Ultraschaluntersuchung wird der Fötus hierbei als 'korrekte' Repräsentation und damit als konkretes (materielles) Phänomen durch das Zusammenwirken unterschiedlicher Agentien (Eltern, Ärzt_innen, Ultraschallgerät, Ultraschallbild, Körper etc.) konstitutioniert [...]. In den Risiko-Kalkulationen [...] wird jedoch etwas ganz anderes realisiert. Hier wird der Fötus auf einen Grenzwert bezogen und als ‚risikohafter' Fötus hervorgebracht – der wirksame Apparat sei nunmehr weniger das Bild als die Risikozahl [...].[12]
>
> (Hoppe/Lemke 2015, 268–269)

As Hoppe and Lemke outline, Schwennesen and Koch's recourse to Barad's term 'int*ra*-action' allows to describe the foetus as ontologically and epistemologically multiple: The (material-discursive) foetus is thus to be understood not as a static and pre-given entity but rather as a procedural phenomenon (Hoppe/Lemke 2015, 269). Knowledge production, as Hoppe and Lemke conclude, therefore strongly depends on the (material) apparatus that brings the foetus into existence in the first place: "der Fötus präexistiert in diesem Sinne nicht; er wird in vielfältiger [intra-aktiver] Weise und unterschiedlichen Relationen in Kraft gesetzt" [Translation: The fetus does not preexist in this sense; rather, it is brought into being through various [intra-active] ways and different relations.] (Hoppe/Lemke 2015, 269). What is more, the foetus, as part of the reproductive body, is not simply 'reflected' but 'refracted' in its ongoing int*ra*-activity with the multidimensional apparatus.

In 2018, Barad emphatically underlines that diffraction is "not a set pattern, but rather an iterative (re)configuring of patterns of differentiating-entangling"; agential cuts therefore do not generate "absolute separation but rather *cut together-apart*" (emphasis added, Barad 2018, 4). They also repeatedly explain the relevance of Bohr's work for their methodology and thus lever out the critique of some of their colleagues who have accused them of focussing too much on this physicist's work. Bohr's interpretation of metaphysics is useful for a material-discursive approach as his thoughts on the mysterious 'wave-particle duality problem' help to understand that "identity is not essence, fixity or givenness, but a contingent iterative performativity" (Barad 2018, 9–10). Like gender 'troubles' identity, diffraction 'troubles' the "onto(epistemo)logy of classical physics" (Barad 2018, 10). Bohr's approach can easily be utilised for a feminist or queer understanding of nature and culture which makes a rethinking of matter possible, as Barad concludes:

> Bohr understood difference in its materiality. Meaning is not an ideality; meaning is material. And matter isn't what exists separately from meaning. Mattering is a matter of what comes to matter and what doesn't. Difference isn't given. It isn't fixed. Subject and object, wave and particle, position and momentum do not exist outside of specific intra-actions that enact

> cuts that make separations – not absolute separations, but only contingent separations – *within* phenomena.
>
> (emphasis in the original, Barad 2018, 11)

In sum, Haraway, Hayles and especially Barad offer a new way not only to think *with* but also *through* the body. These approach helps to find an adequate language to talk about the body and its materiality in the first place. These concepts do not do away with discourse or representationalism altogether. Rather, they enable a possibility to acknowledge the body's material-discursive entanglement with the world.

1.3.6 Synopsis: Thinking through the Body

The previous chapters demonstrate the need for further studies on the history of the reproductive body and also highlight a significant research gap regarding the material-discursive entanglement of the maternal body and its representations. In particular, the research overview shows the necessity to move *beyond* a Foucauldian discourse analysis and extend this approach by making matter more prominent. It is therefore crucial to acknowledge the material practices of knowledge production in order to avoid reaffirming the duality of mind over matter, representation over body or language over 'reality.' As outlined, the current approach certainly does not dismiss language, including metaphors, or representations. This book rather aims at analysing the complex int*ra*-active 'networks of information' and acknowledges the 'multiplicity of material-discursive practices' of reproduction in eighteenth-century Britain (see Fox Keller 1995, 8; Waddington 2011, 83; Buckley 2017, 25).

In this context, Schiebinger's indication that representations of the reproductive body are never "simply the product of the growth of realism in anatomy" cannot be overstated (Schiebinger 1986, 43). Even Jordanova, who focusses on images of gender from the eighteenth century onwards, already hints at the entanglement of (material) medical practices with the "language in which they are expressed," when she strongly criticises Foucault's overtly abstract discourse theory (Jordanova 1989, 6, see also 10–15). What was not yet, however, available to Jordanova and others is an appropriate language to talk about the body and its material-discursive entanglement.

The same holds true for Newman's extremely valuable research that exposes the increasing "erasure of the woman's body" in eighteenth-century medical illustrations and beyond (Newman 1996, 8). She also condemns claims of supposedly 'realistic' images for reproducing the same old binary between representation and reality (Newman 1996, 4). In that respect, McGrath skilfully problematises representations of the reproductive body by riveting on the effects these images had on the material practices of obstetricians who regarded the 'real' maternal bodies as fragmented birth machines (McGrath 2002, 64–66). The obstetrical machines Lieske discusses can thus be understood as the epitome of the fragmented (female) reproductive body (Lieske 2012, 71–72).

The identified gaps hence include the increasing erasure of the reproductive body in eighteenth-century medical representations, its implications for the 'real' (material) body as well as the remaining problem of the representation/reality dualism. In order to acknowledge the body's material discursivity and merge the physical with the historical, it is necessary to make 'matter matter' again and *extend beyond representationalism* as the only key to understanding the material; as Richards points out, there is the need for an appropriate language to talk (and think) about bodies and their materiality (Richards 2018, 25). More precisely, it is necessary to find a way to think *through* the body in order to avoid reaffirming dichotomies between nature and culture or science and gender. New materialism offers an alternative for these dualisms; it not only identifies the body's simultaneous absence and presence in literary and cultural artefacts but also points to the limits of a Foucauldian approach that, regardless of its achievements to recognise the impact of power on the body, still renders the body a passive object (Hillman/Maude 2015, 3–5). In order to make the reproductive body 'visible' (again) and carve out its "*inter*-corporeal" entanglement "*within*" and "*between*" nature and culture or science and gender, it is essential to extend beyond postmodern concepts like performativity and recognise the illusion that 'reality' is prior to representation (emphasis in the original, Shilling 2016, 17, 19, 36, 38).

Haraway's cyborg imagery can be harnessed to conceptualise the reproductive body as a hybrid 'cyborg body' that leads out of the "maze of dualism" (Haraway 2000, 316). Not only is the cyborg body already fragmented and thus simultaneously points towards fragmented (gender) identities and the illusion of the modern self's pregivenness – it also refers to the role technology plays in the shaping and reshaping of the reproductive body as new practices make physical boundaries "newly permeable" through intervention and new forms of visualisation (see Haraway 2000, 299, 302, 306). Moreover, the pregnant body is equally hybrid or 'indeterminate' due to its 'mutability' and 'indivisibility' (see Hanson 2004, 87). Haraway's cyborg imagery is particularly useful for a first attempt at a material-discursive analysis of the reproductive body as it additionally underlines the obvious – that science or medicine and materiality are inextricably linked (see Haraway 2000, 316).

Hayles' critique of the hierarchical representation/reality binary by the example of the "erasure of embodiment" in information technology offers a fruitful way to "put back into the [posthuman] picture the flesh" and recognise that society and the material are entangled with each other (Hayles 1999, 4–5). Hayles particularly criticises the understanding that information and medium are separated; instead, she points to "feedback loops" between reality and representation (Hayles 1999, 13). Hayles' explicit aim is thus to reunite materiality with information by "putting back together parts" (Hayles 1999, 13). In other words, there is no discourse without matter and no matter without discourse – a claim that Barad builds on in their *agential realism*.

Indeed, Barad radically rethinks materiality by thinking *through* it. They extend beyond representationalism and offer performative alternatives by assigning matter agency, not in the form of intentionality or subjectivity but rather in a "cyborgian" sense of a posthuman and performative material-discursive entanglement of matter and meaning (Barad 2008, 144). Barad further discards the term 'reflection' in favour of 'diffraction' which she borrows from the field of physical optics. As opposed to two (or more) preformed entities reflecting each other, the diffraction metaphor 'troubles' seemingly stable ontologies and epistemologies of matter and meaning and turns them into "onto(episteme)olog[ies]" (Barad 2008, 10). Put simply, Barad rethinks reality and representation, matter and performativity, science and culture as well as subjects and objects by reminding us that each of them is always already part of the world's becoming in an ongoing and especially *non-causal* process which they call *intra-activity* (see Barad 2008, 122). Biology and history (and the observation of both) thus simultaneously and 'actively' generate each other; neither materiality nor discursivity is thus given priority, which is why Barad terms the relations between matter and discourse *agential realism* (see Barad 2008, 129).

Barad's material-discursive approach to matter and meaning opens up multiple opportunities to rethink or think *through* the reproductive body. Not only does this framework dissolve the representation/reality hierarchy, but it also allows for shifting the focus from language as the only access point to history to an investigation of material-discursive medical practices of childbirth and obstetrics during the eighteenth century. As Hoppe and Lemke comprehensibly illustrate in their critical evaluation of Barad's agential realism by the example of prenatal risk assessment, the foetus is not a preformed entity passively awaiting inscription by an observer. On the contrary, the material-discursive entanglement of ultrasound image, body, instrument, practitioner and interpretation int*ra*-actively yields both the (material) foetus and (discursive) knowledge in the first place.

To conclude this book's deliberately extensive PART I, I wish to emphasise that what follows in PART II are still discursive analyses of literary and cultural artefacts since the analysed (material) bodies are obviously bygone. Nevertheless, the approach significantly differs from a classic or traditional discourse analysis by making matter matter more. What follows are discussions of selected eighteenth-and early nineteenth-century well-and lesser-known texts in conversation with questions of reproduction. Though all analysis chapters refer back to those in PART I, they can theoretically be read separately or in non-chronological order. Each chapter is divided into four subchapters, whereas the first offers a general introduction. The following three subchapters focus on the context, the actual text at hand, and the final sections stitch the pieces back together again.

Notes

1 With regard to the body and/in history, Richards emphasises that especially the French Revolution "functions as an originating trauma," while the "nearly continuous wars" of the eighteenth century contribute to its "narrative of loss" due to its lack of historical artefacts (Richards 2018, 18). The era of Enlightenment thus "required a narrative of progress, and its wounded bodies [...] were often erased or removed from serious consideration to make room for a cultural history that marginalized loss" (Richards 2018, 18). Wounded bodies, Richards points out, became "less culturally visible" in canonised literature and culture and if they did, they were subject to comedy or satire that "avert our gaze" (Richards 2018, 18–19).

2 See Latour's *Science in Action: How to Follow Scientists and Engineers through Society* ([1987] 2015).

3 The shift from the one- to the two-sex model in the eighteenth century, based on "*distorted* biological differences between the sexes," was later taken up in Simone de Beauvoir's feminist manifesto *The Second Sex* (1949), which famously claimed that "One is

not born but rather becomes a woman" (emphasis in the original, Shilling 2016, 31; see also Braidotti 2013, 3).

4 Such a reading is already implied in the novel's title that aligns the scientist Victor Frankenstein with the Greek god Prometheus who is punished for stealing fire and handing it over to humanity, thus enabling civilisation.

5 See also Barad's *Meeting the Universe Halfway: Quantum Physics and the Entanglement of Matter and Meaning* (2007). "Posthuman Performativity" (2008), in which they cite seven of their own publications, is a revised version of an essay she published in 2003. Barad's article (2008) as well as selected sections from their book (2007) fully suffice for this book's main argument.

6 Physical optics or wave optics is a subfield in physics that deals with the reflection, refraction (bending) and diffraction (dispersion) of light.

7 In physical optics, diffraction refers to wave patterns that are produced. One example for this effect is the dispersion of (monochromatic) light after it passing small apertures in the scope of the so called two-slit experiment. However, water can produce the same pattern after passing small openings. Barad gives further examples such as the indeterminate boundaries of a razor blade's boundaries after being illuminated with monochromatic light or the changing hues of colour in a soap bubble, depending on the observer's position. The point they want to make is that reflection does not suffice to explain differences between representation and 'reality.' By the example of diffraction, Barad emphasises not only the blurry or rather non-existent boundaries between light and particles (or 'non-matter' and matter) but especially that patterns are produced by differences *within*.

8 Barad questions representationalism's conviction that there are several distinct and independent entities: (1) representations (or knowledge), (2) the represented (the known) and (3) the knower ("someone who does the representing") (Barad 2008, 123). According to Barad, this ontological assumption, that ascribes representation a "mediating function," also inevitably leads to "questions of the accuracy of [e.g. scientific] representations" (Barad 2008, 123). They outline how certain science studies have begun to scrutinise representationalism since the 1980s by shifting the emphasis away from knowledge production to the "actual practice of science" (Barad 2008, 124). This "move *beyond* representationalism" reveals the void between representation and referent as a "Cartesian by-product" that upholds the hierachy of word over matter (emphasis added, Barad 2008, 125–126).

9 See also Pickering's *The Mangle of Practice: Time Agency, and Science* (1995).

10 What is more, other than the Cartesian dualism that assumes a preexisting distinction between mind and body, subject and object, word and matter, Barad states that in*tra*-actions produce an "*agential cut*" between observer and observed in the first place (emphasis in the original, Barad 2008, 133): "the agential cut enacts a *local* resolution *within* the phenomenon of the inherent ontological indeterminacy. In other words, relata do not preexist relations; rather, relata-within-phenomena emerge through specific in*tra*-actions. Crucially then, intra-actions enact *agential seperability* – the local condition of *exteriority-within-phenomena*" (emphasis in the original, Barad 2008, 133).

11 Another critique Hoppe and Lemke seize is that of other sociologists and physicists like Trevor Pinch (2011) who laments a lack of sociohistorical context in Barad's work and its limitation to Bohr's understanding of quantum physics (Hoppe/Lemke 2015, 271).

12 Translation: '[...] thus the foetus is produced in various materialities in the practices of knowledge production [...]. In the context of the ultrasound examination, the foetus is constituted as a 'correct' representation and thus as a concrete (material) phenomenon through the interaction of different agents (parents, doctors, ultrasound device, ultrasound image, body, etc.) [...]. In the risk calculations [...], however, something quite different is realised. Here, the foetus is related to a threshold value and produced as a 'risky' foetus – the effective apparatus is now less the image than the risk figure [...].'

References

Alaimo, Stacy, and Susan Hekman, eds. 2008. *Material Feminisms*. Bloomington: Indiana University Press.

Barad, Karen. 2007. *Meeting the Universe Halfway: Quantum Physics and the Entanglement of Matter and Meaning*. Durham, NC: Duke University Press.

Barad, Karen. [2003] 2008. "Posthumanist Performativity: Toward an Understanding of How Matter Comes to Matter." *Signs* 28 (3): 801–831.

Birke, Lynda. 1999. *Feminism and the Biological Body*. Edinburgh: Edinburgh University Press.

Braidotti, Rosi. 2013. *The Posthuman*. Cambridge: Polity.

Buckley, Jenifer. 2017. *Gender, Pregnancy and Power in Eighteenth-Century Literature: The Maternal Imagination*. Basingstoke: Plagrave Macmillan.

Burke, Meghan L. 2009. "Making Mothers Obsolete: Eliza Fenwick's *Secresy* and the Masculine Appropriation of Maternity." *Eighteenth Century Fiction* 21 (3): 357–384.

Butler, Judith. 1990. *Gender Trouble: Feminism and the Subversion of Identity*. Abingdon: Routledge.

Butler, Judith. 1993. *Bodies That Matter: On the Discursive Limits of Sex*. Abingdon: Routledge.

DeMello, Margo. 2014. *Body Studies: An Introduction*. Abingdon: Routledge.

Fox Keller, Evelyn. 1995. *Reflections on Gender and Science*. New Haven, CT: Yale University Press.

Haraway, Donna. [1985] 2000. "A Cyborg Manifesto: Science, Technology, and Socialist Feminism in the Late Twentieth Century." In *The Cybercultures Reader*, edited by David Bell and Barbara Kennedy, 292–324. New York: Routledge.

Hanson, Clare. 2004. *A Cultural History of Pregnancy: Pregnancy, Medicine and Culture, 1750–2000*. Basingstoke: Palgrave Macmillan.

Hayles, N. Katherine. 1999. *How We Became Posthuman: Virtual Bodies in Cybernetics, Literature, and Informatics*. Chicago, IL; London: University of Chicago Press.

Hillman, David, and Ulrika Maude, eds. 2015. *The Cambridge Companion to the Body in Literature*. New York: Cambridge University Press.

Hoppe, Katharina, and Thomas Lemke. 2015. "Die Macht der Materie: Grundlagen und Grenzen des agentiellen Realismus von Karen Barad." *Soziale Welt* 66 (3): 261–280.

Jordanova, Ludmilla J. 1989. *Sexual Visions: Images of Gender in Science and Medicine between the Eighteenth and Twentieth Centuries*. Madison: University of Wisconsin Press.

Kristeva, Julia. 1982. *Powers of Horror: An Essay on Abjection*. New York: Columbia University Press.

Latour, Bruno. 2015. *Science in Action: How to Follow Scientists and Engineers through Society*. Cambridge, MA: Harvard University Press.

Lieske, Pam. 2012. "'Made in Imitation of Real Women and Children': Obstetrical Machines in Eighteenth-Century Britain." In *The Female Body in Medicine and Literature*, edited by Andrew Mangham and Greta Depledge, 16–33. Liverpool: Liverpool University Press.

McGrath, Roberta. 2002. *Seeing Her Sex: Medical Archives and the Female Body*. Manchester: Manchester University Press.

Newman, Karen. 1996. *Fetal Positions: Individualism, Science, Visuality*. Stanford, CA: Stanford University Press.

Pickering, Andrew. 1995. *The Mangle of Practice: Time Agency, and Science*. Chicago, IL: University of Chicago Press.

Richards, Cynthia. 2018. "History without Trauma: Recovering Bodily Loss in the Eighteenth Century." In *The Future of Feminist Eighteenth-Century Scholarship: Beyond Recovery*, edited by Robin Runia, 132–145. New York: Routledge.

Runia, Robin. 2018. "Introduction." In *The Future of Feminist Eighteenth-Century Scholarship: Beyond Recovery*, edited by Robin Runia, 1–10. New York: Routledge.

Schiebinger, Londa. 1986. "Skeletons in the Closet: The First Illustrations of the Female Skeleton in Eighteenth-Century Anatomy." *Representations* 14: 42–82.

Schwennesen, Nete, and Lene Koch. 2009. "Visualizing and Calculating Life: Matters of Fact in the Context of Prenatal Risk Assessment." In *Contested Categories: Life Sciences in Society*, edited by Susanne Bauer and Ayo Wahlberg, 69–87. New York: Routledge.

Sheehan, Paul. 2015. "Posthuman Bodies." In *The Cambridge Companion to the Body in Literature*, edited by David Hillman and Ulrika Maude, 145–158. New York: Cambridge University Press.

Shilling, Chris. 2016. *The Body: A Very Short Introduction*. Oxford: Oxford University Press.

Ursa, Mihaela. 2014. "Giving Birth the Posthuman Way: Technology, Disembodiment, and Cyber-Progenies." *Ekphrasis: Images, Cinema, Theatre, Media* 12 (2): 131–140.

Waddington, Keir. 2011. *An Introduction to the Social History of Medicine: Europe since 1500*. Red Globe Press.

Part II

Science, Sex & Secret Bodies of Knowledge

2.1 Jonathan Swift's *Gulliver's Travels* (1726)

2.1.1 Introduction

Jonathan Swift's *Travels into Several Remote Nations of the World. In Four Parts. By Lemuel, First a Surgeon, and then a Captain of several Ships*, later abbreviated *Gulliver's Travels*, is a prime example of "world literature" and "as familiar to politicians as to infants" until today (Seager 2022, 175). Swift's well-known satire is not only enmeshed with contemporary colonial or political discourses but especially addresses or rather mocks emerging knowledges in the field of (new) science, empiricism in particular. Swift wrote at a time when different discourses and scientific practices existed alongside each other. One dominant debate (still) revolved around the relationship between words and objects, initiated decades earlier by Robert Hooke's *Micrographia* (1665),[1] a book published by the Royal Society as its first significant scientific piece that quickly became a bestseller among both scientists and the public. In order to fully understand the relevance of Hooke's work for the reading of Swift's novel, what follows is a brief discussion of this book.

Hooke's *Micrographia* especially stood out because of its visual components as it "provided engraved illustrations of various objects as they were seen under the microscope" (Morrissey 2017, 237). What strikes the eye is that Hooke, ironically, used his illustrations and descriptions to criticise what society actually stood for: human reason. The first object he examined was not a fly or a grain of dust but a miniature Bible. Under the microscope, this book looked like nothing more than "a great spl[o]tch of London dirt" (Hooke in Morrissey 2017, 237). By adding this description to the "dirty irregularities of texts," Hooke criticised the "messiness of [printed] words" (Morrissey 2017, 237).

Moreover, Hooke urged readers to "turn away from books and towards the instruments through which the natural world might be observed" and thus contributed to a growing distinction between the "study of the physical world from the study of texts" (Morrissey 2017, 237). Yet, Hooke did not argue against human reason as such, but rather against reasoning with the help of words only. In a way, it is possible to understand his approach to science as an early example of entangled meaning with matter; Hooke (unknowingly) brought the instrument's materiality to the fore and thus rendered it not just a 'gateway' to the natural world but entangled it with language.

DOI: 10.4324/9781003467977-6

To return to *Gulliver's Travels*, this chapter discusses Swift's own relationship to scientific discourses of his time, while also asking about how the text int*ra*-links science, sex(uality), secrecy and the reproductive body. It starts with a more general discussion of the novel's ambiguous satire that, however, notably manifests itself in or rather *through* the texts' material-discursive bodies (Seidel 1998; Rivero 2002; Porter 2004; Marshall 2013; McCormick 2013; Morrissey 2017). It then moves on to the role of secrecy in/and science and literature, and the question of how it is intertwined with masculine authority, the female reproductive body and microscopy (Porter 2004, 2021; Rabb 2006; Armintor 2007; Spratt 2012; Ingram 2022). This chapter's final section discusses how Swift's fascination for 'monstrous' female bodies is linked to (the practice of) obstetrics with the aim to demonstrate the still ongoing entanglement of meaning and matter (Flynn 1990; Francus 2012; Girten 2013).

The Anglo-Irish clergyman, political journalist and writer Jonathan Swift (1667–1745) is still celebrated as a "national hero" in Ireland and referred to as a "vigorous defender of liberty" on his tombstone (Noggle 2018, 245–255). As James Noggle elaborates, Swift enjoyed an "excellent education" before he left his country after Ireland's invasion and explored his "astonishing gifts as a satirist" in England that mainly dealt with topics surrounding the "corruptions of religion and education" and, of course, politics (Noggle 2018, 254). After Swift (unwillingly) returned to his home country in his early thirties, he devoted himself fully to politics, defending the Anglican Church and rejecting "all who seemed to threaten it" (Noggle 2018, 254–255). Moreover, he has been described as a blatant misanthrope, a "hater of humanity" (Noggle 2018, 256). This accusation manifests itself especially in *Gulliver's Travels* that blurs the boundaries between the human and the animal and renders 'man' an "*animal rationis capax* ('an animal [simply] *capable* of reason')" (emphasis in the original, Noggle 2018, 256). To this day, Swift is understood as a "master of prose," and his poems are also characterised by a "love of bluntness […] which shock us with their hard look at the facts of life and the body" (Noggle 2018, 256).

Swift did not just mock religion, politics and the *conditio humana* in general, but found an easy target in natural philosophy or what we know today as 'science.' He in particular mocked science's claim to rationality, objectivity and "reliable observation" (Hawes 2020, 188). As Clement Hawes outlines:

> Early science was a threshold phenomenon: a natural philosophy inflected by alchemical fantasies and monster-mongering. In the focus of early science on dubious anomalies Swift spotted satirical daylight: a major opening in the self-legitimating claim to represent the real and the rational.
>
> (Hawes 2020, 188)

It is thus no coincidence that Swift's protagonist Gulliver is both a traveller and a scientist who meticulously records – or 'dissects' – his surroundings in partially "surreal close-up[s], say, of a grainy human breast 16 feet in circumference" (Hawes 2020, 188). The giant breast that Gulliver records in great detail is not only a human breast but a female one in particular. As the subsequent analysis demonstrates, the way Swift constructs the surgeon's encounter with these potentially reproductive body parts echoes obstetrical practices that dismembered the female reproductive body and thus reduced the 'patient' to a conglomerate of pathologised parts.

Gregory Lynall offers a more nuanced view of Swift's relation to science. He argues that it was more "complex" than generally assumed and "often misunderstood" (Lynall 2012, 1). By referencing the English poet Abraham Cowley's ode "To the Royal Society" that praises the society's founder Francis Bacon and his approach of empiricism, Lynall underscores Swift's general scepticism towards "ultimate truth" (Lynall 2012, 2, 6). What is more, Swift mocks Bacon's "fascination with the exotic and monstrous" that takes shape in Gulliver's encounters with giant insects, bodies and especially parts thereof (Lynall 2012, 3). Swift's criticism, according to Lynall, was rather directed at questions of power: "who has the theological, political or cultural authority to speak publicly to disseminate their ideas; from where does this power originate; and what grants some discourses more authority than others?" (Lynall 2012, 6).

Therefore, the new natural knowledges emerging during this period were, for Swift, "themselves related to this wider debate about who has the right to utterance in the public domain" (Lynall 2012, 6). It seems safe to say that Swift was thus ahead of his time and raised questions that sociologists have only relatively recently addressed when scrutinising the "absolute authority of science" (Lynall 2012, 8). As Lynall further remarks, scholars need to acknowledge that natural philosophy "*within* eighteenth-century culture meant that it could not exist independently of the *outside* world"; Swift's aim was to investigate the "wider consequences of experimental enquiries into nature" (emphasis added, Lynall 2012, 8). The division between 'inside' and 'outside,' however, is not unproblematic as it follows the binary logic of representation and reality or meaning and matter. This book rather aims at emphasising the entanglement of all dimensions that are – simultaneously – part of the world's becoming.

2.1.2 Swift & The Problem of Meaning

Jonathan Swift's *Gulliver's Travels* revolves around a trained surgeon who "winds up shipwrecked [...] on several different islands [...] populated with [fundamentally different] types of people" (Morrissey 2017, 259). What especially distinguishes these people are their bodies: They are either "very short" as in Lilliput, "towering giants" as in Brobdingnag or animal-like as in Houyhnhnm-land (Morrissey 2017, 259). The narrative's very first paragraph already contains a pun in terms of a sexualised physical activity when Mr Bates, Gulliver's mentor, is repeatedly called 'Master Bates' by the narrator (Morrissey 2017, 260). In general, the novel is saturated with Gulliver's "fascination with physiological and sexualised details" of female bodies in particular (Morrissey 2017, 261). As Morrissey stresses, "Gulliver's attitudes strike many readers as misogynist"; yet, this interpretation is too sweeping (Morrissey 2017, 261).[2]

At first glance, Gulliver appears to be a version of the "Enlightenment cosmopolitan […] travelling the world and learning from presumed others": A second look, however, reveals that *Gulliver's Travels* "criticises such Enlightenment cosmopolitanism" (Morrissey 2017, 262). As Morrissey stresses, Swift's narrative is in fact constructed as a harsh critique of early British colonialism during the Age of Enlightenment. This becomes especially apparent during Gulliver's voyage to the 'superior' flying island of Laputa whose inhabitants hover over yet another, 'inferior' island, Balnibarbi: The spatial relationship of these two islands, as has been argued, can be read as an allegory to that of Britain and its first colony – Ireland (Morrissey 2017, 262–263).

The genre of *Gulliver's Travels* is equally hard to define. For Albert J. Rivero, it is whatever readers make of it, a "political book, a children's book, a merry book, a mad book, satiric, ironic, perhaps a novel, perhaps not" (Rivero 2002, vii). For many, the centuries-long popularity of Swift's *Travels* can be ascribed to the novel's core narrative; like Odysseus, the protagonist "travels to exotic lands; meets strange people […] and, after many trials, returns home, presumably wiser" (Rivero 2002, vii). Contrary to Homer's main character, Gulliver never really returns from his exile and learns nothing. The narrative ends with a tragic and alienated figure, "ashamed of his body and revolted by the bodies of those who look and smell like him" (Rivero 2002, viii).

As Rivero points out, we are invited to laugh at Gulliver's "untrammeled pride" only to then experience an eerie feeling that the "fun is at our expense" (Rivero 2002, viii). Though Swift's *Gulliver's Travels* is a fairly easy read, one has to factor in that its meanings and allusions cannot be fully grasped without taking into consideration what the reader knows about the eighteenth century (Rivero 2002, ix). Yet, even with this 'knowledge' at hand, it is nearly impossible to agree on one single interpretation of this 300-year-old masterpiece. This said, the following sections focus on the voyages to Brobdingnag and Houyhnhnm-land as these offer insights into the construction of bodies and their relevance for the issue in question: reproduction.

What we do know for sure, is that *Gulliver's Travels* is written in the satiric mode. This raises the question of how satire can be defined and what its relationship is with the body. Roy Porter offers an elaborate answer to this question when he states that

> [s]atire deflates and debases. It is an art which topples greatness, undermines pretension and punishes pride by revealing the low in the pretendedly high, the filth in the pure, the folly in reason. This belittling trick deploys telescopic lenses which picture the human as lesser and lower, or as a machine or beast, driven by depraved desires. Satire reduces what purports to be subtly superior to a repertoire of stigmatizing symbols and cardboard cut-outs, turning character into caricature, signalled by exaggerated physiognomical distortions – the huge nose, gaping mouth and bloated belly, or comparable animalistic traits. In this humbling of the complex into the simplistic, satire finally reduces the mind, soul or spirit to that flesh which always bespeaks inferiority on the Chain of Being.
>
> (Porter 2004, 148)

From a Christian standpoint, as Porter states, satire "bring[s] man down to his true fallen self, a stinking sink of sin" (Porter 2004, 148). This recognition makes even more sense when considering Jonathan Swift's life and works. Not only was he a "clergyman of the Church of England," but also his satire was of the harshest kind when he proposed to solve Ireland's problem of overpopulation and poverty by feeding on its infants in his essay *A Modest Proposal*, in which he saw the problem of Ireland's poor and the responsibility for it (1729) (Porter 2004, 149).[3]

According to Porter, the cruelty of this suggestion can be partially explained by Swift's childhood. Never having met his father who died shortly before he was born in Dublin in 1667, Swift was brought away to North West England by the family's nurse; here, she isolated him from his family for several years before he was sent back to Ireland where he eventually graduated from Trinity College, only for the Protestant Swift to flee to England after the invasion by James II (Porter 2004, 149). Though he experienced "glory days" during the 1710s in London as a Tory supporter and "controversialist," he yet again returned to Ireland after the succession of the Hanoverian King George I and takeover of the Whigs where he accepted a position at the Dublin St. Patrick's Cathedral, leading to "permanent bitterness," as Porter states (Porter 2004, 149).

Not much can be said for certain with regard to Swift's attitudes towards women as he was always very secretive about his love life, but scholars have pointed to his "profound fear both of the feminine and of his own emotional and sexual wants – in short, of intimacy" (Porter 2004, 150). As Porter emphasises, "[m]isogyny marks the searing disgust" prevalent in most of his poems, "which dissect women's defects with unconcealed gusto" (Porter 2004, 150). In his poem "A Beautiful Young Nymph Going to Bed" (1731), for instance, Swift constructs a prostitute, marked by age and illness, whose bodily "horrors" he describes in an almost clinical manner:

> Then, seated on a three-legg'd Chair,
> Takes off her artificial Hair:
> Now, picking out a Crystal Eye,
> She wipes it clean, and lays it by.
> Her Eye-Brows from a Mouse's Hyde,
> Stuck on with Art on either Side,
> Pulls off with Care, and first displays 'em,
> Then in a Play-Book smoothly lays 'em.
> Now dextrously her Plumpers draws,
> That serve to fill her hollow Jaws.
> Untwists a Wire; and from her Gums
> A Set of Teeth completely comes.
> Pulls out the Rags contriv'd to prop
> Her flabby Dugs [breasts] and down they drop.
>
> (Porter 2004, 150; see also Porter 2021, 45;
> see also Jeffares 1992, 155)

Swift here "literally anatomises the body" of his 'nymph,' an eighteenth-century slang word for prostitute (Carter 2004, 149). The "disassembl[y]" of the prostitute's body in her "filthy garret after a hard night's work" renders female physicality, here also associated with sexuality, monstrous (Carter 2004, 149). In a disturbing manner, the 'beautiful' nymph's body is reduced to both disposable but also mercenary parts: "as she pulls out her glass eye, false teeth, and cat-pissed plumpers, [she] dissolves into a pile of commodities" (Rosenthal 2006, 2). As a result, the female subject is erased through a dismemberment of her body into parts. The poem's main effect, therefore, is the blurring of subject and object or meaning and (bodily) matter, but also of desire and revulsion especially towards the female reproductive body.[4]

A critique of reality and appearance, especially in terms of the relationship between the body and the mind and the question of 'man's' identity, seems to be a common thread of Swift's works (Porter 2004, 151). What Porter calls Swift's "'anthropological' satire" also dominates most of *Gulliver's Travels* (1726). The narrator's trip to Lilliput, as Porter explains, is to be understood as an attack on Britain's first Prime Minister and Whig Robert Walpole who Swift blamed for his exile.[5] During this voyage, Walpole's supporters are "reduced to Lilliputian littleness" whose greed and corruption manifest in the "dwarfishness" of their bodies while Gulliver, the prime example of "honest humanity and decency," towers above them (Porter 2004, 151). In Brobdingnag, the island of giants, it is Gulliver whose physicality is reduced. It is this voyage that exemplifies Swift's "disgust at the flesh"; the narrator is here confronted with the "grossness" of the body that was previously hidden to the human eye while Gulliver is degraded to a "baby, pet or mannikin" (Porter 2004, 151). In this scene, the protagonist is degraded to an "object of sexual desire by the lusts of the gigantic bosomy Brobdignagian matrons" (Porter 2004, 152).

Although Gulliver repeatedly seeks to escape the flesh that causes his severe revulsion, his fate is finally sealed during the voyage to Laputa, whose (male) inhabitants try to "rise above […] the flesh" by engaging in "lofty reasoning," only to witness their wives "slip[ping] off to have sex with males from a neighbouring island": As Porter states, "their husbands have lost touch with what makes them human," a foible the Christian Swift had always despised (Porter 2004, 152). Gulliver's revulsion with the flesh – female flesh in particular – culminates during his fourth voyage to the country of the Houyhnhnms, a species of talking horses that reign over the Yahoos, "bestial beings with human traits" (Porter 2004, 155). Here, Gulliver sides with the wise and rational Houyhnhnms while simultaneously distancing himself from the "loathsome Yahoos" whose physicality ironically resembles his own the most (Porter 2004, 155). It is especially the narrative's end portraying a deranged Gulliver who, after returning to England, prefers the presence of horses that causes much discussion to this day.

In this context, Ashley Marshall discusses what she calls the "problem of meaning" regarding *Gulliver's Travels* in her eponymous chapter and emphasises the "long-standing disagreement" over what Swift's satirical narrative means (Marshall 2013, 220). There is even large dissent among scholars on whether *Gulliver's Travels* is a satire at all, and if it is, what the targets are (Marshall 2013, 221). It is, however, safe to say that the narrative is about "order and chaos, reason and unreason, truth and mendacity" (Marshall 2013, 221). Those scholars who have aimed at a more specific interpretation read it as a satire on British colonialism (Hawes 1991), on entrapment (Donoghue 1998), on narcissism (Boyle 2000) or on nationality (Knight 2004), only to name a few (see also Marshall 2013, 221–222).

Marshall stresses that interpretations strongly hinge on the "assumptions and point of view of a particular kind of reader" since not "all readers would or should have been interested in [...] the many 'principal' targets critics have identified as defining the central thrust of the *Travels*" (Marshall 2013, 222). What most critics agree on is Swift's problematic and often ambiguous "attitude toward a particular target: the human race"; this debate led to the formation of two camps, the "[s]oft-liners and hard-liners" in the first half of the twentieth century (Marshall 2013, 222). While for the hard-liners, *Gulliver's Travels* was a "nasty, half-mad misanthrope" that reflects Swift's own mindset, the soft-liners focussed on the narrative's comic aspects and argued that Swift's satire targets Gulliver's own misanthropy instead (Marshall 2013, 222).

Since the second half of the twentieth century, the hard reading has prevailed, though Marshall reminds us that "whether we like it or not, [*Gulliver's Travels*] is essentially opaque, and scholars tend to find in it what they are predisposed to find" (Marshall 2013, 223). Especially the novel's fourth part 'A Voyage to the Country of the Houyhnhnms' has triggered questions about what the Yahoos and Houyhnhnms represent. "How one reads part IV," as Marshall stresses, "has much to do with the assumptions one brings to it" (Marshall 2013, 223). In any case, *Gulliver's Travels* leaves the reader "uncertain," "uncomfortable" and "puzzled" as to what especially the end means (Marshall 2013, 224–225). Marshall concludes that "[*Gulliver's*] *Travels* is probably best understood not as a satire but as a vehicle for a mélange of satiric hits" (Marshall 2013, 225).

Michael Seidel, for instance, argues that *Gulliver's Travels* not only satirises the genre of travel literature but especially the "narrative bona fides" of the emerging novel genre as such (Seidel 1998, 72). What is more, Swift's work is generally characterised by, what Seidel calls, a "satiric deauthentification" that "cuts to the core of self-representation"; other pieces like *A Tale of A Tub* (1704) or *A Modest Proposal* (1729), for instance, challenge "modern consciousness" by rendering its subjects liars, ramblers or – as in the case of *Gulliver's Travels* – narrators who "talk themselves into states of exhaustion of lunacy" (Seidel 1998, 72–73). As Seidel states, Swift "distrusted virtually everything represented in the early novel: its individualistic psychology; [...] its role in the proliferation of knowledge; its success as a product of the increasingly commercial literary industry" (Seidel 1998, 73). The following sections focus on the striking bodily constructions in *Gulliver's Travels*.

The first place Gulliver visits is the island Lilliput. Here, Gulliver is an "outsized version of the new man of his age," and Swift uses this image to satirise the "inflated status of the subject in modern fiction" (Seidel 1998, 74). When Gulliver visits the land of Brobdingnag during his second voyage, the bodily relations are reversed. In this place, he is the one surrounded by giants.[6] According to Seidel, Swift mocks the novel's (and genre's) claim to authenticity by "destabili[sing] the body and then the mind" of the protagonist who ends up as a man who talks to horses in his barn and questions his own humanity: He is the "surgeon who cannot operate" (Seidel 1998, 74). Seidel also asks how the readers can possibly understand the name of the third place Gulliver visits – Laputa. Quite likely, they would read it as the Spanish "*la puta*, or whore," though Seidel understands this wordplay as Gulliver's (or Swift's in this case) satiric critique of "selling one's narrative produce to all comers" (Seidel 1998, 74). In general, *Gulliver's Travels'* narrator "loses credit" as the story unravels – he becomes increasingly "self-infatuated, self-obsessed, and deranged," considers himself a "superior member of an inferior species" and is thus rendered an unreliable narrator (Seidel 1998, 74).

In terms of medicine, one particular aspect looms large in Swift's satire. Seidel points to the "satiric significance of Gulliver's medical mentor," Mr James Bates (Seidel 1998, 74). As implied above, Gulliver calls Mr Bates, a character who recommended Gulliver to become a surgeon and "settle in *London*," "Master *Bates*" (*Travels*, 16; Rivero 2002, 15–16). According to Seidel, this wordplay on masturbation alludes not only to Gulliver's training in surgery and the resulting familiarity with medical texts that were used for masturbatory reasons as well but also to a "sort of narrative onanism" the narrator demonstrates by "ironically [...] invalidat[ing] the literary form that conveys him" (Seidel 1998, 74). Though Seidel mainly focusses on the novel's narrative uncertainties that result in a mockery of the contract of fiction, one can also clearly identify a vilification of the figure of the medical man who seems to be more invested in narcissistic 'master-bation' than in medical responsibility. Viewed in this light, *Gulliver's Travels'* very first chapter, among many other things, therefore already includes an attack on 'modern' science and medicine.

Ian McCormick goes a step further and aims at a queer reading of *Gulliver's Travels* in conjunction with "human reproduction" and male castration angst (McCormick 2013, 278). He states that the "silenced" – or 'secret' – "masturbatory component" of many eighteenth-century texts actually was a "bestseller industry under the guise of medical treatises" (McCormick 2013, 279). McCormick identifies one major "recurring theme" in such literary artefacts – the "fear of contagion: the spectre of a nation overrun by sodomites and onanists" (McCormick 2013, 279). He references *Onania, Or: The Heinous Sin of Self-Pollution, And All its Frightful Consequences, in both Sexes* (1724), an anonymous inflammatory pamphlet that warned against masturbation and might have informed Swift's writing, although he must have almost finished writing "A Voyage to Lilliput" by this time.

According to McCormick, for some readers, *Onania* even seemed to advise against the mere mentioning of the "heinous sin" as it might seduce those who had never heard of it before (McCormick 2013, 279). He concludes that Swift, by installing "masturbatory innuendo from the start," constructs Gulliver not only as a "self-involved character," but establishes an "underlying erotic paradox of how to generate the [human] race without women" by "spilling precious seed" through onanism (McCormick 2013, 280). In other words, one could argue that the simultaneous production and non-production of potential humans implies a male castration angst with regard to (the loss of) population control. This fear unfolds especially in the end of *Gulliver's Travels* that leaves behind an irrational, powerless or impotent surgeon, a male anatomist in crisis who prefers the company of horses to humans.

2.1.3 Secrecy & Microscopical Masculinity Crises

This subchapter deals with the link between literature, science and the reproductive body and focusses on Gulliver's voyages to Brobdingnag, the country of giants, and Houyhnhnm-land, inhabited by animal-like humans and talking horses. Both trips are characterised by a notion of sex and secrecy that can be linked not only to British politics, but also and especially to sexual politics, science and (human) reproduction. In this context, Melinda Rabb draws an explicit connection between "satire, secrecy, and secret history" in *Gulliver's Travels* (Rabb 2006, 165). Interestingly, she identifies a "national crisis of authority" at the beginning of the eighteenth century with Charles II "hav[ing] much to hide"; rumour had it that he pretended to be a Protestant in public, but secretly practised Catholicism (Rabb 2006, 167). It was in this political atmosphere that secret narratives proliferated.

Rabb stresses how such stories potentially "undermine[d] the stability of authority, to establish instead a world of open secrets" (Rabb 2006, 172). The theme of secrecy takes shape especially in Swift's *Gulliver's Travels* when the "'[g]ullible' Gulliver" sets out on a "journey into a world of dangerous secrets," while "[s]ecrecy determines [the] politics in each of the countries" he visits (Rabb 2006, 176–177). Though Gulliver misses most of the major political events in Britain on his voyage between the years 1699 and 1715, in *Gulliver's Travels*, "English politics has been transplanted"; the countries feature "sophisticated foreign courts" that he visits "in the manner of the 'secret' travels of scandal chronicles" (Rabb 2006, 177). Lilliput, for instance, is dominated by scandalous rumours at court, "private Intrigue," threats of "Impeachment," "Treason," deception and secret pockets (capitalisation in the original, *Travels*, 55–56, 59; see also Rabb 2006, 177).

The motif of secrecy runs through all of the following travels, not only in terms of Swift's use of language and meaning but also with regard to the novel's content: In Brobdingnag, Gulliver's offer to the King to share his secret knowledge of gunpowder is rejected; in Balnibarbi, the inhabitants are incapable of keeping secrets; in Glubdubdrib, Gulliver is confronted with secret magic; and in the country of the Houyhnhnms, he feels the need to hide his resemblance to the despised Yahoos (see Rabb 2006, 177–178). In Rabb's view, Swift's satire not only asks the "crucial question about the *essentiality* of secrecy in human behaviour" and what it means not only for the state but also questions the "secrets of generation [reproduction]" by centring on naked and dissected bodies (emphasis in the original, Rabb 2006, 178). In terms of secrecy, gender and power Rabb argues:

> Conflicting versions of truth undermine patriarchal authority, and these effects are tested on Gulliver [...]: Brobdingnag threatens his manhood; he is at various times child, insect, toy, and little animal. When he finishes his several versions of English history, the King considers him briefly as a sexual being, but only to imagine him as a completely disempowered patriarch.
> (Rabb 2006, 185)

As a result, both secrecy and his (sexualised) short stature threaten Gulliver's masculinity. Deborah Needleman Armintor seizes on this threat of emasculation and entangles *Gulliver's Travels'* sexual politics with a particular field of science that is also relevant for questions of reproduction and the body: microscopy.

Armintor builds on Marjorie Nicolson's pivotal 1935 essay on microscopy and English imagination and the argument that Gulliver is metaphorically rendered a microscopist not only in Lilliput, observing "small creatures and object," but especially in Brobdingnag where he sees the bodies he encounters "in magnified detail, as if [...] through a microscope" (Armintor 2007, 619). In general, as Armintor continues, Gulliver is characterised by a "scientific curiosity" that becomes clear through his "dissection of giant Brobdingnagian wasps" and the stingers he collects as a present for the Royal Society (Armintor 2007, 619). With reference to Nichols, Armintor outlines the eighteenth century's "fascination with little worlds made large" that resulted in microscopy and its agents as "popular object[s] of both satire and awe in the age of Enlightenment" (Armintor 2007, 619).

But Gulliver studies both insects and especially female anatomy in "hideously magnified detail" during his visit to Brobdingnag (Armintor 2007, 619). Armintor thus rethinks Nicolson's rather "sweeping" claim that Gulliver is simply rendered a microscopist in this country and spotlights the peculiarity of this observer's reaction to what he sees: Gulliver is not just the enlightened microscopist fascinated by "insects and objects," but severely revolted by the female bodies he is forced to gaze at (Armintor 2007, 620). This becomes especially clear in the following scene.

In chapter I of Part II, Gulliver attends a dinner hosted by the farmer he first meets on his arrival at Brobdingnag, and his wife. Already scared by the giant cat present, a nurse joins the meal, carrying a bellowing one-year-old infant that ogles Gulliver, grabs him and inserts his head into its mouth, happy to have found a "Play-thing" (*Travels*, 76). Gulliver is only saved by the nurse who catches him in her apron after the child, frightened by Gulliver's terrified screams, lets him go. To soothe the child, she is "forced to apply the last Remedy by giving it suck" (*Travels*, 76). Gulliver describes this, for him, utterly revolting moment as follows:

> I must confess no Object ever disgusted me so much as the sight of her monstrous Breast, which I cannot tell what to compare with, so as to give the curious Reader an Idea of its Bulk, Shape and Colour. It stood prominent six Foot, and could not be less than sixteen in Circumference. The Nipple was about half the Bigness of my Head and the Hew both of that and the Dug so verified with Spots, Pimples and Freckles, that nothing could appear more nauseous: For I had a near sight of her, she sitting down the more conveniently to give Suck, and I standing on the table. This made me reflect upon the fair Skins of our *English* ladies, who appear so beautiful to us, only because they are of our own size, and their Defects not to be seen but through a Magnifying Glass, where we find by Experiment that the smoothest and whitest Skins look rough and coarse, and ill coloured.
>
> (emphasis in the original, *Travels*, 77)

As Armintor stresses, Gulliver is not just a "miniature 'seeing object,'" but an observer who cannot "pick and choose" what he sees – the power of the gaze here belongs to his "gigantic and predominantly female owners and manipulators" (Armintor 2007, 620). What is more, Gulliver is reduced to a "small woman-manipulated object with magnified vision" (Armintor 2007, 620). Interestingly, this reading concurs with the history of the microscope which is also a gendered one: In the seventeenth century, the microscope mainly belonged to the male-connoted sphere of science and represented an instrument only very few had access to. As the eighteenth century gave rise to a smaller and portable version of the microscope, it could be carried about in one's pocket and was used especially by upper-class females as a commodity and fashion object (Armintor 2007, 620). In this light, Gulliver is degraded to a "miniature woman-owned seeing object" and devolves "from microscopist to miniature microscope" (Armintor 2007, 620). In addition, Gulliver is equally likened to an animal or even the product of an abortion that is investigated by medical men as if on the dissection table, thus further threatening his masculinity.

In chapter III of the voyage to Brobdingnag, the farmer sells Gulliver to the queen who "presents him to the King" (*Travels*, 84). His little nurse Glumdalclitch carries him to court. There, the king sends for "three great Scholars," "educated in the Study of [natural] Philosophy," to examine and discuss the spectacle (*Travels*, 86). The "Gentlemen" inspect him as follows:

> [...] after they had a while examined my Shape with much Nicety, were of different Opinions concerning me. They all agreed that I could not be produced according to the regular Laws of Nature, because I was not framed with a Capacity of preserving my Life, either by Swiftness, or climbing of Trees, or digging Holes in the Earth. They observed my Teeth, which they viewed with great Exactness, that I was a carnivorous Animal; yet most Quadrupeds being an Overmatch for me, and Field-Mice, with some others, too nimble, they

> could not imagine how I should be able to support my self, unless I fed upon Snails and other Insects, which they offered by many learned Arguments to evince that I could not possibly do. One of these Virtuosi seemed to think that I might be an Embrio, or abortive Birth. But this Opinion was rejected by the other two, who observed my Limbs to be perfect and finished, and that I had lived several years, as it was manifested from my Beard, the Stumps whereof they plainly discovered through a Magnifying-Glass. They would not allow me to be a Dwarf, because my Littleness was beyond all degrees of Comparison; [...] After much Debate, they concluded unanimously that I was only *Relpum Scalcath*, which is interpreted literally, *Lusus Naturae* [freak of nature, *Travels*, 87, fn 8].
>
> (emphasis in the original, *Travels*, 86–87)

Here, it is Gulliver who is treated as the object of scientific enquiry. Swift thus subverts the idea of enlightened (male) science by rendering the male body a 'freak of nature.' Though not explicitly linked to the female reproductive body, this subversion serves as a general critique of male doctors gazing at bodies – tiny, emasculated male bodies in this case.

The situation is again reversed when Gulliver is forced to gaze at yet another what he finds revolting female body. In chapter IV of Part II, the narrator describes the country and the "[a]uthor's way of travelling" through Brobdingnag in a coach (*Travels*, 92). He is accompanied by Glumdalclitch who carries Gulliver in a box and occasionally takes him out to gaze at the surroundings. One day, the coach "stop[s] at several Shops, where the Beggars watching their Opportunity, crouded [sic] the sides of the Coach" and Gulliver is forced to see the "most horrible Spectacles that ever an *European* Eye beheld" (emphasis in the original, *Travels*, 93):

> There was a Woman with a Cancer in her Breast, swelled to a monstrous size, full of Holes, in two or three of which I could have easily crept, and covered the whole Body. [...] But, the most hateful Sight of all were the Lice crawling on their Cloaths. I could see distinctly the Limbs of these Vermin with my naked Eye, much better than those of an *European* Louse through a Microscope, and their Snouts with which they rooted like Swine. They were the first I had ever beheld, and I should have been curious enough to dissect one of them, if I had proper Instruments [...] although indeed the Sight was so nauseous, that it perfectly turned my Stomach.
>
> (emphasis in the original, *Travels*, 93–94)

Not only does the narrator here fragment the female reproductive body by focussing on its details, but the woman's reproductive organs are also represented as revolting which contributes to the woman's otherness. Moreover, the narrator aligns breasts with animals or insects, here lice, therefore amplifying the (female) beggar's status as inhuman. Nevertheless, to argue that what we see here is simply an example of Swift's misogyny manifesting in the narrator's voice is too sweeping. *Gulliver's Travels* is characterised by the protagonist's ambivalence towards the female reproductive body as simultaneously revolting and sexually inviting as the following scene demonstrates.

Furthermore, as Allan Ingram argues in *Swift, Pope and the Doctors* (2022), Gulliver's obsession with perspective is most likely a result of Swift's own health condition as he suffered from a chronic illness today known as Ménière's Disease, causing "physical and mental dizziness," "hearing loss" as well as "deteriorating eyesight" (Ingram 2022, xii, 195). It is thus no coincidence that Gulliver's perspective, despite his profession as a surgeon, towards the bodies he encounters is both literally and figuratively limited:

> Medically qualified Gulliver sees a great deal while on his travels, but his understanding of what he sees is increasingly awry, just as Swift's own trust in the process of seeing, in the widest sense, became more and more self-questioned.
>
> (Ingram 2022, 195).

Ingram reads the "flesh-creeping section" mentioned above as proof of Hooke's influence on the novel that is confirmed by Gulliver's "surprising step back from revulsion to scientific curiosity," similar to the descriptions of the magnified creatures' "strength and beauty" in *Micrographia* (Ingram 2022, 195–196). Yet, the novel emphasises 'ways of seeing' and also 'ways of touching' bodies by constructing them as almost haptic, just like Hooke did in his masterpiece on microscopy. The following scene demonstrates the entanglement of vision and touch in particular.

In chapter V, the queen's maids of honour, who regularly invite Glumdalclitch and her little *homunculus* to their quarters to "have the pleasure of *seeing and touching*" him, not only desire to gaze at this bodily spectacle but also to "strip [him] naked from top to toe" only to then lay the nude little man between their breasts: This and the maid's "offensive" body odour again utterly disgusts Gulliver (emphasis added, *Travels*, 98). Interestingly, what seems to disturb him the most is how the maids use his body:

> THAT which gave me most uneasiness among these Maids of Honor, when my Nurse carried me to visit them, was to see them use me without any manner of Ceremony, like a Creature who had no sort of Consequence. For, they would strip themselves to the Skin, and put on their Smocks in my Presence, while I was placed on their Toylet [dressing table] directly before their naked Bodies, which, I am sure, to me was very far from being a tempting Sight, or from giving me any other emotions than those of Horror and Disgust. Their Skins appeared so coarse and uneven, so variously coloured when I saw them near, with a Mole here and there as broad as a Trencher, and Hairs hanging from it thicker than Pack-threads; to say nothing further concerning the rest of their Persons. Neither did they at all scruple while I was by to discharge what they had drunk, to the quantity of at least two Hogsheads, in a Vessel that held above three Tuns. The handsomest among these Maids of Honor, a pleasant frolicksome Girl of sixteen, would sometimes set me

> astride upon one of her Nipples, with many other Tricks, wherein the Reader will excuse me for not being over particular. But, I was so much displeased, that I entreated *Glumdalclitch* to contrive some excuse for not seeing that young Lady any more.
>
> (emphasis in the original, *Travels*, 98–99)

Armintor maintains that this moment in *Gulliver's Travels* renders Gulliver not only a "miniature microscope" but also a "woman-owned miniature microscope-cum-sexual prop" (Armintor 2007, 621). While this reading of Gulliver as a "sex toy" has already been addressed by scholars such as Ruth Salvaggio (1988), Laura Brown (1990) or Paul-Gabriel Boucé (2001), it is Armintor who merges the sexual politics with microscopy (Armintor 2007, 195). In her view, Gulliver devolves into a "freakish hybrid of pocket microscope and sex toy"; in particular, she argues that

> Swift's joke [is] at the expense of 'enlightened' male scientists who imagine themselves to be far removed from the world of women and commodities but who are themselves […] as affected [by] the newly commodified microscope and what might be called the ultimate object of female 'consumption' – the dildo.
>
> (Armintor 2007, 621)

Armintor's reading makes sense if one turns to the history of the microscope from a feminist viewpoint. By referring to Catherine Wilson's (1995) and Marian Fournier's (1996) studies, she points towards the popularity of the "pocket microscope" among eighteenth-century women who thus could at least remotely participate in the field of scientific enquiry (Armintor 2007, 623). The female use of this new, fashionable instrument did not please everyone, of course. As Armintor continues, it was especially Robert Hooke who blamed the pocket microscope for the "decrease in microscope-oriented Royal Society publication" in the late seventeenth century (Armintor 2007, 623).

Danielle Spratt argues along similar lines and states that Gulliver himself becomes a "type of commodity" who is "denied both human and sexual volition" through the maids of honour who treat him like a "human sex toy" (Spratt 2012, 143). What is more, the way the scientists in Brobdingnag examine his body blurs the boundaries between human and animal; Gulliver is regarded "only in non-categorical terms" and rendered a "spectacular monster" (Spratt 2012, 143). Most importantly, Spratt aligns Gulliver's body with that of Mary Toft who represented a "seemingly monstrous case of human and animal bodies colliding" (Spratt 2012, 143). In her view, *Gulliver's Travels* is especially about population or reproductive control that becomes clear through the king's 'scientific' "breeding scheme" with the aim to pair Gulliver with a female of similar size only to "create [more] spectacle" for the court: "Gulliver's categorization as an uncategorizable monster gives licence to the king to control him sexually through breeding" (Spratt 2012, 145). This reading further makes sense in light of the notion that England's population was regarded as the wealth of the nation, while at the same time, Ireland suffered from overpopulation (or rather the lack of resources to feed its people) that resulted in the "newly emergent field of demographics, including population control" (Spratt 2012, 138).

Needless to say, the most effective way to control reproduction, and hence population growth, would be to pair as many men and women as possible and control their reproduction through marriage: As Spratt outlines with reference to Mary Poovey[7] and Charlotte Sussman,[8] especially "child-bearing women" were regarded as "livestock" in many "political treatises" that linked reproduction with "national productivity" (Spratt 2012, 146). In this context, the new (woman-owned) invention of the pocket microscope posed a threat to both individual masculinity and patriarchal society or the nation as a whole as it potentially endangered reproduction if used as a sex toy according to the (unfounded and absurd) fears of Swift's contemporaries, above all scientists.

Robert Hooke particularly criticised the degeneracy of the formally male-connoted microscope "into a miniaturized plaything in the hands of frivolous amateurs" (Armintor 2007, 624). Armintor reads Hooke's critique as a form of symbolic castration angst, a "metaphorical shrinkage [...] of the worst kind" (Armintor 2007, 624). This fear of emasculation, she argues, is the main target of Swift's satire and manifests itself in the depiction of the "scientifically minded Gulliver" who is rendered a "helpless woman-manipulated microscope" (Armintor 2007, 624). Similar to the earlier scene of Gulliver's encounter with the beggar woman's cancerous breast, during his interaction with the maids Gulliver predominantly focuses not only on female bodies but especially on individual parts. Though much has been said about Swift's misogyny, Armintor seizes on Gulliver's obsession with grotesque and "enormous female bodies"; she aligns his "neurosis" with his scientific ambitions that, together, demonstrate a certain "microscopical masculinity crisis" (Armintor 2007, 627). Gulliver not only fears emasculation through shrinkage but also by the (sexually active) female reproductive body in particular as is demonstrated in the following.

This section revisits Melinda Rabb's notion of satire and secrecy and further links science with sex and reproduction by turning to one major incidence in the country of the Houyhnhnms that poses a special threat to Gulliver's masculinity. This place is populated with rational human-like horses, the Houyhnhnms, who reign over animal-like humans, the Yahoos. Gulliver describes the female Yahoos as particularly revolting: Their breasts ("Dugs") hang between their feet and "often reached almost to the Ground as they walked" (*Travels*, 189). The narrator pictures the people of the Yahoos as a "cursed Brood" consisting of "ugly Monster[s]" who "discharge their Excrements" while he passes under their trees (*Travels*, 190). According to Rabb, especially Gulliver's encounter with a female Yahoo in Houyhnhnm-land resembles "secret 'histories,' 'memoirs,' and 'anecdotes'" in the form of narratives of sex and seduction that proliferated during the eighteenth century (Rabb 2006, 165, 167). As Rabb elaborates, these sexually charged secret narratives usually included the following episode: "the weather is excessively hot; a young woman goes to a river bank or garden and removes her clothes, unaware of the gaze and desiring male who, inflamed by desire, catches her in a surprised embrace from which she struggles to escape" (Rabb 2006, 165).

Rabb adds that readers familiar with Aphra Behn or Eliza Haywood will immediately "recognize the amatory conventions" at play in the following scene in which the protagonist narrates his own "near-rape" (Rabb 2006, 165):

> BEING one Day abroad with my Protector the Sorrel Nag, and the Weather exceeding hot, I entrenched him to let me bathe in a River that was near. He consented, and I immediately stripped my self stark naked, and went down softly into the Stream. It happened that a young Female Yahoo standing behind a Bank, saw the whole proceeding, and enflamed by Desire, as the Nag and I conjectured, came running with all speed, and leaped into the Water within five Yards of the Place where I bathed. I was never in my Life so terribly frighted; the Nag was grazing at some distance, not suspecting any Harm. She embraced me after a most fulsome manner; I roared as loud as I could, and the Nag came galloping towards me, whereupon she quitted her Grasp, with the utmost Reluctancy, and leaped upon the opposite Band, where she stood gazing and howling all the time I was putting on my Cloaths.
> (*Travels*, 225)

As Rabb infers, this satirical scene is not only to be understood as a "reverse of gender roles," but due to its resemblance to secret (amatory) narratives, it also constructs a "clandestine 'other'" in order to maintain the age's patriarchal, "political, social, and religious power" (Rabb 2006, 166–167). This 'other' is not simply a "bestial beings with human traits" (Porter 2004, 155), but particularly female. It represents the sexually unrestrained female other that needs to be controlled. Female sexuality, that potentially leads to pregnancy and childbirth, thus poses a threat that has to be kept in check.[9]

This reading is confirmed by Spratt who argues that this threatening "sexual encounter" not only "further dehumanizes and disempowers Gulliver" and thus contributes to his (sexual) objectification but also represents the "catalyst" for his subsequent suggestion to stamp out the Yahoos in chapter IX: "THE Question to be debated, was, Whether the *Yahoos* should be exterminated from the Face of the Earth [...] as the *Yahoos* were the most filthy, noisome, and deformed Animal which Nature ever produced" (emphasis in the original, *Travels*, 228). For Spratt, this proposal is to be read as "another form of population control" (Spratt 2012, 148). What needs to be emphasised is that the Yahoo who deeply threatens Gulliver's (masculine) identity is not just any kind of 'monster,' but a female one in particular who displays sexual behaviour beyond control. In short, Swift renders female reproduction monstrous, while simultaneously criticising this form of othering the female body through his satire – he is having it both ways, it seems.

2.1.4 Monstrous Reproduction & Entangled Tactility

One common assumption is that Swift's work, including *Gulliver's Travels*, is marked by blatant misogyny. In *The Body in Swift and Defoe* (1990), Carol H. Flynn deals with this very question and aims at a biographical reading of the author. She criticises Swift's inability to "imagine women from the inside" by maintaining an "ironic distance" to what he finds is the "loathsome condition" of the – especially female – flesh (Flynn 1990, 88). She explains:

> The knowledge [Swift] produces is always external and judgemental. For reasons cultural as well as psychological, Swift defines women according to a physicality that is gross, filthy and lasting. Women threaten to scatter reason, waste energy, and destroy the possibility of civilization. [...] In the end, he can only run from the engrossing feminine temptations of unreason that he has both exposed and invented.
>
> (Flynn 1990, 88)

As Flynn argues, this distance to or "ironic detachment" from female flesh at the same time shields him from the "hysterical implications of his misogyny" (Flynn 1990, 88). Swift, however, is simultaneously petrified, horrified and fascinated by the bodies he discovers (Flynn 1990, 88–89). This ambivalence becomes apparent especially in his (fictional) nurse figures that are both affectionate and punishing, caring and nauseous. While scholars have already drawn connections between the nurse figure and Swift's biography, in particular his 'abduction' as a child by an overprotective nurse who educated him while also isolating him from his mother and family, Flynn goes a step further and suggests that Swift's "fascination with the condition of being nursed informs his most fundamental ideas of sexuality [...] for the nurse 'whips' as well as caresses" (Flynn 1990, 105, 101). Against the backdrop of female reproduction and the rise of obstetrics, Swift's literary descriptions align the female reproductive body with eighteenth-century obstetrical representations, both visually and haptically. This makes sense if one recalls what scholars have said about the eroticised illustrations as well as the obstetrical machines or mannikins that at least invite the viewer to voyeurism if not more.

Gulliver's Travels displays further links between reproduction and masculinity. As mentioned earlier with reference to Armintor, the narrative draws a connection between Gulliver's body, the microscope and the dildo. Although not explicitly mentioned in the scene in which the naked young maid of honour "set[s] him astride upon one of her Nipples, with many other Tricks, wherein the Reader will excuse [him] for not being over particular" (*Travels*, 99), this moment "allows the reader to imagine that this enormous woman uses Gulliver – in what can be called the ultimate act of female consumption – as a human dildo, rendering Gulliver's own genitalia both physically and symbolically insignificant" (Armintor 2007, 632).

The portrayal of Gulliver as a pocket microscope/dildo serves as a threat not only to the masculine-connoted field of science but also, and especially, to (male) reproduction, both in the text and its context. As Armintor outlines, contemporaries viewed the dildo as a "reprehensible artificial penis and un(re)productive female plaything (and as contributing to what many wrongly perceived as a nationwide depopulation crisis)" (Armintor 2007, 632). Therefore, the dildo represents "women's appropriation of the male member" and hence a "threat to man's claim to his own genitalia," as well as endangering the initially male-connoted instrument of the microscope and the “enlightened Englishman’ claim to the scientific gaze” (Armintor 2007, 632).

Ultimately, as Armintor concludes, it is (unrestrained) female sexuality that poses a threat to male reproduction: “this new breed of sexually insatiable minded female consumer – as Hooke seems to have feared of the new generation of microscope user – will eventually make English men irrelevant” (Armintor 2007, 633). She ends her investigation by seizing on the apparent misogyny in *Gulliver’s Travels* and relativises this accusation: “‘A Voyage to Brobdingnag’ appears neither misogynist per se but rather as a sexual satirist exposing the gynophobia latent in Enlightenment’s science’s aversion to the new consumerism” (Armintor 2007, 636). The object (microscope) and the subject (microscopist) thus become “virtually interchangeable” – it is this “imagined horror of Enlightenment purists such as Hooke” that Swift satirises (Armintor 2007, 636). Yet, Swift realises his critique at the expense of both female sexuality and the reproductive body that are rendered monstrous.

In *Monstrous Motherhood – 18th-Century Culture and the Ideology of Domesticity* (2012), Marilyn Francus equally identifies a “male disgust with (and fear of) sexuality and reproduction” in eighteenth-century British fiction (Francus 2012, 25). This revulsion with female reproduction can be partially explained from a religious viewpoint, as female physicality “evokes original sin and the punishment of painful childbirth for the initial fall from grace” (Francus 2012, 25). It is therefore not surprising that both eighteenth-century literature and culture were dominated by the “patriarchal fear of that female power” (Francus 2012, 25). Hence, literary female reproductive bodies are often portrayed in “monstrous size, shape, and number” in an attempt to “justify female containment as a social and moral imperative by depicting the catastrophic results of maternal agency and reproduction” (Francus 2012, 26).

Francus suggests two reasons for the “acceleration of maternal misogyny” in the eighteenth century: (1) patriarchal vulnerability due to the political uncertainties during the Glorious Revolution (1688), and (2) “shifting politics of literary culture, as mass publication, literary paternity, and female authorship became sites of conflict during the Restoration”: Put simply, Swift belonged to those writers who dreaded the “reproductive ‘feminization’ of literature” caused by the overproduction of literature, female literature in particular, that would “flood society” with “misshapen texts” – “like excessive fertility, over-production in the literary marketplace,” for them, was regarded as an “act of hubris and monstrosity” (Francus 2012, 26).

This fear of overproduction merged literature with female desire that needed to be controlled: It was this anxiety towards unrestrained reproduction that, according to Francus, rendered the female reproductive body “monstrous” (Francus 2012, 27). In this context, monstrosity or teratology (the study of monsters) served useful as it pointed towards the sexually uncontrolled female that “violates the codes of proper female behavior” (Francus 2012, 26). It was only the “menopausal” or “virgin” who did not “threaten the male sensibility” or “phallic pen,” as Francus stresses with reference to Sandra Gilbert and Susan Gubar (Francus 2012, 33). The "maternal body and its various monstrosities (pregnant, in labor, uncontrollably fertile [...]) increasingly appeared in the context of [eighteenth-century] medicine and science" as well as literary and cultural artefacts (Francus 2012, 41).

As Francus emphasises, especially the rise of the man-midwife or obstetrician and his "invention of the forceps" contributed to the "rhetoric of reproduction" as pathological and disastrous (Francus 2012, 41–42). Ironically, however, "[m]aternal fertility" was regarded not only as a "necessity" but also as a "source of vexation" as population control needed constant supervision, well knowing that it was "ultimately beyond the control of men and state" (Francus 2012, 45). What caused the most concern was the female reproductive body's "inexplicability" and "unpredictability," especially in the context of maternal myths like that of Mary Toft's rabbit breeding, outlined in PART I, which continued to circulate among the population (Francus 2012, 45). Francus concludes that the

> 'monstrous' maternal body could not be hidden, but it could be ignored as is evident in the marginalization of the maternal body in literature, whether through adherence to cultural codes of modesty or as a result of anxiety or physical disgust.
>
> (Francus 2012, 45)

The maternal body's erasure becomes apparent in particular in Jonathan Swift's *Gulliver's Travels* – here, the *pregnant* female body is completely suppressed or erased,[10] despite the many references to sexuality, while at the same time especially parts of the potentially reproductive body are rendered both grotesque and erotic.

This chapter's final sections revisit the connection between science, empiricism, microscopy and the reproductive body one more time with the aim to conclude with an emphasis on matter to demonstrate the material-discursive entanglement of science, literature and the body. In "Mingling with Matter – Tactile Microscopy and the Philosophic Mind in Brobdingnag and Beyond," Kristin M. Girten investigates Swift's assumed distrust in the new sciences of the eighteenth century. She argues that scholars have hitherto neglected one crucial aspect with regard to Swift's scepticism expressed in *Gulliver's Travels*, namely his "disdain [...] for empirical philosopher's investment in tactility" (Girten 2013, 497). As outlined above, Robert Hooke's *Micrographia* did not simply call for the abandonment of words in favour of instruments but rather urged to entangle matter with meaning.

Girten also identifies a shift "from words to things" in eighteenth-century microscopy, although natural philosophers were rather prompted to equally engage in "tactile interaction" with their "specimens" similar to the practice of "surgery and dissection" that was not just based on words in medical handbooks but on the handling and manipulation of actual bodily matter (Girten 2013, 497–498). This procedure enabled an entanglement of haptic and visual perception including new technologies or instruments like the microscope or forceps. Girten criticises that eighteenth-century scholars have largely "blinded" themselves with their "ocularcentrism" (the focus on "Enlightenment vision" alone) instead of acknowledging the "interrelation between vision and touch" (Girten 2013, 499–500). While

Francis Bacon, for instance, aimed at a "divide between human beings and nature" by means of reason, Swift demonstrates that, ironically, "tactile empiricism threatens such separation" (Girten 2013, 500). Girten extends beyond Flynn's critique of "Swift's sexual strategies" by shifting attention to the ways he negotiates "tactile empiricism" in *Gulliver's Travels* (Girten 2013, 501).

Girten continues with Hooke's *Micrographia* and its "'intermingling' of self and object" that was highly problematic in the light of Bacon's previous work, as the latter "envision[ed] a psyche that has [in accordance with the Cartesian dualism] risen above […] the material" (Girten 2013, 501). Hooke, however, merges the eye with the hand or the visual with the tactile in his illustrations by drawing a connection between a certain "mushroom and soft leather" or the "wooliness of [a] fly's face, and the sharpness of its face's protuberances – all tactile, not visual, qualities" (Girten 2013, 504–505). Moreover, as Girten stresses, by literally drawing the objects he investigates "by hand [he] only further emphasizes his engravings' association with touch" (Girten 2013, 505). This, she argues, is the actual power of Hooke's representational practice – it merges eyes and hands, vision and touch and thus "thwarts the separation and hierarchy" of mind over matter (Girten 2013, 505, 509).

It is especially Swift's "A Voyage to Brobdingnag" that subverts Bacon's conviction by entangling object and subject and thus "threatens the legitimacy of empirical discovery" (Girten 2013, 501). The scene in which Gulliver describes the maids of honour's body parts in a "quasi-microscopic" manner not only reduces the distance "between observer and observed" by exchanging it with a "heightened (and regularly disgusting) intimacy of touch," but it also parodies the "relationship between philosopher and specimen produced by tactile microscopy" (Girten 2013, 509). Gulliver goes into so much detail when describing the maid's body parts – female breasts in particular – that it evokes a "haptic sensation" (Girten 2013, 509).

The same holds true for Gulliver's encounter with the beggar woman's giant cancerous breast that has holes so large he could creep into: The "reader experiences the scene not just visually but also via touch […] Swift invites us not only to envision the woman's cancer but to feel its texture" (Girten 2013, 510). By doing this, the text accomplishes a "radical and bizarre intimacy between observer and observed" (Girten 2013, 510). Again, it cannot be overemphasised that Swift's Gulliver is mostly revolted by *female* bodies or parts thereof. This makes sense if one considers the association of femininity with the (material) body that was not only constructed as inferior to the mind but also threatens masculine-connoted reason and thus science. Ultimately, Swift's satire is two-fold: On the one hand, he mocks tactile empiricism's union of eyes and hand or vision and touch, and on the other hand, it exposes Bacon's conviction of mind over matter as well as science's alleged distance between subject and object.

To conclude, some readers of this book may question to what extent Swift's *Gulliver's Travels* negotiates questions of reproduction and medicine. Though actual pregnancy is not mentioned in this eighteenth-century satire, the only exception being the brief mention of Gulliver's pregnant wife whom he leaves behind in the final part,[11] Swift's overly detailed descriptions of (reproductive) body parts merge female physicality with the dissection table. Like the surgeon in the medical theatre, Gulliver dissects and fragments the bodies he investigates – he is a surgeon after all. In fact, the literary bodies' almost tactile aesthetics not only very much resemble those illustrations in Hooke's *Micrographia* but also show similarities to Smellie's and Hunter's obstetrical atlases.

What is more, Gulliver is simultaneously revolted by and fascinated with the gigantic, female body parts. They are at the same time pathologised and invited to voyeurism, especially with regard to the maids of honour's bodies. Bodies in *Gulliver's Travels* are simultaneously rendered grotesque and sexualised, just like the eroticised illustrations, wax models and machine-like mannikins used in eighteenth-century obstetrics as outlined in PART I. Like the medical field of obstetrics and its representatives, Swift seems to contribute to the rising pathologisation of the female reproductive body by treating it as a conglomerate of fragmented parts, thus ridding it of subjectivity or individuality. One could even argue that the female body in Swift is, to a certain degree, ignored or even erased by rendering it repulsive as becomes clear by the examples of both the maids of honour and the female Yahoo that threaten Gulliver's masculinity. All of this might serve as an indicator for the fear of (unrestrained) female sexuality that needed to be kept in check as a form of population control.

Yet, we need to keep in mind that Swift's novel is a satire. The question that still has not been – and can hardly ever be – answered is what Swift's actual target is. In fact, the surgeon-turned-voyager Gulliver is himself investigated by and gazed at by both male and female characters. He is equally rendered a 'freak of nature,' eroticised and used as a sexual 'play thing.' This is one of the main strengths of Swift's *Gulliver's Travels* – it turns the (dissection) table and entangles Gulliver's very own body with that of the female reproductive body scrutinised, pathologised and eroticised in obstetrical visual as well as haptic representations. The greatest potential, however, lies in Swift's ability to mingle meaning with matter. Not only do the detailed descriptions of reproductive body parts reduce the distance between observer and observed, but they also create tactile sensations.

I go a step further and argue that the novel's represented bodies create a *feedback loop* (Hayles) between matter and meaning: They *entangle* (Barad) the textual with the material, haptic reproductive body on the dissection table. Bodies are thus not simply reflected but rather *diffracted* in fictional texts – they simultaneously create the history of the reproductive body they int*ra*-act with. Hence, we need not just to think with but rather *through* the body in literary and cultural artefacts of the eighteenth century. Last but not least, both the fragmented female bodies as well as Gulliver's own dissected body can be conceptualised along the lines of Haraway's metaphor of the cyborg: They defy categorisation and are thus rendered 'monstrous.' At the same time, they open up forms of agency as they bear the potential to criticise science, reproductive medicine and its very real material-discursive practices.

Notes

1 The full title is *Micrographia, Or: Some Physiological Descriptions of Minute Bodies Made by Magnifying Glasses. With Observations and Inquiries Thereupon* (1665).

2 What needs to be considered is that Swift's text is a satire – an art form that for a long time has been linked the "Greek mythological figure [of] the Satyr, half-human and half-animal" (Morrissey 2017, 261). Naturally, one of the main characteristics of satire is also its use of sexual allusions, bawdy language and scatology, the latter a mode that either implicitly or explicitly references excrements. The function of such techniques is to dissolve social ranks and place all human beings on the same level.

3 The full title is *A Modest Proposal For preventing the Children of Poor People From being a Burthen to Their Parents or Country, and For making them Beneficial to the Publick* (1729).

4 In *Intricate Laughter in the Satire of Swift and Pope* (1986), Allan Ingram offers an entirely different reading. He argues that the poem rather "confront[s] the reader[s] successfully with the nature of [their] own laughter" by first "offer[ing]" the prostitute Corinna to the reader as an "always available […] body/machine" and "object of laughter," only to then "dismantle" it again and turn it into, a "body [and mind] habitually in pain": "Having willingly suspended the inclination to sympathise, preferring the poet's offer of easy pleasure through sex and laughter, the reader is now compelled by Swift's change of focus to face up to the possibility of Corinna[] being a real living and feeling person after all" (Ingram 1986, 40–42).

5 As the Swift expert Ingram has pointed out, one has to factor in, however, that Swift voluntarily returned to Ireland and the position of Dean after the death of Queen Anne in 1714, fearing the beginning of Whig rule, but Walpole's political dominance began around 1721. Although he was certainly attacking Walpole and the Whigs in *Gulliver's Travels*, it is more likely it was his continuing exile he blamed them for (cf. Ingram's introduction to the Broadview edition of *Gulliver's Travels* 2012; cf. also David Cody's entry on https://victorianweb.org/previctorian/swift/history.html, last access October 2024).

6 During a personal conversation with the Swift expert Allan Ingram in 2024, he noted something obvious that is, however, rarely emphasised: Gulliver himself never changes in size; it is his context that makes him seem large or small, which then paves the way for this to be switched to moral perspectives.

7 Cf. *A History of the Modern Fact: Problems of Knowledge in the Sciences of Wealth and Society* (1998).

8 Cf. "The Colonial Afterlife of Political Arithmetic: Swift, Demography, and Mobile Populations" (2004).

9 Furthermore, as the next paragraph reveals, the female Yahoo "could not be above eleven Years old," adding to the threat of female sexuality and the problematic issues it might raise within male sexuality (*Travels*, 225).

10 The same holds true for sections after the beginning of Part IV, "A Voyage to the Country of the Houyhnhnms," where Gulliver leaves his children and "poor Wife big with Child," and neither her pregnancy nor the child's birth is ever mentioned again (*Travels*, 187).

11 In the beginning of part IV, it reads: "I CONTINUED at home with my Wife and Children about Five Months in a very happy Condition, […] I left my poor Wife big with Child, and accepted an advantageous Offer made me to be Captain of the *Adventure*, […]" (*Travels*, 187).

References

Armintor, Deborah Needleman. 2007. "The Sexual Politics of Microscopy in Brobdingnag." *Studies in English Literature, 1500–1900* 47 (3): 619–640.

Boucé, Paul-Gabriel. 2001. "Gulliver Phallophorus and the Maids of Honour in Brobdingnag." *XVII-XVIII* 53 (1): 81–98.

Boyle, Frank. 2000. *Swift as Nemesis: Modernity and Its Satirist.* Stanford, CA: Stanford University Press.

Brown, Laura. 1990. "Reading Race and Gender: Jonathan Swift." *Eighteenth-Century Studies* 23: 424–443.

Carter, Sophie. 2004. *Purchasing Power: Representing Prostitution in Eighteenth-Century English Popular Print Culture.* Aldershot: Ashgate.

Donoghue, Denis. 1998. *The Practice of Reading.* New Haven, CT: Yale University Press.

Flynn, Carol H. 1990. *The Body in Swift and Defoe.* Cambridge: Cambridge University Press.

Fournier, Marian. 1996. *The Fabric of Life: Microscopy in the Seventeenth Century.* Baltimore, MD: Johns Hopkins University Press.

Francus, Marilyn. 2012. *Monstrous Motherhood: Eighteenth-Century Culture and the Ideology of Domesticity.* Baltimore, MD: Johns Hopkins University Press.

Girten, Kristi M. 2013. "Mingling with Matter: Tactile Microscopy and the Philosophic Mind in Brobdingnag and Beyond." *The Eighteenth Century* 54 (4): 497–520.

Hawes, Clement. 1991. "Three Times Round the Globe: Gulliver and Colonial Discourse." *Cultural Critique,* No. 18 (Spring). 187–214.

Hawes, Clement. 2020. "Gulliver Effects." In The Oxford Handbook of the Eighteenth-Century Novel, edited by Alan Downie, 523–541. Oxford: Oxford University Press.

Hillman, David, and Ulrika Maude, eds. 2015. *The Cambridge Companion to the Body in Literature.* New York: Cambridge University Press.

Ingram, Allan. 1986. *Intricate Laughter in the Satire of Swift and Pope.* Basingstoke: Macmillan.

Ingram, Allan. 2012. "Introduction." In *Gulliver's Travels,* edited by Allan Ingram, 1–12. Peterborough, ON: Broadview Press.

Ingram, Allan. 2022. *Swift, Pope and the Doctors: Medicine and Writing in the Early Eighteenth Century.* Leiden, Netherlands: Brill Fink.

Jeffares, A. Norman, (ed.) 1992. *Jonathan Swift: The Selected Poems.* London: Kyle Cathie Limited.

Knight, Charles. 2004. *The Literature of Satire.* Cambridge: Cambridge University Press.

Lynall, Gregory. 2012. *Swift and Science: The Satire, Politics, and Theology of Natural Knowledge, 1690–1730.* New York: Palgrave Macmillan.

Marshall, Ashley. 2013. *The Practice of Satire in England, 1658–1770.* Baltimore, MD: Johns Hopkins University Press.

McCormick, Ian. 2013. "Sex, Sodomy, and Death Sentences in the Long Eighteenth Century." In *Sex and Death in Eighteenth-Century Literature,* edited by Jolene Zigarovich, 42–67. New York; London: Routledge.

Morrissey, Lee. 2017. "The Restoration and Eighteenth Century, 1660–1780." In *English Literature in Context,* 2nd ed., edited by Paul Poplawski, 189–273. Cambridge: Cambridge University Press.

Noggle, James. 2018. "The Restoration and the Eighteenth Century." In *The Norton Anthology of English Literature,* 10th ed., edited by Stephen Greenblatt, 3–31. New York: Norton.

Poovey, Mary. 1998. *A History of the Modern Fact: Problems of Knowledge in the Sciences of Wealth and Society.* Chicago, IL: University of Chicago Press.

Porter, Roy. 2001. *Bodies Politic: Disease, Death and Doctors in Britain, 1650–1900.* London: Reaction.

Porter, Roy. 2004. *Flesh in the Age of Reason*. London: Penguin.
Porter, Roy. 2021. *Bodies Politic: Disease, Death and Doctors in Britain, 1650–1900*. London: Reaktion.
Rabb, Melinda. 2006. "The Secret Memoirs of Lemuel Gulliver: Satire, Secrecy, and Swift." *ELH* 73 (2): 325–354.
Rivero, Albert J. 2002. "Preface." In *Gulliver's Travels*, by Jonathan Swift, edited by Albert J. Rivero, vii–xii. New York: Norton.
Rosenthal, Laura J. 2006. *Infamous Commerce: Prostitution in Eighteenth-Century British Literature and Culture*. Ithaca, NY: Cornell University Press.
Salvaggio, Ruth. 1988. "Swift's Disruptive Woman." In *Enlightened Absence: Neoclassical Configurations of the Feminine*, edited by Ruth Salvaggio, 77–102. Urbana: University of Illinois Press.
Seager, Nicholas. 2022. "Jonathan Swift, Gulliver's Travels (1726)." In *Handbook of the British Novel in the Long Eighteenth Century*, edited by Katrin Berndt and Alessa Johns, 279–301. Berlin; Boston, MA: De Gruyter.
Seidel, Michael. 1998. "Samuel Richardson: Fiction and Knowledge." In *The Cambridge Companion to the Eighteenth-Century Novel*, edited by John Richetti, 131–150. Cambridge: Cambridge University Press.
Spratt, Danielle. 2012. "Gulliver's Economized Body: Colonial Projects and the *Lusus Naturae* in the Travels." *Studies in Eighteenth-Century Culture* 41: 137–159.
Sussman, Charlotte. 2004. "The Colonial Afterlife of Political Arithmetic: Swift, Demography, and Mobile Populations." *Cultural Critique* 56 (1): 96–126.
Swift, Jonathan. 2002. *Gulliver's Travels*. Edited with an introduction by Albert J. Rivero. New York: Norton.
Wilson, Catherine. 1995. *The Invisible World: Early Modern Philosophy and the Invention of the Microscope*. Princeton, NJ: Princeton University Press.

2.2 John Cleland's *Fanny Hill* (1749)

2.2.1 Introduction

John Cleland's *Memoirs of a Woman of Pleasure*, also known as *Fanny Hill* (1749), is one of the best-known examples of eighteenth-century erotic literature. It is thus all the more surprising that it at the same time ranks among the most underrated and under-analysed novels of the period. What follows are renditions of various introductions to the narrative (Plumb 1965; Gautier 2001; Sabor [1985] 2008), while the subsequent sections focus on studies that deal with medicine, sex, bodies and gender (Harvey 2004, 2010) prostitution (Rosenthal 2006; Lewis/Ellis 2016) and pornography (Peakman 2012, 2016) in eighteenth-century literature and culture. The aim is to discuss selected aspects of Cleland's life and works with an emphasis on *Fanny Hill* as well as an investigation of how erotica is entangled with science, sex and the reproductive body. Special attention is given to metaphors that derived from the fields of science and society and were int*ra*-linked with (material) discourses of sex and gender during the Enlightenment in Britain.

John Cleland is mainly known for his first novel *Fanny Hill* which has been sold "both above [...] and under the counter" in English-speaking continents including America and Europe (Plumb 1965, vii). First released "anonymously and under false imprints," Cleland wrote an erotic novel that deals with the "pleasures of the flesh" and brought the then 40-year-old man in need of financial stability "immortality and infamy" (Plumb 1965, vii; Sabor 2008, vii). Since its publication, *Fanny Hill* has survived multiple "bannings [and] burnings," while "[d]emand for it has never ceased" (Plumb 1965, vii). This "constant suppression" is all the more surprising given that *Fanny Hill* lacks even a "trace of obscenity or a flicker of guilt," a trait that will be taken up again later (Plumb 1965, vii).

Nevertheless, Cleland's erotic novel did not cause public outrage until a "disreputable publisher" by the name Drybutter added an "explicitly homosexual [lesbian] scene" to it in 1757 that attracted the authorities' attention (Plumb 1965, viii). After returning to London from his many travels abroad, Cleland was "arrested for an £840 debt [...] and committed to Fleet Prison, where he remained for over a year" and wrote *Fanny Hill* (n.n. *The Secret Bookshelf* 2014, 5; Gautier 2001, vi). The erotic novel was published in two volumes, the first in 1748 and the second in 1749, the year he left prison, only to be arrested again "along with the publishers

DOI: 10.4324/9781003467977-7

and printer of *Fanny Hill,*" Fenton Griffiths (n.n. *The Secret Bookshelf* 2014, 5; Gautier 2001, vi; Sabor 2008, ix–x). After their publication, Cleland and Griffiths released a shorter fig-leaf version titled *Memoirs of Fanny Hill*, while *Memoirs of a Woman of Pleasure* "remained an illicit but much sought-after text" across Europe and became an "underground bestseller" (Sabor 2008, x; Gautier 2001, vi).[1] Apparently, after his release from prison, Cleland was also employed by the government to make better use of his talents and furthermore received an annual pension to do so before he died in 1789, but none of this has ever been proven (Plumb 1965, x). Historians largely agree, however, that he "died impoverished and forgotten" (Gautier 2001, vi).

What can be said for sure is that *Fanny Hill* ranks among "one of the most remarkable books of the eighteenth century" due to its originality: "For the first time in English literature the sexual act, in all its diversity, is frankly and joyously described" (Plumb 1965, x–xi). *Fanny Hill* emerged at a time when "elements of puritanism" were still circulating among the population and the Christian "cult of virginity" was still strong (Plump 1965, xi). Needless to say, writing a novel that "reiterated [the] theme [...] that in copulation lies the one sure human bliss" was a risky endeavour (Plumb 1965, xi). As a result, *Fanny Hill* can (also) be understood as a biting satire about the "sexual morality of the age in which it was written" (Plumb 1965, xi).

Yet, eighteenth-century England was "robustly coarse about the physical side of life": Especially London hosted a "multitude of brothels," while "[c]ountry girls, quickly seduced, [...] provided a never-ending stream of young prostitutes for the metropolis" (Plumb 1965, xi). In fact, erotic texts proliferated with William Hogarth's series of engravings *A Harlot's Progress* (1730–1732) but also novels, ranging from Daniel Defoe's *Moll Flanders* (1722) and *Roxana* (1724) to Samuel Richardson's *Pamela* (1740) and *Clarissa* (1748). What needs to be kept in mind, however, is that these erotic or erotically charged narratives were so successful because they "touch[ed] the lives of *men*" (emphasis added, Plumb 1965, xiii). This becomes especially clear by the example of the eponymous character Fanny who is the embodiment of male fantasy:

> [Fanny is the] ideal erotic companion – tender, loving, discreet, always animated by the most delicate sentiments yet sexually uninhibited, capable of any variation of technique, enjoying an almost unquenchable appetite, guiltless, randy, preoccupied with the climax of love and obsessed by the size and power of its engine: in fact, a male dream.
>
> (Plumb 1965, xiii)

In other words, Fanny is a product of male desire – it is thus no coincidence that Cleland wrote the novel from a first-person perspective (Plumb 1965, xiii). As Plumb states, Fanny represents the manifestation of Cleland's "unconscious fantasies" that do not require "justification" since "male human nature has a strong erotic streak, so why should it not have artistic expression?" (Plumb, xiv). Plumb, though, was born in 1911 and wrote in the 1960s which partly explains the essentialist notion of 'male human nature.' Yet, his somewhat questionable statement stresses erotic literature's main target group – male readers – and explains the masculine perspective on female sexuality and bodies.

Fanny Hill's (alleged) status as a profane pornographic piece has undergone significant changes since it was released in the eighteenth century. In 1966, the United States Supreme Court "ruled that *Fanny Hill* was not obscene" which led to a scholarly re-evaluation of the text (Gautier 2001, vi; Sabor 2008, vii). Furthermore, as V. S. Pritchett notes:

> The disconcerting thing about the book – as a piece of 'pornography' – is that it has its charm [...] Fanny goes into prolonged, detailed descriptions of several kinds of sexual adventure and intercourse. In doing so, however, she never utters an obscene word [...]; she indeed writes an elaborate literary language that would do credit to any master of baroque and poetic utterance [...] spoken in the drawing room.
>
> (Pritchett in Gautier 2001, vi-vii)

Gary Gautier shifts attention away from Cleland's life to the "rise of capitalism and the bourgeois world view" in the eighteenth century and argues that bodies and sexuality were reduced to "relations between things" (Gautier 2001, xiv). It is thus possible to read *Fanny Hill* as a "conservative critique of bourgeois commercialism", as intercourse is repeatedly represented as an "act between autonomous sexual organs" (Gautier 2001, xiv). Gautier identifies a "movement from aestheticized body to commodified body" in the eighteenth century that also manifests itself in Fanny's relationship to her own body which she regards as "so many units of product" (Gautier 2001, xv). The novel achieves this link between human flesh and commodified "raw material" especially through a "repeated conflation of nature, body and business" (Gautier 2001, xv).

As Peter Sabor notes, despite *Fanny Hill*'s status as a considerable contribution to the emergence of the British novel, "it has been [largely] ignored by many literary historians [...] reluctant to pronounce his name" (Sabor 2008, vii). In spite of this neglect, the novel ranks "among the most frequently reprinted translated and illustrated of all English novels" (Sabor 2008, vii). Yet, until the 1960s, *Fanny Hill* was "widely read but scarcely considered in formal criticism" (Sabor 2008, xiv). Scholars such as Peter Quennel, who wrote an introduction to a new Putnam edition in 1963, insisted on the lack of vulgarity in Cleland's novel and praised its sophisticated style (Sabor 2008, xv). Although the following two decades witnessed a substantial amount of scholarship on *Fanny Hill*, most of them were "bibliographical and biographical studies" or "accounts of its legal battles" in Europe and the US (Sabor 2008, xvi).

Scholarship gained momentum in the 1980s when (feminist) critics such as Erica Jong (1978), Janet Todd (1980), Nancy Miller (1980) or Anne Robinson Taylor (1981) debated whether *Fanny Hill* was simply a "subterfuge for glorifying masculine authority" or a celebration of female pleasure (Sabor 2008, xvii). Ultimately, as Sabor concludes: "*Memoirs of a Woman of Pleasure* has crossed the barriers of critical silence and condescending recognition to confront the challenges and dissenting views that a significant work of literature demands" (Sabor 2008, xvii). The following chapters redirect attention from topics such as early capitalism to eighteenth-century erotic culture, the function of the prostitute figure as well as the entanglement of pornography with science.

2.2.2 Cleland & Erotic Culture

Not much information is available on John Cleland's life, despite the fact that his father William Cleland, a tax collector, was befriended by the English poet and satirist Alexander Pope, the Irish writer and politician Richard Steele as well as the writer and art historian Horace Walpole and was thus "well-known and well-liked in social and literary circles" (Plumb 1965, vii; Gautier 2001, v; Sabor 2008, viii). John Cleland was born in Surrey, South East England, in 1709, visited Westminster school but dropped out in 1723 "at the age of thirteen" for unknown reasons that "must have been personal: either rebellion or sin or both" (Plumb 1965, vii–viii; Gautier 2001, v). Though there is "no certainty" as to the rest of Cleland's life, historians agree that he spent a significant amount of time abroad, first in Turkey, then in Bombay, where he served the East India Company, and in Europe, most probably France, before he returned to London (Plumb 1965, viii). Rumour has it that he led a difficult life and was also addicted to gambling before he wrote *Fanny Hill* in 1749 (Plumb 1965, viii).

The society Cleland lived in was characterised by a clash between politeness as a form of disciplining the individual and the disentanglement of sexuality with sin. It was erotic culture that merged sexuality with pleasure but also embodied an ambiguous representation of sex. As Karen Harvey points out, "unbridled pleasure" ran counter to the eighteenth-century culture of politeness and restraint, which is why "erotic material rendered depictions of sex and bodies hazy" and hid them under "cloaks of metaphor": The effect was a modest "distance between reader and text" (Harvey 2004, 1). Yet, erotic literature often included explicit (visual) illustrations, usually of naked women, which certifies a male obsession with female physicality (Harvey 2004, 2).

Harvey further urges us not to regard erotic texts as marginalised – they were rather entangled with economic, social, cultural, literary and scientific developments of the time (Harvey 2004, 3). In terms of the latter, erotica was particularly int*ra*-linked with "new bodies of knowledge" that emerged as a result of scientific exploration abroad, most importantly geography and botany (Harvey 2004, 3). Authors of erotica, in contrast, did not randomly reflect new scientific or medical ideas in their works; instead, they chose them very carefully, which becomes especially clear by the example of "sexual difference," based on "male superiority," that was repeatedly mocked in erotic literature (Harvey 2004, 3). Eighteenth-century erotica is, in fact, very well-suited for a discussion of gender, the body and sexual difference as the period – apparently – witnessed significant changes in human sexuality (Harvey 2004, 4).

In this context, Harvey references Laqueur's *Making Sex* ([1990] 1992), based on the claim that "opposite sexes were born in the eighteenth century"; according to Laqueur, this period saw a major shift from a one- to a two-sex model as already mentioned in chapter 1.2. Though Laqueur's work is pivotal in terms of the history of gender and the body, Harvey agrees with those scholars who have criticised his central statement of sudden and especially linear change (Harvey 2004, 6–7). She reminds us that culture is never a "monolith [and] rarely one-dimensional" and calls for acknowledging the "plurality of [...] bodies" that "complicates" Laqueur's book (Harvey 2004, 8). Another problem Harvey addresses is the "limitation [of] evidence" regarding representation and lived experience that "remains murky" at best (Harvey 2004, 8).

Harvey builds on Foucault's discourse-oriented work, while she already seems to draw attention to the problem of causality or correlation between discourse and "sexual science," though she does not (yet) consider the body's materiality or material medical practices such as dissection: In any case, she reminds us to avoid over-simplification when talking about relationships between texts and the world that can be more complicated than generally assumed (Harvey 2004, 9). Most importantly and with regard to represented bodies, Harvey calls for regarding them as "both products of cultural, social and political debate and screens onto which cultural, social and political concerns were projected" (Harvey 2004, 10). Although I largely agree with Harvey, I disagree with the understanding of bodies as (passive) screens since it equally evokes the idea of linearity and causality. I rather argue that bodies, texts and the world simultaneously 'produce' one another – in Barad's words, they are int*ra*-linked or *entangled* with the world's becoming. Interestingly, a couple of pages later Harvey admits herself that a "language of 'representativeness' [...] is inappropriate for a study of meaning," thus confirming the concept of non-causal entanglement (Harvey 2004, 12). Yet, Harvey's research largely focusses on recurring themes in erotica.

One dominant theme in eighteenth-century erotic culture certainly is prostitution. Sophie Carter states that sex and sexuality were "central to the imagining of eighteenth-century culture" with "chief female [...] fictional and factual characters", ranging from Moll Flanders to Fanny Hill to Georgina Duchess of Devonshire (Carter 2004, 1). However, Carter criticises the still "lingering rose-tinted" assumption that prostitution was an accepted practice and simply part of eighteenth-century everyday life: On the contrary, the practice of prostitution was "more complex" than generally assumed and especially "underpinned by a perception of female sexuality as a malevolent force that enslaves and emasculates men" (Carter 2004, 1–2). Prostitution rather evoked "extreme anxiety and fear" and ranked among one of the contemporaries' main concerns regarding "urban culture" (Carter 2004, 2). Yet, prostitution models were anything but universal – different discourses existed alongside one another.

Laura J. Rosenthal identifies two main models of prostitution – for pleasure and for business (Rosenthal 2006, 1). While the first model has had a long tradition, the second gained more importance in eighteenth-century early capitalism (Rosenthal 2006, 29). The prostitute's "economic meaning" gained such relevance because she could either "empower or threaten the individual through self-control, self-sacrifice, and self-division in marketplace exchanges" (Rosenthal 2006, 2). What is more, the figure of the prostitute entangled the public with the private sphere since sex and sexuality were believed to belong to the latter (Rosenthal 2006, 2, 4). Representations of prostitution could be either "disturbing" or "comically liberating" (or both); this becomes clear by the example of Cleland's *Fanny Hill* which features a young woman who "trades poverty for comfort through infamous commerce" and eventually "retires to wealth, love, and happiness" (Rosenthal 2006, 2, 8).

With reference to J. G. A. Pocock, Rosenthal reads the prostitute figure as the embodiment of the feminised marketplace that threatens the notion of individualism (Rosenthal 2006, 3). The prostitute as a trope can thus both question capitalist ideology and simultaneously serve as a "scapegoat of an irrational, feminized 'other'" (Rosenthal 2006, 3). In both cases, the female body is rendered an object, a thing to be owned, used or disposed of. As Rosenthal outlines, this form of objectification also manifested itself on a linguistic level: "In less polite circles, 'commodity' functioned as a slang for female genitalia [...] prostitutes were 'jades' or 'hacks'" (Rosenthal 2006, 6). What is more, the prostitute posed a threat not only to the individual's identity (and integrity) but also to the nation as a whole and the question of what it means to be "truly British" (Rosenthal 2006, 7). Hence, the prostitute figure was (and still is) a highly "ambiguous" and "disturbing" figure that entangles the private with the public while embodying an "unpredictable commercial economy" (Rosenthal 2006, 7).

Nevertheless, eighteenth-century prostitution is not to be understood in negative terms only (Rosenthal 2006, 8). Most importantly, it must also be read against the backdrop of changing perceptions of the female body (Rosenthal 2006, 8). Rosenthal equally references Laqueur and stresses that the construction of "modern prostitution" is entangled with shifting medical discourses which, by 1800, had established the female body "as distinct from the male and thus capable of – even inclined to – experience[ing] sexual activity without bodily pleasure" (Rosenthal 2006, 9). Still, the female prostitutes posed a "threat to masculine authority" due to the financial independence some of them enjoyed, the "temptation of commercial sex" they evoked and the "traditional bonds" they dissolved (Rosenthal 2006, 10, 15).

Ann Lewis and Markman Ellis build on Rosenthal's work and confirm that the prostitute "subverts all the approved modes of behaviour of normative gender roles for women: passive politeness, public invisibility, sexual submissiveness, social domesticity, linguistic refinement" (Lewis/Ellis 2016, 3). They do remind us that the "voice of the prostitute is largely missing from the historical record" – first-person recollections by prostitutes themselves are, for example in Cleland's *Fanny Hill*, rather "imitated and imagined" (Lewis/Ellis 2016, 3). Lewis and Ellis add that the prostitution trope was also entangled with both "new science," such as botany, anatomy or medicine, and the eighteenth-century Libertine movement that rendered female physicality a thing to be "used," "essentially disposable" and "monstrously sexualized" (Lewis/Ellis 2016, 10). In terms of erotic literature, they argue that

> [e]ven in the polite 'pornotopia' of Cleland's *Memoirs of a Woman of Pleasure*, in which both the prostitute's sex work is clean, safe, healthy and pleasurable, and the language of the novel abjures sexual vulgarity, the echo of

> the libertine whore can be seen. Although Cleland depicts his heroine Fanny Hill as a sex worker who finds her self and prosperity through prostitution, libertine literature was not liberationist.
>
> (Lewis/Ellis 2016, 10)

This raises the question of whether Cleland's novel is simply an example of (soft) erotica or if it belongs to the genre of (more violent) pornography that usually sexually objectifies especially female characters and their bodies. Most importantly, the following sections discuss how erotic literature and culture are intr*a*-linked with contemporary knowledges of the reproductive body.

Julie Peakman deals with "what we would now call 'pornography'" in eighteenth-century literature and culture and is especially interested in its entanglement with the world (Peakman 2012, 1). Though she investigates a plethora of material ranging from poems to print to memoirs, the following section attempts to focus on the question of how erotica was entangled with (material) discourses of science. Since the eighteenth century is also the period of the Scientific Revolution, new knowledges in natural philosophy, medicine and exploration intr*a*-acted with people and the world (Peakman 2012, 1). As Peakman stresses, "new findings" played a large role in the emergence of bawdy texts that frequently mocked "new scientific terminology" (Peakman 2012, 1). Erotica's main themes included "[p]rocreation, disease and degeneration" that echoed "very real" anxieties of the period: Hence, what characterised erotica, despite its subversive potential, was a tendency towards conservatism and a fear of 'leaky vessels' and uncontrollable bodies, female in particular (Peakman 2016, 2). But how *is* erotica defined and what distinguishes it from pornography?

In short, Peakman explains that traditionally, pornography is understood as the "explicit depiction" of the sexual act including the participants' genitalia with the goal to evoke arousal (Peakman 2016, 5). Erotica, however, tends to hide "sexual matters" especially by use of metaphor (Peakman 2016, 7). Peakman emphasises, though, that boundaries between erotica, pornography or bawdy illustrations are blurry; ultimately, the very term 'pornography' was not coined until the second half of the nineteenth century and runs the danger of creating an anachronistic view on eighteenth-century erotic material (Peakman 2016, 5–6). To avoid confusion, Peakman follows a common definition and uses the term pornography to describe texts that "contain graphic description[s] of sexual organs and/or action [...] written with the prime intention of sexually exciting the reader" (Peakman 2016, 6). She situates it as "one genre within a superfluity of other texts of erotica," while the latter is used as an umbrella term for "all books on sex" (Peakman 2016, 7).

As mentioned above, prostitution was a common theme in eighteenth-century erotica, while female sex workers' portrayals were ambiguous; they either represented (passive) victims of their profession or were constructed as (active) "powerful and sexually threatening" figures (Peakman 2012, 8). What most of these texts had in common, however, was their interconnectedness with (male) "anxieties about female sexual desire" (Peakman 2012, 8). Satire played an important role for erotica as it enabled a subversion of dominant sexual discourses (Peakman 2012, 9). In addition, many authors of erotica also produced scientific or "pseudo-medical" texts, further blurring the demarcations between science, medicine and erotic literature (Peakman 2012, 24).

Peakman stresses the "multiplicity of images" in erotica; she rejects a dichotomous approach to such texts in favour of one that is "multi-layered" and thus enables "more complex visions" (Peakman 2012, 11). Though Cleland does not utter one vulgar word in *Fanny Hill*, the novel has been regarded as "one of the first major [pornographic] pieces" of the age alongside Thomas Stretser's *A New Description of Merryland* (1741), an erotic text that uses topographical metaphors to describe the female body and was published by the "pornographer Edmund Curll," or Payne Knight's *A Discourse on the Worship of Priapus* (1786), a book that deals with sexuality and religion (Peakman 2012, 21, 39). It is therefore difficult to assign *Fanny Hill* to either category – the boundaries between erotica and pornography remain blurred. In any case, as Peakman concludes, by 1800, Britain had undergone a development "from being an occasional producer of bawdy humour to a society awash with erotica" (Peakman 2012, 44). The following sections discuss the strategies of displaying explicit sexual acts and organs that mainly involved the use of metaphors.

2.2.3 Mechanical & Botanical Metaphors

As mentioned above, not only are literary genres as such blurred, but this holds especially true for the demarcations of erotic fiction. This gave Cleland the opportunity to play with "strict generic boundaries" (Harvey 2004, 19). What needs to be kept in mind is that although scholars today distinguish between literature and pornography, both "grew from common roots" (Harvey 2004, 19). Yet, eighteenth-century English culture differentiated between certain text forms as Harvey outlines: "[I]t meant one thing to read an erotic poem with some claims to refinement, and quite another to read a pornographic novel in which people fucked" (Harvey 2004, 19). I claim that Cleland's *Fanny Hill* sits astride the two: On the one hand, it avoids vulgar language, but on the other hand, it is clearly written to evoke arousal through its quite explicit descriptions of sexual organs and acts, despite its coding through the use of metaphors.

Fanny Hill is Cleland's first novel and, according to Sabor, interested in the "texture of everyday life" (Sabor 2008, xxi). It is divided into two long letters or volumes, narrated by the eponymous character Fanny ("Francis Hill," *Memoirs*, 1). In these letters, the protagonist, now happily married, narrates her life retrospectively to an unknown female friend, "Madam" (*Memoirs*, 1). She announces a recollection of the "scandalous stages" and "loose part" of her life and how she is now blessed with the "power of love, hearth and fortune" despite her "unhappy profession" (*Memoirs*, 1). Fanny also assures her friend that what she will learn in the following is the "stark naked truth," and that she will "paint situations such as they actually rose," thus adhering to the eighteenth-century novel's typical truth claim (*Memoirs*, 1). Fanny will also not show consideration for the "violation" of the "laws of decency" and reminds her 'Madam' that she, too, has "much knowledge of the *originals* themselves, [than] to snuff prudishly, and out of character, at the *pictures* of them" (emphasis in the original, *Memoirs*, 1).

The first volume consists of her "personal history" (*Memoirs*, 1): Fanny was born in the country into an extremely poor family, badly educated, and orphaned at a very young age. In search of fortune, she ventured on a journey to London at the age of 15, accompanied by her friend Esther who told her stories about

> how several maids out of the country had made themselves and all their kin for ever, that by preserving their VARTUE, some had taken so with their masters, that they had married them, [...] and lived vastly grand, and happy.
> (emphasis in the original, *Memoirs*, 3)

On her arrival, Fanny was lured into a brothel by a female bawd. Here, she first secretly observed people having sex, was seduced by the 25-year-old Phoebe, while struggling with "ideas of pollution," pleasure and "violent emotions," and only narrowly escaped rape by an utterly revolting customer she repeatedly calls "monster" in her recollection of events (*Memoirs*, 12–13, 16, 18, 21). Before she became a prostitute herself, Fanny was 'saved' by the handsome young gentleman Charles who was the first man she (voluntarily) had intercourse with in a bloody scene of pain and pleasure. After less than one year Charles suddenly had to leave for business reasons. Again, Fanny was confronted with poverty while the text suggests she was also pregnant ("I was three months gone with child by him," *Memoirs*, 54) when Charles left her, but she miscarried shortly after (*Memoirs*, 56).

In volume II, Fanny tells her friend how she finally found longer-term accommodation in Mrs Cole's "house of conveniency" (*Memoirs*, 88). Though Fanny engaged in impressive "practice[s] of pleasure" for a duration of nearly three years, pleased mostly older customers and seemed to have enjoyed her work, she never forgot her lover, Charles (*Memoirs*, 91). She eventually inherited a significant amount of money from one of her elderly clients, gained financial independence (at least momentarily), regretted her past and realised how much she loved Charles (*Memoirs*, 176). Shortly after her lover returned, she handed over her fortune to him as a compensation for his 'damaged honour.' Both married, Fanny regained her 'virtue,' she could leave the brothel, and both lived happily ever after.

In short, *Fanny Hill* is about a young woman "who progresses from [a helpless and] naïve, fifteen-year-old country girl to [a] nineteen-year-old bride" (Sabor 2008, xxi). Sabor notes that Cleland's novel contains many "detailed descriptions" including the amount of money Fanny owns in the beginning and the end as well as with regard to "clothing, hairstyle, food and drink, furniture and means of transportation," thus adhering to the realistic mode of the emerging eighteenth-century novel (Sabor 2008, xxi). Moreover, Cleland satirises the "distasteful pursuit of deflowering virgins" in various instances (Sabor 2008, xxi). Though *Fanny Hill* is partially of "idyllic, incandescent quality," the novel still does not quite fit the genre of "pornotopia," a term coined by the literary critic Steven Marcus[2] in the

1960s, that describes a utopian fantasy world in which men are always potent and women always willing to have sex with them (Sabor 2008, xxi).

On the contrary, in Cleland's universe, men are more often than not impotent, women also lack "sexual desire" and characters are repeatedly haunted by "jealousy, possessiveness and anger" (Sabor 2008, xxii). These factors distinguish *Fanny Hill* from the "mainstream" eighteenth-century novel as it connects romance with realism, while at the same time displaying a strong interest in "explicit and obsessive" descriptions of sexual acts, organs and effects: "Not until Sterne's *Tristram Shandy* [...] did another English novel render physiological responses so graphically" (Sabor 2008, xxii–xxiii). These and other issues lead to the question of how gender, femininity in particular, was constructed during the British Enlightenment. Most importantly, the following subsections discuss what kind of metaphors Cleland uses in *Fanny Hill* to describe sexual acts and bodies. One aim is to demonstrate how gender, sex and the (reproductive) body were entangled with both early capitalism and new knowledges and practices in the fields of science (and technology), including botany, anatomy or medicine.

As Gautier outlines, eighteenth-century Britons not only engaged in a "remapping [of] world territories" abroad but were also involved in the reconstitution of categories like 'womanhood' in their home country, while simultaneously "exposing that [kind of] remapping as ludicrous" (Gautier 2001, xi). Against the backdrop of early capitalism, the re-formation of 'woman' was especially achieved by the use of certain metaphors such as "prospects" or "flowers," thus "aestheticiz[ing] and commodif[ying]" the "sexual body" (Gautier 2011, xi). Gautier continues that through *Fanny Hill*, Cleland equally "remaps [...] concepts of sexuality [and] female identity." At the same time, however, he links this reconstitution to an "emergent bourgeois ideology" only to then take on the position of an "antagonist to that ideology" by ridiculing it (Gautier 2001, xi). In other words, Cleland attacks "bourgeois constructions of gender" through satire (Gautier 2011, xi). Yet, it is misleading to assume that Cleland can therefore be understood as a proto-feminist (Gautier 2011, xi). On the contrary, his point of departure is rather that of conservatism as he wrote in the tradition of Tobias Smollett or Henry Fielding – both well-known and conservatist eighteenth-century novelists and satirists (Gautier 2001, xii).

With regard to the entanglement of gender, sex, the body and capitalism, Gautier believes the word "prospect" to be central to *Fanny Hill*. For him, it is used metaphorically and has "three meanings" in Cleland's text: (1) "a view of nature," meaning an "aesthetic appreciation of natural scenery," (2) a perspective of the "sexual body" and (3) "a view of change in material conditions" (Gautier 2001, xii). Gautier argues that these three dimensions – nature, the body and the material – together result in an aestheticisation and commodification of the sexual body, both female *and* male (Gautier 2001, xii). Gautier stresses emphatically that the "metaphorical use of 'prospects,'" that first becomes evident during Fanny's 'defloration,' is anything but "gender-specific" (Gautier 2001, xii):

> After breakfast, *Charles* [...], with a smile full of meaning, took me gently by the hand, and said: "Come, my dear, and I will show you a room that commands a fine prospect over some gardens:" and without waiting for an

> answer, in which he relieved me extremely, he led me up into a chamber airy and lightsome, where all seeing of prospects was out of the question, except that for a bed, which had all the air of having recommended the room to him.
>
> (emphasis in the original, *Memoirs*, 39)

The morning after her 'defloration,' Fanny gazes at Charles' "body of the most perfect form" and equally describes it in great detail (*Memoirs*, 44):

> The plat-form of his snow-white bosom, that was laid out in a manly proportion, presented on the vermillion summet [sic] of each pap, the idea of a rose about to blow. Nor did his shirt hinder from observing that simmetry [sic] of his limbs, that exactness of shape, in the fall of it towards the loins, where the waist ends, and the rounding swell of the hips commences, where the skin, sleek, smooth, and dazzling white, burnishes on the stretch over firm, plump-ripe flesh, that crimpled and run into dimples at the least pressure, or that the touch could not rest upon, but slid over as on the surface of the most polish'd ivory. [...] Then the growth of hair, in short and soft curls round its roots, its whiteness, branch'd veins, the supple softness of the shaft, as it lay foreshorten'd, roll'd and shrunk up into a squob [sic] thickness, languid, and born up from between the thighs, by its globular appendage, that wondrous treasure-bag of nature's sweets, which rivell'd round, and purs'd up in the only wrinkles that are known to please, perfected the prospect; and all together form'd the most interesting moving picture in nature [...].
>
> (spelling in the original, *Memoirs*, 44–45)

The way Fanny gazes at Charles' body is almost clinical; she describes his "proportions," the "simmetry [sic] of his limbs," "exactness of shape" but also mingles her descriptions with botanical metaphors such as "rose" or "branch'd" and links his body with "nature." The focus lies on his "flesh," "firm" and "plump-ripe," that evokes a "perfected [...] prospect." As Gautier notes, the text not only sexualises and objectifies but also aestheticises the body to cater for the "needs of the commercial world" (Gautier 2001, xiii). In other words, the body needs to become an object, a thing, before it "can be readily mapped into the bourgeois world of commodity values" (Gautier 2001, xiii). I argue, however, that the body is not simply objectified by fragmentation, but that this form of verbal dismemberment is also, albeit remotely, reminiscent of actual dissection practices of the period that equally dismembered the body. Therefore, the sexual body is entangled with both early capitalism and scientific or (material) medical practices. What strikes the eye with regard to this passage is the fragmented body's gender: male. Gautier argues that the text makes no distinction between female or male bodies – both are subject to the same form of sexualisation and aestheticisation. This argument will be seized upon again later.

For the moment, this section lingers on the question of how the text entangles metaphors of nature, production and machinery. According to Gautier, Cleland's novel not only uses traditional "erotic topography" but also seems to almost exchange it with mechanical metaphors (Gautier 2001, xiii). The effect, however, is that "all individuals, regardless of class or gender, become interchangeable units in some gigantic sociosexual machine" (Gautier 2001, xiii). As the text reveals, Cleland indeed uses botanical and mechanical metaphors to describe the sexual body. In volume I, Fanny recalls how she watched one of the (unnamed) girls in the brothel serve a customer. The scene is described as follows:

> As he stood on one side, for a minute or so, unbuttoning his waist-coat and breeches, her fat, brawny thighs hung down, and the whole greasy *landskip* [sic] lay fairly open to my view; a wide open-mouth'd gap, overshaded with a grizzly *bush*, seemed held out like a beggar's wallet for its provision. But I soon had my eyes called off by a more striking object, that entirely engross'd them. Her sturdy stallion had now unbutton'd, and produced naked, stiff, and erect, that wonderful *machine*, which I had never seen before, and which, for the interest my own seat of pleasure began to take furiously in it, I star'd at with all the eyes I had: however, my senses were too much flurried, too much concenter'd in that burning spot of mine, to observe any thing more than in general the make and turn of that *instrument* […].
>
> (emphasis added, *Memoirs*, 24–25)

This scene demonstrates Cleland's use of botanical metaphors to describe sexualised bodies. The prostitute's body is rendered a "landskip" (landscape) and her pubic hair a "bush" that covers her "gap." As this example clearly shows, it is also connoted with a degree of disgust – the landscape is "greasy" and the bush "grizzly." The vulva resembles a "beggar's wallet" – an association that recalls both 'factual' and fictional encounters of men with 'revolting' reproductive bodies of beggar women in texts such as Paré's *Monsters and Marvels* or Swift's *Gulliver's Travels*. Moreover, the girl's body stands in stark contrast with the male sexualised body that is portrayed as a "more striking object," a "wonderful machine" and "instrument," thus evoking images of machinery, technology but also anatomy or dissection. This scene in particular contradicts Gautier's implied claim that all bodies – regardless of gender – are aligned with the same metaphors. This might hold true for images such as "prospect," as discussed above, that interlink the body with early capitalism, but it certainly does not apply to the use of botanical and mechanical metaphors.

Without doubt, Cleland's novel is saturated with sexualised bodies and parts thereof. The text not only objectifies bodies through fragmentation but also utilises plant and machine imagery. The following section seizes upon Gautier's claim that botanical and mechanical metaphors are applied to both female and male bodies alike. Though this might be true in (very) few cases, I argue that in general, female and male bodies are neatly divided and assigned to either the feminine connoted sphere of nature or the masculine connoted realm of machinery with only very few exceptions (See Figure 15).

As these examples demonstrate, Cleland's text seems to separate female and male genders by assigning them with either botanical or mechanical metaphors. On the one hand, this contradicts Gautier's claim that all characters, regardless of

botanical (f)	mechanical (m)
- "greasy landskip" (24) - "grizzly bush" (24) - "my virgin-flower was yet uncrop'd" (40) - "he had crop't its richest flower" (105) - "I deflower myself" (107) - "downy spring-moss" (115) - "luxury of the landscape" (115) - "mouth of nature" (116) - "symptoms of defloration" (132)	- "wonderful machine" (25) - "instrument" (25) - "enormous machine" (27) - "fierce erect machine" (31) - "engine of love-assaults" (40) - "largeness of his machine" (40) - "terrible spit-fire machine" (45) - "over-siz'd machine" (73) - "in-driven engine" (74) - "monstrous machine" (76) - "formidable machine" (77) - "machine so siz'd for its destruction" (79) - "plenipotentiary instrument" (113) - "true-siz'd instruments" (123) - "torpid machine" (151) - "man-machine" (163) - "brute-machine" (164) - "curious engine" (165) - "his own engine" (168) - "in-driving machine" (169)

Figure 15 Gendered botanical and mechanical metaphors in Cleland's *Fanny Hill* (1749).

gender, meld into a "gigantic sociosexual machine" – female bodies, or rather parts thereof, are obviously relegated to the sphere of nature or plants, and not machinery. On the other hand, Gautier correctly argues that the text's erotic topography is almost exchanged with mechanical metaphors: However, he overlooks that this mostly holds true for male characters. To my knowledge, there are only a few exceptions where botanical metaphors are used to picture masculine body parts. Apart from the above-mentioned metaphor "wondrous treasure-bag of nature's sweets" that Fanny uses to describe Charles' physicality, there are further noteworthy instances that entangle the male body with nature: When Fanny curiously watches a couple engaging in sexual intercourse in volume I, she constructs the "texture of that capital part of man" by use of a botanical metaphor and describes the "shrub-growth of curling hair" she sees, only to then immediately resort to mechanical metaphors such as "enormous machine" (*Memoirs*, 26–27).

During a similar scene in volume II, Fanny first verbally dismembers a prostitute's body by focusing on her "winking eyes, [...] her lips, and cheeks" and then continues to describe how "she was now as meer [sic] a machine, as much wrought on, and had her motions as little at her own command" (*Memoirs*, 165). These two examples, however, do not suffice to support the argument that Cleland's text disregards gender when it assigns its sexualised bodies with metaphors. In fact, this erotic novel is imbued with a multitude of metaphors, while many of them also evoke images of war. This becomes clear when Fanny describes sexual activities or male body parts such as "terrible weapon," "weapon of pleasure," "murderer of my virginity," "his drawn weapon" or "furious battering-ram" (*Memoirs*, 28, 33, 41, 68, 82).

With regard to botanical and mechanical metaphors, however, Cleland makes sure to enable his male characters an examination of the "sweet secret of nature, in order to make room for a stately piece of machinery," thus neatly assigning female physiology to the realm of plants, and male bodies to the sphere of machines (*Memoirs*, 169). Nevertheless, it has to be noted that in eighteenth-century anatomy and medicine, the mechanical metaphor was used to describe all bodies. Yet, Cleland's text constructs the female reproductive body as an eroticised landscape to be mapped and conquered by powerful (masculine) machines or instruments. In this context, the following concluding subchapter discusses in more detail the implications of such botanical metaphors especially with regard to female reproductive bodies and female sexuality. For this reason, it is necessary to yet again turn to the history of science and sexuality and ask how it is linked to erotic literature.

2.2.4 Botany, Erotica & Reproduction

In the course of the Scientific Revolution and the emergence of new knowledges, especially in the fields of botany and anatomy, natural philosophers began to entangle metaphors of reproduction with their studies. Scientists aimed at solving the mysteries of nature and thus systematically categorised the objects of investigation they encountered, from plants to insects to bodies. In order to understand nature's mechanisms, anatomists, for instance, resorted to mechanical metaphors of the body; all bodies, both female and male, were understood as machines or clockworks that could be dismembered and their components dissected. These parts were then assigned to specific boxes, thereby enabling a system of categories. The same form of categorisation held true for the world of plants: Botanists singled them out of their natural surroundings and equally put them into neat little boxes. As a result, metaphors of nature and the body inevitably overlapped. But the masculine connoted field of science not only entangled knowledges of nature and the body, it especially contributed to the link between nature and femininity and the strengthening of the Cartesian dualism of mind over matter.

As outlined in PART I, the eighteenth century brought about a plethora of contradicting theories with regard to reproduction, both in terms of human/animal or plant reproduction. The main questions that were asked are: How many sexes are there? How does reproduction work? What role do the sexes play in reproduction? In terms of human reproduction, the question of who is responsible for 'monstrous births' played a particularly large role and was hotly debated. The Royal Society of London, mainly consisting of wealthy gentlemen, published widely on these questions. Some authors of fiction, however, considered these studies to be "useless miscellanea," and many of the published theories were just what satirists of the age were waiting for (Peakman 2012, 70–71). Especially authors of erotica utilised these 'new knowledges' to mock some of the ideas emanating from the Royal Society.

Julie Peakman offers valuable insight into how especially writers of erotic literature satirised reproductive theories in her two monographs *Mighty Lewd Books* (2012) and *Amatory Pleasures* (2016). In her chapters on botanical metaphors, she focusses on two well-known, frequently printed, imitated and "easily accessible" texts: "Arbor Vitae, Or: The Natural History of The Tree of Life Verfify'd" and "Natural History of the Frutex Vulvaria," both probably published in 1732 by Thomas Stretser, first as a poem and then "along with prose," only a few years before Cleland's *Fanny Hill* (Peakman 2012, 71). Nothing much can be said about Stretser, the author, only that he was a member of the *Royal Society of Gardeners* and "one of Edmund Curll's hacks" (Peakman 2012, 71). Curll was a publisher of pornography and "often used false imprints, including false dates to avoid detection" (Peakman 2012, 71). The poem "Arbor Vitae" reads as follows:

> The Tree of which I fain would sing
> If the kind Muse her Aid would bring,
> In *Arbor Vitae*; but in brief,
> By vulgar Men call'd – *Tree of Life*
>
> That is, to take especial Care,
> Not to set *Vulvaria* near;
> Of them two Sorts are frequent found,
> One helps, and t'other spoils the Ground;
>
> (emphasis in the original, Stretser in Peakman 2012, 71)

This poem is not about the biblical 'tree of life' but instead uses sexualised botanical metaphors to describe the penis (tree) and vulva ([*Chenopodium*] *vulvaria*, also known as 'stinking goosefoot'). As Peakman stresses, botanical metaphors were everywhere in erotica as a result of science's attempts to categorise the world of plants (Peakman 2012, 71). In this case, the erotic poem equally describes the sexual behaviours of humans by applying botanical terminology. The text appropriates these terms and uses them as "satirical analogies" to human sexuality and reproduction; "botanical metaphors were used as a device to communicate openly about sex" and open up a "new erotic world" (Peakman 2012, 71–72). As Peakman outlines:

> In this 'other world', secret gardens, hidden valleys and cavernous holes contain mysterious erect plant life, furry thickets and bushy knolls, which mirrored the sexual nature of bodies constructed elsewhere. This gendered space was made recognisable for the readership through graphic imagery in the form of trees as penises, caves as vaginas, and so on, in the creation of a "landscape of desire."
>
> (Peakman 2012, 72)

Peakman adds another excerpt from Stretser's "Arbor Vitae" to her 2016 monograph to further highlight the (wide) use of sexualised botanical metaphors:

> Arbor Vitae, *or* the Tree of Life, *is a succulent Plant; consisting of one straight Stem, on the Top of which is a* Pistillum, or Apex… *Its* Fruits, *contrary to most others, grow near the Root; they are usually no more than two in Number.*
>
> (emphasis in the original, Peakman 2016, 145)

Stretser used "gendered terminology" not only to reconstruct the sexual life of plants; at the same time, this text described "male genitalia," in the above case the "dimensions of a perfect penis," in a way that "reflected the content and style of popular medical handbooks" (Peakman 2016, 150). The appropriation of field-specific terms, however, worked both ways: Not only did satirists and authors of erotica use botanical terms to describe human sexuality and reproduction – botanists equally borrowed gendered terms to explain how plants procreate; words such as "'nuptuals' [weddings] of living plants and 'bridal beds' of flower petals" demonstrate this strategy (Peakman 2012, 73, 2016, 149). These metaphors lead to an "eroticisation of plants" and even more so "expressed conservative attitudes and relegated the female to a secondary role" (Peakman 2012, 73). As Peakman emphasises:

> Plant sexuality lay at the core of the eighteenth-century revolution in the study of the plant kingdom. Gender was a main principle in attempting to organise revolutionary views on nature and gave rise to the emergence of sexual difference in plant terminology in the late seventeenth and eighteenth century. Nature's laws were perceived as a reflection of social and sexual relations between men and women, and within this model, nature was firmly linked with femaleness.
>
> (Peakman 2012, 73)

The link between nature and femininity was further fostered by well-known botanists of the eighteenth century. Carl Linnaeus (1707–1778), for instance, equally participated in the categorisation of nature and not only "chang[ed] the views of the world" with regard to the plant kingdom, but also in terms of (human) sex and sexuality (Peakman 2012, 73). Linnaeus was in fact one of the "first to recognise the sexual reproduction of plants" (Peakman 2012, 73). What he did, in fact, was compare plant sexuality to that of human reproduction by "labelling the parts of the plant as parts of the male or female body" (Peakman 2016, 149).

Linnaeus' work was good fodder for satirists who especially mocked his patriarchal language and use of "phallic terms," as Peakman outlines with regard to Linnaeus' *Systema Naturae* (1735); here, plants and parts thereof were "described as 'naked,' 'erect,' […], 'hairy' […] and even 'pubescent'" (Peakman 2016, 149–150). Equally, terms such as "'marriage beds' of plants" further evoked hierarchical (and heteronormative) relations between the sexes (Peakman 2012, 73). Ultimately, Linnaeus' system of classification "reflected the contemporary gender hierarchy" through the use of sexualised metaphors (Peakman 2012, 73). By reference to Londa Schiebinger's work,[3] Peakman states that this hierarchy also presented itself in the plant world on two levels; *implicitly*, meaning the adoption of "traditional notions of sexual hierarchy" with the male as the "most important," and *explicitly*, meaning the "use of sexual metaphors" to describe "plant reproduction" (Peakman 2012, 73).

Unsurprisingly, this sexualised language became an "obvious target for humorists of erotica" (Peakman 2012, 73). Nevertheless, the advantage of erotic satire was that it contributed to a subversion of gender hierarchies, thus "challenging patriarchal assumptions," and also offered the opportunity to represent "women as sexually powerful, and even dominant" (Peakman 2012, 73). This might be one of the reasons why, according to Peakman, "botanical metaphors in erotica are neatly divided into two sets of material, the male and the female, otherwise loosely termed as the trees and the shrubs" (Peakman 2012, 74). In fact, the botanical metaphor "Flowering Shrub" was used as a synonym for female genitalia and pubic hair which becomes especially clear in "Frutex Vulvaria," "Arbor Vitae"'s counterpart:

> *The* Frutex Vulvaria *is a flat low Shrub, which always grows in a moist warm Valley, at the Front of a little Hill, which is constantly water'd by a Spring, whose Water is impregnated with very saline Particles, which nevertheless agree wonderfully well with this* Shrub.
>
> (emphasis in the original, Peakman 2016, 145)

Contrary to Linnaeus' patriarchal language he applied to plants, this example, although it clearly links femininity with nature, does not render the female reproductive body inferior (Peakman 2016, 152). What is more, venereal diseases were blamed on both sexes and satirised by the use of botanical metaphors that described the "withering plants of the realm" (Peakman 2016, 153). Furthermore, erotica mocked quacks and well-known "medical practitioners" such as Sir Richard Manningham in relation to the infamous Mary Toft case (Peakman 2016, 155). Topics like "embryology and procreation," prostitution, "uncontrollable female desire" and its regulation or "manly men" were equally satirised in erotica; it is no coincidence that Cleland's Fanny describes a penis she touches as a "sensitive plant," thus ridiculing the "man of sensibilities" (Peakman 2016, 153–154; see also *Memoirs*, 162).

Eventually, as Peakman concludes with one more reference to Schiebinger, by 1800, erotica and botany had further amalgamated and resulted in more complex metaphors such as the "erotic garden" (Peakman 2016, 156). The greatest advantage of botanical metaphors in the eighteenth century was that they allowed for public discussions of sex and sexualised bodies "without use of graphic detail" (Peakman 2016, 158). Yet, erotica also expressed contemporary fears, especially with regard to "women's sexual inconsistency" that might result in "medical problems" such as venereal diseases or pregnancy (Peakman 2016, 158). But how exactly might we (int*ra*-)link Cleland's *Fanny Hill* not just with botany but also with pregnancy and medicine or obstetrics?

Karen Harvey, whose research on visualisations of reproduction was mentioned earlier, focusses on the pornographic mode in medical illustrations and argues that, in contrast, the erotic mode is usually characterised by a an "illusion of concealment and distance" towards the body that is often achieved through metaphors which seems to confirm the claim that Cleland's *Fanny Hill* rather belongs to erotic fiction than pornography (Harvey 2010, 43). In the context of childbirth, however, Harvey stresses that erotic texts frequently "drew on midwifery and medical texts as raw material for innuendo" – this makes sense if one considers that, according to her, there are "[s]everal accounts of eighteenth-century sexuality" that "reproduce the example of a young bachelor masturbating while reading a midwifery book" (Harvey 2010, 43). In turn, medical illustrations of female reproductive body parts such as those including a "female torso and pudenda, with upper arms and thighs sliced and the abdomen played open to reveal the reproductive organs" were suggested for erotic texts like Stretser's *A New Description of Merryland: Containing, a Topographical, Geographical, and Natural History of that Country* (1741) (Harvey 2010, 43–44). This further demonstrates the entanglement of the female reproductive body with topography, botany, medicine and erotica.

Having said all this, the question still remains what Cleland's *Fanny Hill* might actually mean. Though Gautier correctly observes that the metaphor of 'prospects' is applied to female and male characters alike and thus renders both genders – and gendered bodies – commodities to be consumed, it is still quite clear that Cleland neatly divides and assigns his sexualised body parts to two spheres; that of machinery and that of botany. At first glance, Cleland serves the traditional (and sexist) stereotypes of female-connoted nature versus male-connoted science and technology. Yet at a second, he also plays with these associations as he sometimes exchanges these metaphors to fit all genders.

Trying to come to a single interpretation of this satire is a matter of impossibility as was also demonstrated with regard to *Gulliver's Travels*. Gautier emphasises that, ultimately, *Fanny Hill* is a text that "glorifies the phallus"; at the same time, however, it "deliberately mocks *bourgeois* strategies of privileging the phallus" (emphasis in the original, Gautier 2001, xxviii). Yet, female bodies in *Fanny Hill* are subject to a world of "patriarchal coding": "The female, in such a world, has only quasi-identity which must be 'finish'd' by male penetration. She is a sort of *vagina rasa* awaiting male inscription" (Gautier 2001, xviii). Bonnie Blackwell argues along similar lines and confirms the "author's failure to capture female subjectivity authentically" (Blackwell 2013, 49).

What certainly remains unclear is if Cleland's division of female and male bodies and parts thereof by means of machine and plant imagery actually fed into the patriarchal discourse of masculine connoted science and technology that constructed female bodies as flowers to be picked or landscapes to be ploughed. What also cannot be fully answered is whether Cleland's readership was in fact able to recognise Cleland's humour, though some scholars argue that most eighteenth-century readers of erotic texts were indeed familiar with such metaphors. One of the novel's greatest potentials lies in the praise of female desire – yet, we should not forget that it is female desire constructed by a male author for a largely male readership:

Ultimately, the novel is a narrative about a female character first gazing at other women having sex – a typical plotline to be found in (mainstream) pornography across all (sub)genres and timelines – and whose own sexuality is initiated by another woman before she engages sexually with other men, either against her will or voluntarily, only to then be 'saved' by one of her clients who finally 'restores' her 'virtue' through marriage. The subversive potential of *Fanny Hill* in terms of gender stereotypes thus remains unclear.

The greatest achievement of Cleland's novel is that it offers itself for a discussion of how erotica is entangled with science, sex and the reproductive body. Though the text avoids any use of vulgar words and veils its quite explicit descriptions of sex and sexual organs through metaphors, it nevertheless draws a stronger connection between femininity and nature by reserving its machine imagery especially for male reproductive bodies. Whether this satirical strategy strengthened or weakened gendered stereotypes is for the reader to decide. Yet, Cleland's novel confirms the problem of causality expressed by scholars such as Karen Barad who prefers the term 'entanglement' over the more linear concept of 'representation.' The question of whether erotica influenced botany and medicine or vice versa is not only impossible to answer but also quite irrelevant: All of these (material) discourses were, and still are, int*ra*-linked with one another.

What needs to be stressed nevertheless is that the prostitute figure posed a threat to eighteenth-century patriarchy for a variety of reasons. This fear manifested itself especially in the unrestrained reproductive female body. It not only threatened masculine authority through its embodiment of a feminised marketplace as outlined by Rosenthal but also represented the danger of pregnancy due to the uncontrollable sexual desire associated with it. In order to keep these 'leaky vessels' in check, the female body was, to use Lewis and Ellis' words, monstrously sexualised. This becomes especially clear in Cleland's *Fanny Hill* where female genitalia are no powerful machines but all too often constructed as hairy monsters or greasy landscapes. At the same time, male bodies and parts thereof are repeatedly rendered impotent, thus subverting the mode of a (utopian) pornotopia.

In any case, all bodies in *Fanny Hill* are remapped and commodified. Still, female reproductive bodies fall behind their male counterparts by reducing them to sexualised landscapes that are mapped, conquered and most importantly examined by powerful 'machines' and 'instruments.' I argue that this mode of fragmentation and investigation int*ra*-links the literary and cultural female reproductive bodies with the very real, material body of the dissected female on the surgeon's table: Both are simultaneously dismembered, pathologised and eroticised with the aim not only to 'know' the 'secrets of nature' but also to control (female) reproduction.

Due to the multitude of these ambiguities, it is certainly also possible to understand the prostitute body as a cyborg body as it evades masculine control. Like the cyborg, the body of the prostitute poses a threat to individualism through its own bodily multiplicity. Moreover, the prostitute's (potentially reproductive) body can also be conceptualised as the ultimate obstetrical machine – grotesque and sexualised, sometimes machine-like, but mostly associated with the plant world, both passive and active. Ultimately, the prostitute body is not simply represented in fictional texts, but it *diffracts* the boundaries between science and society, literature and medicine, botany and erotica. Most notably, the prostitute body in Cleland's *Fanny Hill* is equipped with agency as its own ontology criticises male-dominated scientific discourses. This is mainly achieved through ridicule that manifests itself especially in bawdy botanical and mechanical metaphors.

To conclude, as with *Gulliver's Travels*, *Fanny Hill* is what we make of it. Since research on this text is still surprisingly scarce, it will be the task of literary and cultural scholars to further engage with its meaning. In light of reproduction, however, it is safe to say that Cleland's text int*ra*-links science and the sexual body. Yet, by appropriating patriarchal metaphors and applying them to the world of botany, scientists not only reflected but also reinforced rigid gender relations. As a result, the male-dominated field of botany equally contributed to the idea that the female body – like nature – needs to be studied, categorised, dissected and neatly divided into boxes. In this context, erotic literature functioned as a potential bastion of resistance to these stereotypes. This section ends with one more erotic poem. What follows is an earlier piece written by Edward Ward in 1725 that satirises the link between the female reproductive body and the landscape. The poem is called *The Riddle or A Paradoxical Character Of An Hairy Monster* (1725):

When full 'tis round, when empty long,
Sometimes a Hole, sometimes a Slit,
Hairy when old, and bald when young,
Too wide for some, for others fit.

It justly may be stil'd a Well,
At each Spring-Tide it overflows;
Its Depth no mortal Man can tell;
That none but he that made it knows.

It Lies obscurely in a Clift,
That's fenced with Brambles around it.

(Ward in Peakman 2012, 76)

Notes

1 Rumour also has it that Cleland was "summoned before the Privy Council" based on a complaint by the Bishop of London who accused him of "obscenity" (Plumb 1965, x; Gautier 2001, vi). In response to these charges, Cleland tried to deny he had ever written such a piece and branded it as a text to be ignored (Gautier 2001, vi). Cleland's later novels including *Memoirs of a Coxcomb* (1751), *The Surprise of Love* (1764), *The Woman of Honor* (1768), his plays *Titus Vespasian* (1755), *The Ladies Subscription* (1755), *Tombo-Chiqui* (1758) as well as his poems, pamphlets and studies in linguistics, however, never met the success of *Fanny Hill* (Gautier 2001, vi).

2 See Steven Marcus' (ed.) *The Other Victorians: A Study of Sexuality and Pornography in Mid-Nineteenth-Century England* ([1966] 2009).
3 Cf. *Nature's Body. Sexual Politics and the Making of Modern Science* (1993) and "Gender and Natural History" ([1996] 2004).

References

Blackwell, Bonnie. 2013. "Corkscrews and Courtesans: Sex and Death in Circulation Novels." In *Sex and Death in Eighteenth-Century Literature*, edited by Jolene Zigarovich, 81–98. New York; London: Routledge.

Carter, Sophie. 2004. *Purchasing Power: Representing Prostitution in Eighteenth-Century English Popular Print Culture*. Aldershot: Ashgate.

Cleland, John. [1751] 2005. *Memoirs of a Coxcomb*. Edited by Hal Gladfelder. Peterborough, ON: Broadview Press.

Cleland, John. [1749] 2008. *Memoirs of a Woman of Pleasure*. Edited with an introduction by Peter Sabor. Oxford: Oxford University Press.

Defoe, Daniel. [1724] 2008. *Roxana: The Fortunate Mistress*. Edited by John Mullan. Oxford World's Classics. Oxford: Oxford University Press.

Defoe, Daniel. [1722] 2011. *Moll Flanders*. Edited by G. A. Starr and Linda Bree. Oxford World's Classics. Oxford: Oxford University Press.

Gautier, Gary. 2001. "Introduction: Fanny Hill's Mapping of Sexuality, Female Identity, and Maternity". John Cleland. *Fanny Hill Or, Memoirs of a Woman of Pleasure*. Notes by Audrey Bilger, xi-xxxiii. New York: The Modern Library.

Harvey, Karen. 2004. *Reading Sex in the Eighteenth Century: Bodies and Gender in English Erotic Culture*. Cambridge: Cambridge University Press.

Harvey, Karen. 2010. "Visualizing Reproduction: A Cultural History of Early-Modern and Modern Medical Illustrations." *The Journal of Medical Humanities* 31 (1): 37–51.

Jong, Erica. 1978. *Introduction to Fanny Hill*. New York: Erotic Art Book Society.

Knight, Payne. 1974. *A Discourse on the Worship of Priapus, and Its Connection with the Mystic Theology of the Ancients: To Which Is Added an Essay on the Worship of the Generative Powers during the Middle Ages of Western Europe*. New Foreword by O. V. Garrison. New York: University Books.

Laqueur, Thomas. 1992. *Making Sex: Body and Gender from the Greeks to Freud*. Cambridge, MA: Harvard University Press.

Lewis, Ann, and Markman Ellis, eds. 2016. *Prostitution and Eighteenth-Century Culture: Sex, Commerce, and Morality*. Oxfordshire; New York: Routledge.

Linnaeus, Carl. [1735] 1964. *Systema Naturae*. London: Coronet Books.

Marcus, Steven, ed. 2009. *The Other Victorians: A Study of Sexuality and Pornography in Mid-Nineteenth-Century England*. New York; London: Routledge.

Miller, Nancy K. 1980. *The Heroine's Text: Readings in the French and English Novel, 1722–1782*. New York: Columbia University Press.

Peakman, Julie. 2012. *Mighty Lewd Books: The Development of Pornography in Eighteenth-Century England*. Houndmills, Basingstoke, Hampshire: Palgrave Macmillan.

Peakman, Julie. 2016. *Amatory Pleasures: Explorations in Eighteenth-Century Sexual Culture*. London; New York: Bloomsbury Academic.

Plumb, J. H. 1965. "Introduction." In *Memoirs of Fanny Hill*, by John Cleland, v–xv. New York: Signet.

Richardson, Samuel. [1740] 2008. *Pamela: Or, Virtue Rewarded*. Edited by Thomas Keymer and Alice Wakely. Oxford World's Classics. Oxford: Oxford University Press.

Richardson, Samuel. [1748] 2010. *Clarissa: Or, The History of a Young Lady*. Edited by Toni Bowers and John Richetti. Peterborough, ON: Broadview Press.

Rosenthal, Laura J. 2006. *Infamous Commerce: Prostitution in Eighteenth-Century British Literature and Culture*. Ithaca, NY: Cornell University Press.

Sabor, Peter. [1985] 2008. "Introduction." In *Memoirs of a Woman of Pleasure,* edited by John Cleland, vii-xxxiii. Oxford: Oxford University Press.

Schiebinger, Londa. 1996. "Gender and Natural History." In *Cultures of Natural History*, edited by N. Jardine, J. A. Secord, and E. Spary, 163–177. Cambridge: Cambridge University Press.

Schiebinger, Londa. 2004. *Nature's Body: Gender in the Making of Modern Science*. New Brunswick, NJ: Rutgers University Press.

Stretser, Thomas. [1741] 1932. *Merryland*. New York: Robin Hood House.

Swift, Jonathan. 1726. *Gulliver's Travels*. Edited by Albert J. Rivero. New York: Norton, 2002.

Taylor, Anne Robinson. 1981. *Male Novelists and Their Female Voices: Literary Masquerades*. New York: Troy.

Todd, Janet. 1980. *Women's Friendship in Literature: The Eighteenth-Century Novel in England and France*. New York: Columbia University Press.

2.3 Laurence Sterne's *Tristram Shandy* (1759)

2.3.1 Introduction

Sterne's *Tristram Shandy* is both one of the best-known eighteenth-century novels and a narrative that explicitly engages with questions of reproduction. Before turning to the text's 'opinions' on childbirth, this analysis chapter starts with a short introduction to the text, its precursors and status as a 'new literary species', its fragmented structure, and 'birth themes' (Keymer [2002] 2018; Hawley 2019; Hawes 2020). The following subchapters take a closer look at Sterne's constructed bodies and the text's entanglement with eighteenth-century (material) discourses of reproduction, childbirth and obstetrics (Martin 1991; Blackwell 2001; Porter 2004; Vanderbeke 2006; Sprang 2008, 2013; Ross 2009; Harries 2009; Morrissey 2017; Noggle 2018). Particular attention is also given to metaphors as well as moments of agency that are mainly achieved through the refusal of reproduction.

The full title of Laurence Sterne's well-known satire and so-called anti-novel is *The Life and Opinions of Tristram Shandy, Gentleman.* Not only do most first-time readers find the novel's name odd – *Tristram Shandy* is also and especially renowned for its peculiar form and style.[1] Sterne wrote at a time when the novel as we know it today was still in formation. As Thomas Keymer outlines, the "conventions of fictional representation" were "fluid, ill-defined, and keenly contested," for instance during the "Richardson–Fielding" dispute that revolved around a variety of contradictions from "narrative strategies" to "religion and ethics" or "gender and class" (Keymer 2018, 521). Many scholars have viewed especially *Tristram Shandy*'s unusual opening sequence in which Tristram, who is both the protagonist and narrator of his own life story, contemplates his own begetting by his parents, as "novelistic" in the sense that it indeed "pointedly disrupt[ed] the norms of the genre" (Keymer 2018, 521). *Tristram Shandy* therefore inevitably raised – and still raises – the question 'what *is* the novel, anyway'? Most dictionaries define this genre as an extended narrative, as fictional or simply as prose (cf. Baldick 2015, 173). These definitions, however, prompt even more questions: What differentiates prose from, for instance, epic poetry? Is realism the decisive factor that distinguishes the novel from other, fantastic narratives? In other words, "what is the relation between fiction and the real" (Morrissey 2017, 228)? What role does realism play for the emergence of this literary form?

DOI: 10.4324/9781003467977-8

The rise of *Tristram Shandy* and the novel genre in the eighteenth century can be better understood against the backdrop of its predecessors that reach back to the Middle Ages. One of the novel's precursors is Miguel de Cervantes' *Don Quixote* or *The Ingenious Gentleman Don Quixote of La Mancha* (part one published in 1605 and part two in 1615), a Spanish epic novel that parodies the genre of the medieval or chivalric romance. One well-known example of this form is Sir Thomas Malory's *Le Morte d'Arthur* (1485); this Arthurian narrative, written in the chivalric mode, features a knight who embarks on a journey or quest during which he has to face various challenges in the hope of winning the love of a virtuous lady. The protagonist of *Don Quixote*, however, has read too many of these chivalric romances; he is portrayed as a deranged character who wears a basin instead of a helmet, rides a lame horse called Rosinante and embarks on his journey without even having met his object of love.

Sterne is indebted to Cervantes as *Tristram Shandy* contains references to both *Don Quixote* and the chivalric romance which both authors mock.[2] The intertextual links also serve as a satire of the further emerging novel as well as various contemporary discourses including theories of reproduction, childbirth and medicine as will be discussed later in this chapter. What can be said for certain is that *Tristram Shandy* is especially characterised by its hybridity as it borrows from many (sub)genres such as the chivalric romance, the adventure novel as well as modes like the Menippean satire of Francois Rabelais. It is already very similar to the modern novel as we know it today, "this being the medium *par excellence* of generic hybridization and polyglossia" (Keymer 2018, 524). As Judith Hawley states in her preface to the 2019 Norton edition: "When *Tristram Shandy* burst anonymously on the London reading public at the end of 1759, it dazzled readers with its originality and daring. A reviewer […] continued: 'what shall we call thee? – Rabelais, Cervantes, What?'" (Hawley 2019, viii).

Last but not least, *Tristram Shandy* also exhibits intertextual references to Swift's *Gulliver's Travels*. Not only is reality rendered absurd in both narratives, but the novel's protagonists equally suffer from a masculinity crisis – while Gulliver is emasculated by the maids of honour who use him as a miniature pocket-microscope-turned-dildo, Tristram nearly "experience[s] an accidental penectomy," also by the hands of a female character, Susannah (Hawes 2020, 195). Impotence is the novel's leitmotif: "Sexual disability becomes the governing metaphor in *Tristram Shandy*," a novel that already starts "with an act of coitus interruptus" and ends "[e]ven [with] the Shandy family bull [being] infertile" (Hawes 2020, 196). The following sections continue with selected aspects of Sterne's life, a discussion of Sterne's 'new literary species' and then transitions to an investigation of contesting theories and (material-discursive) practices of reproduction the novel is enmeshed with.[3]

2.3.2 Sterne & The New Species of Writing

Like Swift, Laurence Sterne was an (Anglo-)Irishman. Born in 1713 in Clonmel, a small town in the County Tipperary, Sterne's early years were characterised by several "removals […] from Ireland to England and back again" (Ross 2009, x). At the age of about 10, Sterne moved to Yorkshire and never saw his father, an army officer, again as he died a decade later in Ireland (Ross 2009, x–xi). In Cambridge, Sterne "received a traditional humanist education" in subjects such as Latin, Greek, classic literature and philosophy; in 1737, he joined the "Church of England as a deacon" and later clergyman, "quickly acquired a parish of his own," and later engaged in political writing under the supervision of his uncle Dr Jacques Sterne (Ross 2009, xi). After renouncing politics, he started a second life in Stillington, North Yorkshire, and married a woman called Elizabeth Lumley with whom he had several children of which only one survived: Lydia (Ross 2009, xi). It took another two decades before his breakthrough with *Tristram Shandy* while he continued to function as a preacher and writer of sermons (Ross 2009, xi).

Sterne's *The Life and Opinions of Tristram Shandy, Gentleman* (1759–1767) was the "most talked-about book of the age," as Ian C. Ross points out in his introduction to the 2009 Oxford edition (Ross 2009, vii). *Tristram Shandy* was aimed at the youthful, "unlearned" reader in particular who had no sturdy knowledge of "polite letters" or epistolary narratives: This makes sense, as Ross continues, since the novel form at the time was (still) not to be "taken too seriously" and rather existed for entertainment (Ross 2009, vii). Yet, as he also stresses, Sterne "took the 'new species of writing' very seriously indeed" predominantly by mocking it, although this claim remains debatable (Ross 2009, vii). In this context, Keymer argues that Sterne's "status as a witty parodist [...] of the 'new species of writing' [...] is so self-evident that demonstration would be pointless" (Keymer 2018, 522). In *The Rise of the Novel* (1957), Ian Watt praises Sterne for his "remarkable literary originality" mainly due to his mastery of formal realism, while at the same time "break[ing] with the tyranny of chronological order" (Watt [1957] 1959, 290–292). As Jonathan Lamb outlines, by doing this Sterne actually parodies the "conventions of realism" entrenched by his literary predecessors Samuel Richardson and Henry Fielding (Lamb 1998, 153).

The first two volumes of *Tristram Shandy* were published in 1759 and the following seven between 1761 and 1767 (Ross 2009, xiii). The reception was, unsurprisingly, marked by a sense of "bewilderment," and critics were not sure what to make of this hero/narrator who was "unable even to get himself born in the first two volumes" only to then let a man-midwife "disastrously [...] bring him into the world" (Ross 2009, xiii). The novel's wit and humour, however, was "much praised" (Ross 2009, xiii). Those who celebrated his novel, including Edmund Burke and David Hume, called it "the best book that has been writ by any Englishman," while others, who did not, such as Samuel Richardson, Oliver Goldsmith or Horace Walpole, dismissed the book's bawdiness, "'dirty wit,' or obscenity" (Ross 2009, xiv). This critique actually pleased Sterne and only increased the sales of his book.[4]

As of 1762, Sterne undertook various voyages through Europe, especially to the "warmer shores of the Mediterranean" in the hope to cure the effects of his tuberculosis from which he had suffered "since his student days at Cambridge" (Ross 2009, xv). He travelled to Paris, Toulouse, back to Yorkshire, then Rome and back to France while finishing *Tristram Shandy*'s final volume (Ross 2009, xvi).

Unfortunately, this "final instalment" did not continue its predecessor's success (Ross 2009, xvi). Yet, this lack of success left Sterne unruffled for two reasons: First, his plan to write a second novel, *A Sentimental Journey through France and Italy*, was already underway, and second, he had deeply fallen for the married 23-year-old Eliza Draper with whom he spent three months before she returned to her husband, an "official to the East India Company" (Ross 2009, xvi). Though visibly deteriorating, Sterne completed his second book, *A Sentimental Journey*, in two volumes that was published in 1768, the year he died in London at the age of 54 (Ross 2009, xviii).

As James Noggle outlines, Sterne seemed to have forbode his own death by making Yorick, the narrator of *A Sentimental Journey*, refer to his cough at the end of this book (Noggle 2018, 863). Yorick evokes a multitude of associations in this sense – not only is this character's death indicated in *Tristram Shandy* in the form of a completely black page, but the figure also immediately evokes images of Shakespeare's *Hamlet*, contemplating life and death at a cemetery while holding Yorick's skull (Noggle 2018, 863). Sterne's Yorick, in fact, can be understood as "one of literature's great portraits of vitality and vibrant feeling" (Noggle 2018, 863). What is more, as Noggle briefly hints at, the "novel narrates his [Yorick's] sensations in near microscopic detail, from the individual beating of his heart to the sensitive pressure of his fingertips" (Noggle 2018, 863). Noggle finally points to Sterne's addition to a "new 'sentimental' focus to literature" that merges action with affect such as "sympathy, [the] erotic, desire, [and] pathos" (Noggle 2018, 863).

As with both *Gulliver's Travels* and *Fanny Hill*, it is up to the reader what to make of Sterne's satire: For example, as implied above, it is impossible to assign *Tristram Shandy* to one genre only as it summons various literary modes such as the "classical epic [...], classical romance [...] Renaissance tragedy [as well as] romance [and] autobiography" (Ross 2009, ix). Ross outlines that Sterne deliberately amalgamated these models to "teas[e] his readers" (Ross 2009, x). Scholars still debate the question of whether Sterne's *Tristram Shandy* contributes to the "tradition of 'learned wit,'" is simply satire or if it is a novel at all (Ross 2009, x). The latter question triggers particularly intense discussions due to *Tristram Shandy*'s non-chronological, fragmented narration and constant interruptions and diversions that alternate with "bawdy humour, serious reflection, and frequently poignant sentiment" (Ross 2009, x). The disorderly narration is the main reason why Sterne's *Tristram Shandy* is commonly described as an anti-novel.

Sterne's *Tristram Shandy* already stands out in comparison to other eighteenth-century texts by its title alone: While most authors wrote about the "fictional 'lives' – like 'histories' and 'adventures,'" Sterne chose to offer the reader Tristram's "opinions" (Ross 2009, viii). Unsurprisingly, this led to "considerable confusion among the book's first critics" since his novel seemed like an "autobiography of no common kind" (Ross 2009, ix). The narrative's 'hero' does not, as in Defoe's *Robinson Crusoe* (1719) or Swift's *Gulliver's Travels* (1726), begin by briefly stating his date and place of birth before he embarks on an adventure to far-away places – in Sterne's *Tristram Shandy*, it takes him one-third of the novel to get born in the first place (Ross 2009, ix).

From the very beginning, then, the novel makes clear what it is about: birth and copulation, in short: reproduction (and the failures thereof) (Harries 2009, 111). Williams even calls the novel the "most celebrated cultural artefact" of medicine, motherhood and reproduction; it resorts to a common eighteenth-century satirical strategy that ridicules questionable theories such as *animalculism* by "putting them in the mouth of an obsessive fool," Walter Shandy (Williams 2012, 21). Tristram's father-to-be not only tries to make a "legal argument" for Elizabeth Shandy's "lack of seed" in an attempt to grant himself "greater authority over his children," but the text also mocks the myth of maternal imagination by discussing the "effect of the mother's thoughts on the unborn child" (Williams 2012, 21).

Undoubtedly, Sterne's *Tristram Shandy* is perfectly suited for a discussion of contesting theories and material discourses of reproduction. This also includes the power struggle between traditional midwifery and institutionalised obstetrics that manifests itself in characters like Walter and Elizabeth Shandy. Last but not least, the (anti-)novel can be understood as a critique of eighteenth-century medical discourses and practices; bodies in *Tristram Shandy* are, among other things, constructed as machines or fragmented into pieces and hence material-discursively entangled with the body on the eighteenth-century dissection table.

2.3.3 Contesting Theories & Practices of Reproduction

As mentioned above, *Tristram Shandy* is hard to define. To begin with, the novel "attempts" to narrate the narrator's own conception that is immediately interrupted. Tristram, who is both the protagonist and the narrator of his own 'coming into life,' continues to share his thoughts on "naming children" and his 'opinions' on childbirth (Noggle 2018, 863). After reflecting on his father Walter's customs, he introduces other characters like his "good-natured" uncle Toby, a "wounded veteran" who re-enacts how his groin injury that came about during battle, and later the talkative soldier Corporal Trim as well as the household servant Obadiah, Parson Yorick and Dr Slop, the obstetrician (Ross 2009, xviii; Noggle 2018, 863).

Female characters include Elizabeth Shandy, Tristram's mother, Widow Wadman – who wishes to marry uncle Toby but first needs to know "exactly *where* uncle Toby was wounded in the groin" – and Wadman's maid Bridget (emphasis in the original, Ross 2009, xviii). Tristram also feels the need to tell us about the terminally ill soldier Le Fever and the story of Slawkenbergius' "tale of the stranger who astounds all Strasbourg with the size of his nose" (Ross 2009, xix). The narrative is, in fact, saturated with noses: Not only is Tristram's own nose injured during his birth, but he also circumcises himself as a young boy in an accident that involved a "falling sash window" (Ross 2009, xix). Noses are everywhere in this novel, and it is not hard to guess what they stand for. As Elizabeth W. Harries argues, the meaning of Tristram's (injured) nose is obvious: It stands for the "symbolic phallus, as the Freudian theorist Lacan would say" and is "part of his [Tristram's] obsessive quest both to hide and to reveal his uncertainties, uncertainties that Sterne is eager to exploit and explore" (Harries 2009, 117). This subchapter, however, focusses less on the phallus and more on the question of how the absurd and non-linear anti-novel *Tristram Shandy* entangles (material) discourses of reproduction, midwifery, obstetrics and the body. For this reason, we need to start at the very beginning: Tristram's conception.

On the novel's first pages, Tristram tells us how his parents "begot" him (*TS*, 5). From the outset, the narrator laments his disastrous birth and regrets that he "should have made a quite different figure in the world," had his parents considered that "miscarriages" not only depend on the "animal spirits, as how they are transfused from father to son, &c. &c." but also on their parents' "motions and activity" during conception (*TS*, 5–6). He criticises that these spirits otherwise "go cluttering like hey-go-mad" (*TS*, 6). Tristram the narrator then reconstructs in great detail what exactly happened between his mother Elizabeth and his father Walter during intercourse:

> *Pray, my dear*, quoth my mother, *have you not forgot to wind up the clock? – Good G –!* cried my father, making an exclamation, but taking care to moderate his voice at the same time, *– Did ever woman, since the creation of the world, interrupt a man with such a silly question?* Pray, what was your father saying? – Nothing. [...] – Then positively, there is nothing in the question, that I can see, either good or bad. – Then let me tell you, Sir, it was a very unseasonable question at least, – because it scattered and dispersed the animal spirits, whose business it was to have escorted and gone hand-in-hand with the *HOMUNCULUS*, and conducted him safe to the place destined for his reception.
>
> (emphasis in the original, *TS*, 6)

On the very first pages, the text already alludes to dominant discourses of reproduction that circulated during the eighteenth century. Put simply, his mother's question led to a 'coitus interruptus' that not only "scattered and dispersed the animal spirits," a comment that refers to the reproductive theory of *animalculism* involving the idea that each sperm contains a whole miniature embryo, but has severe consequences for the formation of the 'little man,' the *homunculus,* a concept relating to the discourse of *homunculism*. Tristram goes into great detail when describing not only the *homunculus*' (material) nature but also emphasises his legal rights:

> The HOMUNCULUS [is] a BEING guarded and circumscribed with *rights*: – The minutest [natural] philosophers, who, by the bye, have the most enlarged understandings, [...] shew us incontestably, That the HOMUNCULUS is created by the same hand, – engender'd in the same course of nature, – endowed with the same loco-motive powers and faculties with us: – That *he* consists, as we do, of skin, hair, flesh, veins, arteries, ligaments, nerves, cartilages, bones, marrow, brains, glands, genitals, humours, and

> articulations; – is a Being of as much activity, – [...] *He* may be benefited, *he* may be injured, – *he* may obtain redress; – in a word, *he* has all the claims and *rights of humanity* [...].
>
> (emphasis added, capitalisation in the original, *TS*, 6)

Sterne here not only further mocks the theory of *homunculism*, but he also endows this 'little man' with the right to personhood by likening especially his bodily characteristics – skin, hair, flesh, etc. – to that of an already born human baby. This entanglement of body and personhood is, in a way, already ironic if we consider the hierarchical Cartesian dualism of body and mind that favours the latter over the former. One can thus safely say that Sterne ridicules theories of reproduction such as *animalculism* and *homunculism* as well as the political implications of such concepts, i.e., the endowment of foetuses with the right to personhood, a debate that is as topical as ever even in the twenty-first century.

The informed reader will recognise yet another reproductive discourse Sterne seems to be mocking when Tristram concludes his narration of his flawed conception:

> Now, dear Sir, what if any accident had befallen him in his way alone? – or that, thro' terror of it, natural to so young a traveller, my little gentleman had got to his journey's end miserably spent; – his muscular strength and virility worn down to a thread; – his own animal spirits ruffled beyond description, – and that in this sad disorder'd state of nerves, he had laid down a prey to sudden starts, or a series of melancholy dreams and fancies for nine long, long months together. – I tremble to think what a foundation had been laid for a thousand weaknesses both of body and mind, which no skill of the physician or the philosopher could ever afterwards have set thoroughly to rights.
>
> (*TS*, 7)

Not only is the "traveller" or "little gentleman" here equipped with masculine connotations such as "muscular strength and virility," despite his "ruffled" animal spirits, but he seems to be plagued by "melancholy dreams and fancies for nine long, long months" as well as a "weakness both of body and mind" whose fatal consequences no "physician or [...] philosopher" can amend after he is born. It is not difficult to read these descriptions as hints towards his mother Elizabeth's nine-month long pregnancy during which she apparently had "melancholy dreams" that further complicate Tristram's formation in the womb. In fact, this episode quite directly addresses, or rather mocks, the myth of the maternal imagination that was still very much alive at the time Sterne published his novel.

Yet, one could also understand these descriptions as not (only) referring to the mother's harmful imagination, but equally to the father's melancholic spermatozoon. This results in a subversion of the patriarchal idea that it is the mother who is predominantly responsible for the birth outcome, let alone a ridicule of the myth of maternal imagination as such. Buckley reads the "notoriously interrupted opening" as a "counterpoint" to the discourse of maternal imagination that involves the idea of "*paternal* imagination," an additional myth assuming the capability of the father's mind to "affect the foetus at the point of conception" (emphasis in the original, Buckley 2017, 131–132).

In general, as Dirk Vanderbeke emphasises with reference to Robert Adams Day, the novel mocks "some of the latest scientific developments in obstetrics" in the eighteenth century (Vanderbeke 2006, 183).[5] Vanderbeke points to the text's construction of the obstetrician Dr Slop who is not only rendered a quack, but also damages Tristram's nose by using one of the new instruments: forceps. In Vanderbeke's view, the novel blames the "medical handyman" who treats Tristram's body "as a machine [...] with mechanical tools" (Vanderbeke 2006, 183). This makes sense if we reconsider Elizabeth Shandy's disruptive question during intercourse: "*Pray, my dear,* [...] *have you no forgot to wind up the clock?*" (emphasis in the original, *TS*, 6).

Vanderbeke further draws a connection between this scene and the eighteenth-century essay *Man a Machine*, published by the French surgeon and philosopher Julien Offrey de La Mettrie in 1748. La Mettrie opposed the Cartesian dualism of body versus mind, and he also wrote about the process of conception:

> The body is but a watch, whose watchmaker is the new chyle [milky bodily fluid]. Nature's first care, when the chyle enters the blood, is to excite in it a kind of fever which the chemists, who dream only of retorts, must have taken for fermentation. This fever produces a greater filtration of spirits, which mechanically animate the muscles and the heart, as if they had been sent there by order of the will.
>
> (transl. Vanderbeke 2006, 183; see also La Mettrie 1996, 186)

La Mettrie thus not only compares the body to a mechanical clock but also describes the process of conception in chemical terms: Once the chyle, a milky bodily fluid of what we know today contains lymph and liquid fats, can here be understood as seminal fluid. It enters into the mother's blood stream, causes a fever that leads to a sort of fermentation and in turn triggers the foetus' heart to "mechanically animate" itself. By allowing Elizabeth to interrupt her husband with the question of whether he has wound up the clock, Vanderbeke outlines that Sterne's novel both "stresses – and satirizes – this mechanistic approach to the mysteries of life" (Vanderbeke 2006, 183). The text thus merges dominant eighteenth-century discourses of the body including both metaphors of the body as a machine as well as "latest ideas about embryology" (Vanderbeke 2006, 188). But what about midwifery, man-midwifery and the rivalry between the two? What role does this power struggle play in the novel?

Felix Sprang seizes on this question. He points to the "rivalry of authority" between Tristram's parents Elizabeth and Walter: While Elizabeth represents the traditional sphere of midwifery, Tristram's father Walter is fascinated by Dr Slop's "new school of obstetrics" (Sprang 2013, 137). This contradiction becomes especially clear in the scene in which the married couple argue over where Elizabeth should give birth: London. Though regulated in their marriage settlement, Elizabeth prefers the midwife over the obstetrician who shall assist her in London.

In addition, Walter scolds his wife after a false alarm that had forced them to take a costly and eventually unnecessary trip to London. Tristram narrates the incident as follows:

> From *Grantham*, till they had cross'd the *Trent*, my father was out of all kind of patience at the vile trick and imposition which he fancied my mother had put upon him in this affair. – "Certainly", he would say to himself, over and over again, "the woman could not be deceiving herself; – if she could, – what weakness!" – tormenting word! which led his imagination a thorny dance, and, before all was over, play'd the deuce and all with him; – for sure as ever the word *weakness* was uttered, and struck full upon his brain, – so sure it set him upon running divisions upon how many kinds of weaknesses there were; – that there was such a thing as weakness of the body, – as well as weakness of the mind, – and then he would do nothing but syllogize within himself for a stage or two together, How far the cause of all these vexations might, or might not, have arisen out of himself.
>
> (emphasis in the original, *TS*, 31–32)

The term "weakness" is used five times in this paragraph. In combination with the "weakness of the body" and "weakness of the mind," one can infer that the text here repeatedly alludes to the myth of maternal imagination and the idea that women's bodies and minds are feeble and especially untrustworthy. Readers acquainted with the scandalous Mary Toft case will most likely also immediately recognise this allusion. Yet, we need to always factor in that Sterne is a satirist, which leads to the conclusion that he is mocking men's gullibility with regard to such spectacular birth myths.

Reading this episode as an allusion to both the Mary Toft case and the power struggle between midwifery and obstetrics becomes even clearer when turning to the following chapter xviii in which Elizabeth, now actually in labour at Shandy-Hall, is determined to call the midwife and rejects being assisted by an obstetrician:

> As the point was that night agreed, or rather determin'd, that my mother should lye-in of me in the country, she took her measures accordingly; for which purpose, when she was three days, or thereabouts, gone with child, she began to cast her eyes upon the midwife, whom you have so often heard me mention; and before the week was well got round, as the famous Dr. *Maningham* was not to be had, she had come to a final determination in her mind, – notwithstanding there was a scientifick operator within so near a call as eight miles of us, and who, moreover, had expressly wrote a five shilling book upon the subject of midwifery, in which he had exposed, not only

> the blunders of the sisterhood itself, – but had likewise superadded many curious improvements for the quicker extraction of the foetus in cross births, and some other cases of danger which belay us in getting into the world; notwithstanding all this, my mother, I say, was absolutely determined to trust her life and mine with it, into no soul's hand but this old woman's only. [...] the old midwife had really some little claim to be depended upon, – as much, at least, as success could give her; having, in the course of her practice of near twenty years in the parish, brought every mother's son of them into the world without any one slip or accident which could fairly be laid to her account.
>
> (emphasis and spelling in the original, *TS*, 32–33)

The text here explicitly refers to the Mary Toft case by adding the name "Dr. Maningham" – an allusion to the historical Sir Richard Manningham, a member of the Royal Society and the "most famous man-midwife of his day" who is also mocked in William Hogarth's graphic satire *Cunicularii* (1726) (Ross 2009, 545).

What this passage also does, however, is evoke the power struggle between the fields of midwifery and man-midwifery. Elizabeth represents the sphere of midwifery by demanding to be assisted by the hands of the "old woman's only," despite the fact that she has heard of a "scientifick operator" whose book both exposes the "blunders of the sisterhood" and most probably promotes the use of new instruments such as forceps to enable a swifter extraction of the foetus in case of a difficult birth. Her preference thus demonstrates her trust in female midwifery. By emphasising the midwife's long-term experience and success in childbirth, Sterne equally seems to favour traditional knowledge over male-connoted new scientific practices. He constructs Elizabeth's husband, Walter, in quite a different manner. In contrast to Tristram's mother, Walter is more fascinated by the new field of obstetrics and continues to quarrel with his wife, as the narrator tells us:

> For all these reasons, private and publick, put together, – my father was for having the man-midwife by all means, – my mother by no means. My father begg'd and intreated, she would for once recede from her prerogative in this matter, and suffer him to choose for her; – my mother, on the contrary, insisted upon her privilege in this matter, to choose for herself, – and no mortal's help but the old woman's.
>
> (*TS*, 35)

In general, Walter seeks control over his wife's reproduction, including the way she gives birth, which aligns him with the eighteenth-century obstetrician who equally sought to usurp the traditional sphere of midwifery as previous scholars have emphasised. Harries argues along similar lines when she states that Walter "is always eager to deny that women play any part in the reproductive process, [...]

Walter would like to claim everything parental for men, from the moment of conception on" (Harries 2009, 117). As she continues:

> Women, on this theory, are scarcely necessary. From Walter's point of view, women upset the sovereign male patriarchal applecart: they are sexually aggressive and sly, they have no interest in following his arcane theoretical arguments, and they always ask questions at just the wrong time.
>
> (Harries 2009, 118)

Sterne's novel not only engages in a discussion about the power struggle between midwives and man-midwives, represented by Elizabeth and Walter Shandy, but also constructs characters that further contribute to a reading of his novel as a critique of the emerging field of obstetrics and its agents. In volume 2, chapter iii, the text introduces the absurd character Dr Slop, an obstetrician with a telling name who breaks Tristram's nose (a symbol for the phallus) during childbirth and also injures uncle Toby's hands with his forceps. When Obadiah, the household servant, is ordered by Walter to bring "Dr. Slop, the man-midwife" to Shandy-Hall to assist his wife who is in the midst of labour in chapter ix, the text describes the obstetrician, who arrives by horse, as follows:

> Imagine to yourself a little, squat, uncourtly figure of a Doctor *Slop*, of about four feet and a half perpendicular height, with a breadth of back, and a sesquipedality of belly, which might have done honour to a Serjeant in the Horse-Guards. Such were the out-lines of Dr. Slop's figure, which, – if you have read *Hogarth*'s analysis of beauty, and if you have not, I wish you would; – you must know, may as certainly be caracatur'd, and convey'd to the mind by three strokes as three hundred. Imagine such a one, – for such, I say, were the out-lines of *Dr. Slop*'s figure, coming slowly along, foot by foot, waddling thro' the dirt upon the vertebrae of a little diminutive pony – of a pretty colour; – but of strength, – alack! – scarce able to have made an amble of it, under such a fardel, had the roads been in an ambling condition. – They were not. – Imagine to yourself, *Obadiah* mounted upon a strong monster of a coach-horse, prick'd into a full gallop, and making all practicable speed the adverse way.
>
> (emphasis in the original, *TS*, 69)

It is obvious that Sterne here alludes to or rather mocks the novel's literary predecessors such as the medieval chivalric romance featuring a knight in shining armour who embarks on a heroic quest on his steed in the hope of winning the first prize – the love of a beautiful and virtuous lady. In particular, Sterne uses the same bodily metaphors that his seventeenth-century precursor Miguel de Cervantes employed in his satire *Don Quixote* with the only difference that here, he utilises these intertextual references not only to mock the chivalric mode but also to satirise the foolish *obstetrician* Dr Slop. Sterne, in fact, pulls this physician to pieces and highlights Dr Slop's 'sloppiness' and his new instruments especially in volume 2, when the narrator scolds him for forgetting his tools as he enters the birthing room: "Thou has come forth unarm'd […] — thy new-invented *forceps* — thy *crotchet*, — thy *squirt*, and all thy instruments of salvation and deliverance behind thee. —— By heaven!" (emphasis in the original, *TS*, 88). Walter eventually acknowledges the obstetrician's incompetency and consents to let the midwife take over in chapter xviii when he tells Dr Slop the following:

> I have ordered, answered my father, the old midwife to come down to us upon the least difficulty; – for you must know, Dr. *Slop*, continued my father, with a perplexed kind of smile upon his countenance, that by express treaty, solemnly ratified between me and my wife, you are no more than an auxiliary in this affair, and – and not so much as that, – unless the lean old mother of a midwife above stairs cannot do without you. – Women have their particular fancies, and in points of this nature, continued my father, where they bear the whole burden, and suffer so much acute pain for the advantage of our families, and the good of the species, in whose hands, and in what fashion, they chuse to undergo it.
>
> (emphasis and spelling in the original, *TS*, 92)

Though this seems like an act of solidarity towards female agency, Walter quickly changes his mind. After the attempt to self-educate himself on childbirth by turning to obstetrical handbooks and the apparent advantages of C-sections that Elizabeth, however, rejects, by the end of volume 2, he still sides with Dr Slop and his practice of using forceps:

> nay, he did not believe, in natural births […] When my father had got so far, – what a blaze of light did the account of *Caesarian* section, and of the towering geniuses who had come safe into the world by it, cast upon this hypothesis? Here, you see, he would say, there was no injury done to the sensorium; – no pressure of the head against the pelvis; no propulsion of the cerebrum towards the cerebellum […] and, pray, what were the happy consequences? Why, Sir, you Julius Caesar, who gave the operation a name; and – […] all came side-way, Sir, into the world. […] This hypothesis of the abdomen and uterus, ran for six weeks together in my father's head; – he had read, and was satisfied, that wounds in the epigastrium, and those in the matrix, were not mortal; so that the belly of the mother might be opened extremely well to give a passage to the child […] Of all men in the world, Dr. *Slop* was the fittest for my father's purpose; – for tho' his new-invented forceps was the armour he had proved, and what he maintained, to be the safest instrument of deliverance.
>
> (emphasis in the original, *TS*, 97–98)

The irony of this male alliance between 'men of science' is, of course, that Dr Slop's forceps injure Tristram's nose – a symbol for his phallus. In addition, Walter is more concerned about the wellbeing of his son than his wife: "we see Walter Shandy prostrate across his bed, mourning the injury that Slop's forceps have done to Tristram's nose, rather than Mrs Shandy on her own bed of pain" (Harries 2009, 114). But this is not all: Before he injures Tristram's nose/phallus, Dr Slop knocks out his own teeth (*TS,* 108–109) and brutally tears off the skin from uncle Toby's hands (*TS*, 120) with his "vile instruments" (*TS*, 136). Sterne thus satirises the field of obstetrics that heavily relied on instruments as opposed to the sphere of midwifery that was mainly based on the use of hands as outlined in PART I of this book. The outcome of Dr Slop, the sloppy obstetrician, is disastrous: crushed noses, broken teeth and hands and a protagonist whose bodily injury is the very cause for his narration.

As Harries confirms, *Tristram Shandy* is saturated not only with questions of reproduction but also with reproductive bodies or parts thereof: "Almost any paragraph can make us think of sex, genitalia, male and female organs" (Harries 2009, 111). At first glance, she argues that the novel's "fixed, repetitive attention to sexed bodies and to crudely represented body parts" coincides with rigid eighteenth-century gender constructs as male characters take centre stage and do most of the talking, while "women, their hopes, and *their opinions* are relegated to the margins" (emphasis added, Harries 2009, 114). Yet, it is also possible to read the text as an investigation of their masculinity crises:

> All the disasters of Tristram's first five years – his interrupted conception; his birth, with the damage to his nose; his bungled christening; his accident with the sash-window that circumcises him (or worse) – call his full masculinity and his origins into question. […] like the Shandy bull […], he has to endure 'suspicions' about his 'character' or reputation as a potent male […].
>
> (Harries 2009, 117)

Based on these reflections, I go a step further and argue that the text's constructed masculinity crises function as a critique of both the eighteenth-century obstetrician's pride as well as his material medical practice that often involved dismembering or cutting into pieces female genitals as outlined in PART I of this study. In a way, Sterne's novel can be conceptualised as a backlash against obstetrics' "anatomy butchery" done to female reproductive bodies in the medical theatre (see also Newman 1996, 101–102). As a result, *Tristram Shandy* quite literally turns the dissection table by exposing the arrogance of seemingly enlightened men seeking total control over reproduction from conception to birth. The following final section ties the pieces back together again, concludes that both the form and content of Sterne's masterpiece are entangled with the fragmented material body, and ends with a reflection on the persistence of patriarchal metaphors of reproduction.

2.3.4 (Re)Producing (Material) Metaphors of Conception

Sterne's *Tristram Shandy* negotiates the power struggle between two contesting areas of knowledge – the female-connoted sphere of midwifery and the male-dominated field of obstetrics. The reproductive body plays a central role in this piece of fiction as it functions as a critique of the new field of obstetrics. *Tristram Shandy's* fragmented form not only mocks the emerging novel and its literary predecessors but also satirises enlightened science by fragmenting its reproductive bodies and thus rendering them impotent. As outlined, Tristram's squashed (phallic) nose by the hands of the obstetrician, his accidentally circumcised penis as well as his father's inability to name his son correctly suggest a form of masculinity crisis in terms of sexuality and reproductive power. Elizabeth Shandy's pregnant body and *coitus interruptus* allude to the image of the body as a (malfunctioning) machine. Dr Slop's own overweight body, his dangerous instruments and 'sloppy' medical practice pose a threat to the integrity of other bodies.

Toby Shandy's wounded groin and hands, crushed by the obstetrician Dr Slop, equally evoke images of male impotency. Last but not least, Susannah's body, the "leaky vessel," that gets Tristram's name wrong and triggers a series of calamities, satirises the stereotypical image of the weak female mind and body (*TS*, 184). Furthermore, not only does the novel implicitly and explicitly refer to spectacular birth myths such as the Mary Toft case by referencing the name Dr Maningham – the obstetrician Dr Slop is also modelled after the historical and actually quite competent man-midwife but "suspected Jacobite Dr. John Burton [...] whose Tory politics the Whig Sterne intensely disliked," thus adding another political dimension to the narrative (Ross 2009, 555).

Fragmentation is *Tristram Shandy*'s leitmotif. As Sprang emphasises, by bringing the body and its parts to the fore, Sterne spotlights the systematic fragmentation of the body that dominated eighteenth-century anatomy in order to categorise body types, illnesses and functions (Sprang 2008, 171). This form of dismemberment also manifests in the novel's form – *Tristram Shandy* satirises this endeavour by systematically breaking all the rules of the conventional novel (Sprang 2008, 171): The 'plot' is constantly disrupted, events are narrated in non-chronological order, and the narrator engages in a range of narrative diversions that render the novel absurd. In accordance with Vanderbeke, Sprang infers that the fragmented narrative structure meticulously negotiates contemporary theories of reproduction and practices of childbirth (Sprang 2008, 176).

Tristram Shandy achieves this critique especially through the narrator-protagonist's own, disastrous conception. The descriptions of the *homunculus'* 'ruffled' animal spirits, triggered by Elizabeth's question whether her husband Walter had 'wound up the clock,' recall both mechanical images of the body as well as (contradicting) reproductive theories such as *homunculism* and *animalculism* that still circulated during the eighteenth century and existed alongside each other. As Porter outlines, while Greek or Hippocratic medicine was based on a more holistic philosophy that "presumed the unity of body and behaviour" and regarded the "physical and the psychological" as "two sides of the same coin," the metaphor of the body as machine prevailed during the Enlightenment; this "mechanical philosophy" rendered the body a "*machina carnis*, a machine of the flesh" and raised the question "[w]hat makes bodies tick?" (Porter 2004, 47–52). Was the body like a clock that could be wound up, or did it require some form of "vital flame" to animate its 'soul' (Porter 2004, 54, 57)?

The idea of the 'vital spark' played a particular role in sexual reproduction. One "fashionable London physician" and member of the Royal Society, Thomas Willis (1621–1675), believed in the soul's corporeality (a conviction not so different from that of the Greeks) which he called "animal soul" or "animal spirit" (Porter 2004, 55–56). This 'animal spirit,' an "outgrowth" of the 'vital flame' that flowed from the brain into the entire body and was regarded as a "'little animal soul, not yet kindled' – lay in the seminal fluid"; during conception, the seminal fluid would find a suitable place to rest where the soul was 'ignited,' just like one flame ignites another (see Porter 2004, 57).

It is not hard to see that *Tristram Shandy* plays with these reproductive theories by letting Elizabeth interrupt the 'little man's' voyage to his final destination, the egg, a more modern metaphor that will be taken up again below. What needs to be kept in mind, however, is that Willis' reproductive theory was based on the assumption that the human body had two souls – one corporeal, mortal, material, animal and thus inferior, and one rational, immortal and especially superior soul, hence reinforcing the mind-body dualism (Porter 2004, 57–58).[6] Man, as Porter concedes, was thus a "bi-souled biped" with two hierarchically structured souls – again, an idea similar to that of the (patriarchal) theory of the king's two bodies or the Cartesian dualism (Porter 2004, 58).

As mentioned in PART I of this book by reference to Keller, the mind-body dichotomy posed a very real problem for women due to its gendered associations of (masculine connoted) mind over (feminine connoted) body. It is thus possible to read Tristram's disastrous conception as a critique of this sexist stereotype – in the end, it is no coincidence that the *homunculus* is equipped with a gender from the very beginning and travels through Elizabeth's reproductive body as a 'little gentleman' well before its little 'soul' is 'ignited.' What is more, Sterne also seems to ridicule the *homunculus'* status as a person since he claims him to possess "all the claims and rights of humanity" (*TS*, 6).

Sterne's critique with regard to theories and practices of reproduction does not stop with his mockery of the *homunculus*. He not only renders the obstetrician incompetent, but his attack is especially directed towards Dr Slop's new and 'vile' obstetrics instruments, his forceps, that first break Tristram's (phallic) nose and then crush Toby's hands. Both Sterne and his character Dr Slop fragment the (reproductive) bodies they engage with. *Tristram Shandy* thus ridicules the very real (material) scientific fragmentation of the body that took place on the eighteenth-century dissection table. Sterne's novel also functions as a critique of medical men's – obstetricians in particular – claims to objective truth by referencing the myth of maternal imagination or the Mary Toft case.

The greatest subversive potential arguably lies in Elizabeth's 'reproductive interruption' of Tristram's conception. Sterne therefore allows female physicality a certain form of agency since the body, at least for a moment, refuses to reproduce. As a result, Elizabeth's body can equally be conceptualised as a cyborg body that is both machine (or clockwork) and human. Yet, the ambiguous cyborg is always also 'monstrous' and hence poses a threat to seemingly stable and especially hierarchical distinctions between categories like man and/over woman, science and/over nature or medicine and/over the body. The cyborg body, (cf. Haraway). however, blurs these boundaries and unsettles patriarchal authority.[7]

At the same time, Sterne's novel elevates the foetus' status and constructs the *homunculus* as an autonomous little man with legal rights. The effect is yet again the erasure of embodiment (cf. Hayles) at the cost of the mother. It is astonishing that nearly three centuries later, the discussion with regard to the question of whether a foetus is a (legal) person with (more) rights is still very much alive given the current debates over reproductive rights in English-speaking countries such as Ireland or the US. Most importantly, these discussions reaffirm that representations of reproduction are inextricably *entangled* (cf. Barad) with very real, material (medical) practices not just across place but also time: Sterne's *Tristram Shandy* both forecasts and reflects on material-discursive phenomena such as conception, childbirth, medicine and reproductive rights; they create one another simultaneously. Last but not least, representations (of the body) are always bound up in practice, medical in this case. The novel thus forces us to think of reproduction not with, but *through* the body.

In this context, the final section ends by turning to *Tristram Shandy*'s ongoing topicality as well as continued metaphors of reproduction that (still) have very real, material consequences for (discursive) gender constructs and (material) reproductive bodies. As Bonnie Blackwell states, *Tristram Shandy* was already a very timely book when it was published in the 1760s, a time that witnessed the "culmination of the most important four decades in obstetrics history" (Blackwell 2001, 81). As mentioned in PART I, in the first half of the eighteenth century, man-midwives were only called in case of difficult births and mostly delivered dead infants. By the second half of the century, the "dissemination of the forceps patent" enabled obstetricians to "unite their instrument-practice with the delivery of a living child," allowing them to stress their profession's "humanitarian" aspect, as the development of forceps not only ruined but also saved lives (Blackwell 2001, 81). This strategy repeatedly demonstrates how material practice and discursive meaning are int*ra*-linked with one another.

Tristram Shandy seizes on the "private and political revolution" in the field of obstetrics; yet, it also seems to call for the acknowledgement that (female connoted) midwifery still exists (Blackwell 2001, 81). Along the lines of Sprang, Blackwell equally argues that Sterne satirises the power struggle and lampoons the obstetrician's "ardent propaganda [of the] instrument-wielding man-midwife" in favour of the more competent midwife: In fact, as Blackwell stresses, "everyone in the book passionately comments, in the languages available to them, upon the obstetric revolution" (Blackwell 2001, 81). By rendering orthodox reproductive theories as well as the figure of the obstetrician absurd, Sterne mocks the idea of "scientific progress" and the "plot of triumphal enlightenment" (Blackwell 2001, 124).

Especially Walter's contemplation on the benefits of the C-section that completely disregards the mother's physical wellbeing while instead focussing on the 'undamaged good'– the (male) child – represents the beginning of the "control of women" and childbirth from the early eighteenth century onwards (Blackwell 2001, 125). Blackwell particularly addresses the treatment of Elizabeth Shandy's body "like a clock, or an automaton" that aligns her literary body with the haptic bodies of the obstetrical machine (Blackwell 2001, 126). Sterne seems to express sympathy towards the birthing mother who, by interrupting her husband during intercourse, and as stated above, refuses to function like a clock, a passive, inert and mechanical object (Blackwell 2001, 126–127). That said, what relevance does *Tristram Shandy* have for our modern age in terms of reproduction and gender?

As early as the 1990s, Emily Martin published the well-known and groundbreaking essay "The Egg and the Sperm: How Science Has Constructed a Romance Based on Stereotypical Male-Female Roles" (1991). In short, Martin argues that modern "scientific accounts of reproductive biology [still] rel[y] on stereotypes central to our cultural definitions of male and female" (Martin 1991, 485). In order to investigate the rhetoric of reproduction in biology, for instance, we need to turn to the language and the metaphors used in this field. Martin particularly criticises the idea of the passive egg that is fertilised by the active sperm, a dichotomy that also has cultural as well as political consequences. Martin offers a number of examples as discussed in the following.

The story of reproduction has for a long time resembled a "scientific fairy tale" (Martin 1991, 486). We are told that menstruation is a "failure" as the uterus expels dead tissue, "products of no use" (Martin 1991, 486). Male physiology, on the contrary, is rendered "quite differently"; while the egg passively "sits on the shelf," awaiting fertilisation, the sperm is described as an active traveller (just like the *homunculus* in *Tristram Shandy*) that "penetrate[s]" the egg once it arrives (Martin 1991, 487, 489). The egg depends on the sperm – like a "Sleeping Beauty" or "damsel in distress," it awaits its "rescue" by the sperm whose "prize" is fertilisation (Martin 1991, 490–491). Classic biology textbooks use terms such as "thrusting forward" to describe the penetration of the egg's outer surface (Martin 1991, 493).

In the second half of the twentieth century, however, biologists developed new theories of reproduction that, at first, rendered the egg more active: Scientists argued that the egg, in fact, "trap[s] the sperm" due to "adhesive molecules" on its surface that stick to that of the sperm's (Martin 1991, 492–493). Nevertheless, instead of using language that would emphasise the egg and sperm's cooperation, scientists rather described the egg as an "aggressive sperm catcher" (Martin 1991, 493). Other terms that were used include metaphors of courtship and mating that further strengthened the idea of "woman as the hard-to-get prize" (Martin 1991, 497). As the chapter on *Fanny Hill* revealed, such gendered (heteronormative) metaphors prove to be persistent as they were also utilised to describe the reproduction of plants, while botanical metaphors were in turn applied to female bodies and parts thereof that rendered female physicality a passive landscape awaiting active (usually male) plucking or ploughing.

The metaphor I would like to draw particular attention to is that of 'interruption.' While, in biology books, the egg was continuously described as a "dangerous and aggressive threat" that "'captures and tethers' the sperm with its sticky zona, rather like a spider lying in wait in her web," it eventually "'interrupts' the sperm's dive with a 'sudden and swift' rush by which she [the egg] 'clasps the sperm and guides its nucleus to the center'" (Martin 1991, 498). Not only does this imagery render the egg a "femme fatale who victimizes" the sperm, but this stereotypical image is also still used to describe active, independent and thus threatening women (Martin 1991, 498).

Interestingly, the egg that apparently interrupts the sperm's activity bears a striking resemblance to the very first conception episode in Sterne's *Tristram Shandy* when Elizabeth interrupts her husband and thus the 'animal spirit.' As outlined, Sterne targets were, among many other things, orthodox reproductive theories that blamed mothers for the outcome of their pregnancies, further estabilishing the seminal fluids as active and the female body as a passive vessel waiting to be penetrated and fertilised. The end product, so to speak, in *Tristram Shandy* is a *homunculus,* a little *man*, whose nose – a symbol for this phallus – is crushed by the hands of an obstetrician, thus pointing to the arrogance of enlightened male science.

Sterne would have taken much pleasure in Martin's analysis of the egg and the sperm in mocking these metaphors. Her research demonstrates that gendered metaphors are not only long-lasting but also shape our reality: Eventually, they enable social control by evoking images of the "passive female" and the "strong male" (Martin 1991, 500). This acknowledgement underlines the argument that meaning (metaphors) and matter (bodies) are inseparably entangled with one another. Changing technologies such as dissection, its medical representations or simply the modern sonogram still contribute to ideas of little *homunculi* equipped with personhood that need to be 'saved,' regardless of the mother's needs (Martin 1991, 500). In the face of abortion rights that are now again at stake, it is our task as literary and cultural studies scholars to challenge these images and "[w]ake up such metaphors by becoming aware" of their very real, material implications (Martin 1991, 501). Only by doing this, Martin concludes, will we be able to "rob them of their power to naturalize our social conventions about gender" (Martin 1991, 501). Analysing Sterne's *Tristram Shandy* is a good way to start.

Notes

1 Scholars have called it a "parodic anti-novel or sophisticated meta-novel" due its unusual orthography, quirky narration, various interruptions of the 'plot,' narrational diversions and whimsical additions of squiggles, scribbles and even blank or black pages (Keymer 2018, 522).

2 *Don Quixote* not only parodies a literacy predecessor, but the deluded voyager and adventurer can also be read as a critique of colonialism, a topic that is equally debated in Aphra Behn's *Oroonoko, or the History of the Royal Slave* (1688), Defoe's *Robinson Crusoe* and Swift's *Gulliver's Travels* (1726).

3 For more general information, see also Gurr's "Laurence Sterne, *The Life and Opinions of Tristram Shandy, Gentleman* (1759–1767)" in Katrin Berndt and Alessa John's volume *Handbook of the British Novel in the Long Eighteenth Century* (2022) as well as his monograph *Tristram Shandy and the Dialectic of Enlightenment* (1999).

4 A further marketing strategy was to engage the satirist William Hogarth who contributed to the second edition with an illustration, portraying key scenes of the book (Ross 2009, xiv). The novel's popularity also affected Sterne's sermons which were widely purchased and read due to the success of *Tristram Shandy*. As Ross emphasises, "during his lifetime and for many years afterwards, Sterne's literary reputation rested as much on his sermons as on his fiction" (Ross 2009, xiv).

5 See also the more recently published paperback edition of Anja Müller's (ed.) *Fashioning Childhood in the Eighteenth Century: Age and Identity* (2016) that includes Vanderbeke's chapter as well.

6 Undoubtedly, this conviction shows many similarities with the 'king's two bodies,' a theory popularised by Edmund Plowden in the sixteenth century, ascribing the sovereign's body a (mortal) 'body natural' and a (immortal) 'body politic' to justify the king or queen's rule on earth as God's anointed (see also Kantorowicz [1957] 2016).

7 See also William C. Mottolese's paper "Tristram Cyborg and Toby Toolmaker: Body, Tools, and Hobbyhorse in *Tristram Shandy*" (2007) that explores the disconnect between body and mind and highlights how the novel's characters use hobbyhorses as metaphors for tools that bridge physical limitations and mental aspirations. According to Mottolese, the Sterne's novel ultimately anticipates a post-Cartesian worldview, blurring distinctions between self, body and mind (Mottolese 2007, 697).

References

Baldick, Chris. 2015. *The Oxford Dictionary of Literary Terms*. 4th ed. Oxford: Oxford University Press.

Behn, Aphra. [1688] 1997. *Oroonoko*. New York: W. W. Norton.

Blackwell, Bonnie. 2001. "Tristram Shandy and the Theatre of the Mechanical Mother." *ELH* 68 (1): 81–133.

Buckley, Jenifer. 2017. *Gender, Pregnancy and Power in Eighteenth-Century Literature: The Maternal Imagination*. Basingstoke: Palgrave Macmillan.

Cervantes, Miguel de. [1605] 2020. *Don Quixote*. New York: W. W. Norton.

Defoe, Daniel. 1994. *Robinson Crusoe*. New York: W. W. Norton.

Gurr, Jens Martin. 1999. *Tristram Shandy and the Dialectic of Enlightenment*. Heidelberg: Winter.

Gurr, Jens Martin. 2022. "Laurence Sterne, The Life and Opinions of Tristram Shandy, Gentleman (1759–1767)." In *Handbook of the British Novel in the Long Eighteenth Century*, edited by Katrin Berndt and Alessa Johns, 365–389. Berlin; Boston: De Gruyter.

Harries, Elizabeth W. 2009. "Words, Sex, and Gender in Sterne's Novels." In *The Cambridge Companion to Laurence Sterne*, edited by Thomas Keymer, 112–127. Cambridge: Cambridge University Press.

Hawes, Clement. 2020. "Gulliver Effects." In *The Oxford Handbook of the Eighteenth-Century Novel*, edited by Alan Downie, 179–194. Oxford: Oxford University Press.

Hawley, Judith. 2019. "The Anatomy of Tristram Shandy." In *Tristram Shandy*, edited by Laurence Sterne and Judith Hawley, 203–215. New York: Norton.

Keymer, Thomas. 2018. "Sterne and the New Species of Writing." In *Tristram Shandy*, edited by Laurence Sterne and Judith Hawley, 89–101. New York: Norton.

Kantorowicz, Ernst H. 2016. *The King's Two Bodies: A Study in Medieval Political Theology*. Princeton, NJ: Princeton University Press.

La Mettrie, Julien Offray de. 1996. *Machine Man and Other Writings*. Edited by Ann Thomson. Cambridge: Cambridge University Press.

Lamb, Jonathan. 1998. "Sterne and Irregular Oratory." In *The Cambridge Companion to the Eighteenth-Century Novel*, edited by John Richetti, 147–163. Cambridge: Cambridge University Press.

Malory, Thomas. [1485] 2008. *Le Morte d'Arthur: The Winchester Manuscript*. Oxford: Oxford University Press.

Martin, Emily. 1991. "The Egg and the Sperm: How Science Has Constructed a Romance Based on Stereotypical Male-Female Roles." *Signs* 16 (3): 485–501.

Morrissey, Lee. 2017. "The Restoration and Eighteenth Century, 1660–1780." In *English Literature in Context*, 2nd ed., edited by Paul Poplawski, 136–149. Cambridge: Cambridge University Press.

Mottolese, William C. 2007. "Tristram Cyborg and Toby Toolmaker: Body, Tools, and Hobbyhorse in *Tristram Shandy*." *SEL Studies in English Literature 1500–1900* 47 (3): 679–701.

Newman, Karen. 1996. *Fetal Positions: Individualism, Science, Visuality*. Stanford, CA: Stanford University Press.

Noggle, James. 2018. "The Restoration and the Eighteenth Century." In *The Norton Anthology of English Literature*, 10th ed., edited by Stephen Greenblatt, 176–215. New York: Norton.

Porter, Roy. 2004. *Flesh in the Age of Reason*. London: Penguin.

Ross, Ian Campbell. 2009. "Introduction." In *The Life and Opinions of Tristram Shandy*, edited by Laurence Sterne and Ian Campbell Ross, ix–xxviii. Oxford: Oxford University Press.

Sterne, Laurence. [1749] 2019. *Tristram Shandy*. Edited with an introduction by Judith Hawley. New York: Norton.

Sprang, Felix. 2008. "Tristram Shandy und die *Anthropologia Nova*: Systematik in Literatur und Medizin." In *Medizinische Schreibweisen: Ausdifferenzierung und Transfer zwischen Medizin und Literatur (1600–1900)*, edited by Nicolas Pethes and Sandra Richter, 135–153. Tübingen: Niemeyer.

Sprang, Felix. 2013. "Let Me See the Child, and Die: The Medicalization of Childbirth in Eighteenth- and Nineteenth-Century Novels." In *The Writing Cure: Literature and Medicine in Context*, edited by Alexandra Lembert-Heidenreich and Jarmila Mildorf, 135–153. Zurich: Lit Verlag.

Swift, Jonathan. 1726. *Gulliver's Travels*. Edited by Albert J. Rivero. New York: Norton, 2002.

Vanderbeke, Dirk. 2006. "Winding up the Clock: The Conception and Birth of Tristram Shandy." In *Fashioning Childhood in the Eighteenth Century: Age and Identity*, edited by Anja Müller, 179–188. Aldershot: Ashgate.

Watt, Ian. 2015. *The Rise of the Novel: Studies in Defoe, Richardson and Fielding*. London: Bodley Head.

Williams, Carolyn. 2012. "Difficulties, at Present in No Degree Clear'd Up: The Controversial Mother, 1600–1800." In *The Female Body in Medicine and Literature*, edited by Andrew Mangham and Greta Depledge, 16–33. Liverpool: Liverpool University Press.

2.4 Eliza Fenwick's *Secresy, Or: The Ruin on the Rock* (1795)

2.4.1 Introduction

As opposed to the previous three analysis chapters that dealt with novels published by mainly well-known male authors, the following three turn to texts produced by female novelists and philosophers. This chapter discusses a lesser-known novel that addresses questions of secret sexualities, secret pregnancies and the role of hygienic motherhood during the eighteenth century. It begins with a general introduction to the text and its historical context including the culture of sensibility (Todd 1989; Grundy 1998; Isaac 1999; Close 2004) and continues with an investigation of Fenwick's family relations and proto-feminist politics before turning to the concept of hygienic motherhood, mechanical mothers and possible forms of reproductive (cyborgian) agency (Rousseau [1789] 1969; Furniss 1992; Gubar 1994; Emsley 1999; Porter 2004; Cannon 2008; Burke 2009; Buchan [1769] 2014; Woods/Galley 2014; Speck 2016). The analysis builds on a modest number of selected secondary texts on the novel; as to this day, Eliza Fenwick's *Secresy* belongs to one of the most underrated and under-researched narratives of the period. This is surprising given that this epistolary text offers a quite "interesting critique of [...] the roles available to women" during the eighteenth century (Isaac 1999, 115).

In order to fully grasp the novel's meaning, it is essential to turn to selected aspects of its context. Janet Todd begins her introduction to the Pandora edition of Fenwick's *Secresy* with two quotes by Mary Wollstonecraft, one taken from her novel *Mary, A Fiction* (1788), and the other from her political essay *A Vindication of the Rights of Woman* (1792). Both quotes deal with the notion of sensibility but seem to contradict one another to a certain degree: The first quote praises sensibility as the "most exquisite feeling" that, for instance, enables a recognition of the sublime, but the other claims that "over-exercised sensibility" weakens "[c]ivilized women['s] [...] reason [and] cultivation of mind" (Todd 1989, vii). Todd chooses these two very different quotes – one that emerged before and the other after the beginning of the French Revolution – to "summarize the debate[s] over women's nature" in the course of this major historical event, debates that both Wollstonecraft and Fenwick participated in through their works (Todd 1989, vii–viii).

DOI: 10.4324/9781003467977-9

A dominant and hotly debated question was whether females were "naturally more sensitive and tender than men – as well as more irrational and stupid," or whether such stereotypes stood in the way of equality between the sexes (Todd 1989, viii). Another question addressed education: Should men and women enjoy the same form of (practical) education or should women be "raised 'innocently' in nature," isolated from (corrupt) society, to become "virtuous, supportive and obedient wives" (Todd 1989, viii)? Fenwick explores these very questions in *Secresy*; she asks what might happen if a young woman resisted such an isolated education and simply "followed her sensitive and compassionate feelings into forbidden sexual activity" (Todd 1989, viii).

The narrative is divided into three volumes and revolves around the intimate friendship between two young women, Caroline Ashburn, born into a wealthy family, and Sibella Valmont, who is imprisoned in a (Gothic) castle by her capricious, misanthropic and misogynist uncle Mr Valmont. He denies his niece's education and tries to cut her off from the outside world to turn her into a docile future wife, but the highly intelligent Sibella continues to communicate with Caroline through letters. Sibella demonstrates her rational but also romantic voice when she writes of her childhood friend Clement Montgomery, whom she is also in love with. What follows is a series of tragic events that involve Mr Valmont's attempt to arrange a marriage between Sibella and a (supposed) stranger. This prompts Sibella and (the untrustworthy) Clement to pledge their love and loyalty through sex, which Sibella regards as equivalent to marriage. Afterwards, Clement travels to London where he continues his affair with the mistress Janetta, while Sibella strolls through Valmont Park with her pet fawn Nina and writes letters to her friend.

The eponymous word 'ruin' refers to an old hermitage near Valmont Castle where Sibella encounters a mysterious hermit: He is later revealed as Arthur Murden, one of Caroline's friends who is supposed to secretly look after Sibella but then falls in love with his protégé. Arthur saves Sibella from the attempted abduction by Lord Filmar, who hopes to inherit her fortune, only to discover that she is with a child. Filmar eventually manages to abduct Sibella but returns her, as the pregnant woman is of no use to him. In the end, Mr Valmont reveals that it was Clement, who turns out to be his adopted son, who he had had in mind as Sibella's husband all along, but Clement is already married to another woman, Caroline's wealthy mother. The novel ends with three deaths in a birth room: Sibella, her still-born child, and Arthur who crawls into her bed and dies with her.

Against the backdrop of *Secresy*'s bleak ending and the question of the novel's feminist potential, Isobel Grundy argues that Fenwick's text can be understood as a "tragedy, whose plot offers no utopian promise of improvement" (Grundy 1998, 28). What is more, the novel "remains arguably reformist rather than [...] revolutionary" as it eventually confirms patriarchal gender ideology by 'punishing' the female protagonist for her illegitimate pregnancy through death (Grundy 1998, 28). The unhappy end is especially brought about by the narrative's manifold secrets: Mr Valmont conceals his true plans to marry his adopted son Clement to Sibella to inherit the wealth she does not yet know about, Montgomery "lies to everyone he meets", and Caroline and Sibella "slide into secrecy" when they converse about the latter's secret sexual 'marriage' to Clement and the secret pregnancy that results from it (Grundy 1998, 29). What also distinguishes this novel in terms of gender is its reversal of stereotypical roles: Male characters succumb to 'hysteria,' bodily frailty and fall victim to their "secret love," while female figures excel in "psychical toughness" and "icy stoicism in face of emotional loss" (Grundy 1998, 29). It is thus hard to assign this narrative to a particular genre or subgenre as Grundy concludes: "None of the available labels – epistolary, gothic, sentimental, radical, novel of manners, or novel of social conscience – can package this stunning single work" (Grundy 1998, 30).

Secresy's reception was mixed and ranged from "cursory," "outraged" and "approving" to "amusing and interesting," "not very original" or simply "novel," while other reviews described the narrative as a "lighter species of literary composition" (Grundy 1998, 9; Close 2004, 52). The tendency, however, was rather negative due to Fenwick's "public reputation": She was known as an "established radical" who later divorced her husband and was also "accused of sympathising" with proponents of the French Revolution (Close 2004, 52). To this day, *Secresy* remains strikingly under-analysed. Grundy largely blames Fenwick's "absence of an *oeuvre*," which surprises given the narrative's "heavyweight" as a novel of ideas, its "world of idealism, of resistance to accepted ideology" and its negotiations of "multiple psycho-socio-political debates of the 1790s" such as class and gender (Grundy 1998, 25).

Anne Close adds that the "negative reaction" to *Secresy* was also one of the reasons why the text was not reprinted for over two centuries and was consequently scholarly neglected (Close 2004, 52). Ever since the Pandora (1989) and the Broadway View (1998) editions were published, it is now finally possible to revisit this text. This book's aim is to contribute to the still scarce scholarship on Fenwick's *Secresy* by focussing on feminism, reproduction, medicine and motherhood, not least because the novel's title already contains a pun in this respect; it alludes to secret pregnancies and (female) knowledges as well as the tragic outcomes of such secrets.

2.4.2 Fenwick, Family & Feminism

The feminist potential of Eliza Fenwick's work might become clearer by turning to selected aspects of her life, which was marked by a difficult marriage, motherhood and death. As with Cleland, however, relatively little was known about Fenwick's biography until quite recently, when Lissa Paul published her biography *Eliza Fenwick: Early Modern Feminist* in 2019. Paul's impressive book mainly engages with "Eliza's colonial immigration success story: from Britain via the Caribbean to North America" in the early 1810s, nearly 20 years after the "one-hit wonder" Fenwick published her novel *Secresy* (Paul 2019, 3, 8). The following passages, however, are less interested in her "immigration success story" and more in how her biography might have shaped this hitherto underestimated literary masterpiece (Paul 2019, 5).

Born as Eliza Jeco in 1766 in Pelynt, Cornwall, she married Sir John Fenwick, an English Jacobite and "political idealist, Irish patriot, member of the London

Corresponding Society," the latter a democratic reform association or debating club, who was also in debt and an alcoholic (Grundy 1998, 7–8; Paul 2019, 3). There is no information on her education. There are also no surviving images of her, only a photograph of her granddaughter Elizabeth Rutherford Savage from 1876 (Paul 2019, 13). What is known is that Fenwick and her husband moved to London in the 1790s, where she became acquainted with the "who's who" of the time, from Samuel Taylor Coleridge, William Godwin, Elizabeth Inchbald, Charlotte Smith to Mary Wollstonecraft, whose birth of her daughter Mary (Shelley) she attended, to name but a few (Paul 2019, 10). As Paul emphasises, the "sampling of people who made up the everyday community of Eliza's social and cultural life in Britain speaks to her intellectual vitality and accomplishment" (Paul 2019, 10).

In terms of her literary work, Fenwick was mainly known for her children's books characterised by "heavy didacticism" such as *The Story of Little Mary and her Cat* (1804) or *The Life of Carlo, the Famous Dog of Drury-Lane Theatre* (1804) (Grundy 1998, 12). Identifying Fenwick's authorship, however, is not always easy due to the frequent absence of her name or initials, especially with regard to her earlier works, as Grundy states in her introduction to the Broadview edition in which she calls Fenwick's *Secresy* her sole "novel for adults": "*If* she ever wrote anything else of the scope and ambition of *Secresy*, it is not known to survive" (emphasis in the original, Grundy 1998, 7).

In general, Fenwick's writings did not gain much "attention or recognition" from her contemporaries, unlike her husband's publications that were "immortalized" by the criticism of his drinking companion, the English poet and writer Charles Lamb (Grundy 1998, 7). A heavy drinker himself, John Fenwick plunged his family, including his joint children Eliza Anne (born 1789) and Orlando (born 1798), into debt; this forced his wife to take refuge and work as a governess for several employers both in England and Ireland in addition to her activities as a writer (Grundy 1998, 8, 10; see also Paul 2019, 3). Fenwick's relationship with her children, her daughter in particular, was very close, and so she followed Eliza Anne to Barbados to attend her first-born's wedding and "settle permanently" (Grundy 1998, 16–18). Though Fenwick founded a school for girls together with her daughter, she never felt at home in the Caribbean and was plagued by homesickness (Grundy 1998, 18).

The family's later years abroad were marked by misfortune, illness and death: After several physical accidents, "losses to the school" and hurricanes, Fenwick's son Orlando died of yellow fever, which triggered intense "mourning and depression" with her only to then witness her daughter's health deteriorating between 1818 and 1820 (Grundy 1998, 18–19; see also Paul 2019, 4). Fenwick decided to leave Barbados with her family and first moved to West England and then New York where Eliza Anne died in 1828 "leaving her children to her mother's care" (Grundy 1998, 19–20). After moving to Canada, two of her grandchildren, Thomas and William, "drowned in Lake Ontario" (Grundy 1998, 20; see also Paul 2019, 1–2). Eliza Fenwick spent her final years with her granddaughter Elizabeth in Rhode Island "where she died in 1840" aged 74 (Grundy 1998, 20).

Fenwick was a talented writer of letters and frequently corresponded with her children and female friends, including the intellectual, poet and novelist Mary Hays as well as the proto-feminist Mary Wollstonecraft (Todd 1989, x).[1] Especially during the second half of her life abroad, "she had little time to write" due to responsibilities that involved "teaching, running schools, and childrearing," so she resorted to letter-writing: "Her letters became the place where she could exercise her talents when her need to earn a living crowded out the literary life she had started to live in the 1790s and early 1800s" (Paul 2019, 4–5). It is thus rather "unsurprising" that her only novel was written in the epistolary form and equally "unsurprising that her letters should be read as fiction" (Paul 2019, 7). Fenwick's surviving letters demonstrate her status as a "thinker, [...] radical [and] romantic" with a strong "sense of human solidarity" (Grundy 1998, 22). She especially found "comfort in female friendship," a motif that also dominates *Secresy*'s construction of female solidarity in a "threatening male world" (Todd 1989, x). Yet, to argue that Fenwick was a proto-feminist or that her ideologies resembled those of her close friend Mary Wollstonecraft is rather far-fetched since her "feminism [was] in [constant] tension with a self-sacrificial ideal of motherhood" (Grundy 1998, 23).

Fenwick's inherent contradictions became most visible in her attitudes towards slavery. When she joined her daughter Eliza Anne in Barbados, she wrote letters to Mary Hays describing her inner conflicts regarding the "house slaves" whom she both hated and pitied, though she seems to have (correctly) understood slavery as a project of patriarchy:

> To kindness & forbearance they return insolence & contempt. Nothing awes or governs them but the lash of the whip or the dread of being sent into the fields of labour. [...] It is a horrid & disgraceful System. The female slaves are really encouraged to prostitution because their children are the property of the owner of the mothers. These children are reared by the Ladies as pets [...] till grown up, when they are at once dismissed to labour & slave-like treatment. – What is still more horrible, the Gentlemen are greatly addicted to their women slaves, & give the fruit of their licentiousness to their white children as slaves. [...] It is a common case & not thought of as an enormity. It gives me disgusted antipathy & I am ready to hail the Slave & reject the Master.
>
> (Grundy 1998, 24)

Fenwick equally describes her protagonist Sibella as "held in the bondage of slavery" and thus seems to criticise patriarchal systems (*Secresy*, 73). To compare the imprisonment of a (white, British) young woman with actual slavery is, of course, far from unproblematic. The following segments, however, shift attention from slavery to feminism as this requires a longer discussion that would exceed the limits of this book; instead, the subsequent sections focus on sexuality and/as forms of gendered agency in *Secresy*.

According to Close, Fenwick's novel features sexually experienced heroines who "challenge familial and cultural mandates of gendered behaviour" by "foregrounding [their] rational sincerity" as well as their powerful female friendship

(Close 2004, 35). The novel utilises the Gothic mode to investigate "radical [proto-feminist] politics"; it allows its female characters to "resist cultural expectations dictating [female] passivity and docility" and thus exposes "destructive gender ideology" (Close 2004, 38). The (gendered) resistance to social control becomes particularly apparent by the example of the novel's two heroines, Caroline Ashburn and Sibella Valmont; these two young women rebel against the narrative's tyrannical patriarch, Mr Valmont, by refusing his "faith in seclusion" through self-education as well as self-defined sexuality. These female characters thus "contest the system of gendered education" put forward by Swiss philosopher Jean-Jacques Rousseau in his conduct book *Émile, Or: On Education* (1762), through which he defended women's dependence on and obedience towards men, their exclusion from public life and concentration on the family and the home rather than the acquisition of knowledge (Grundy 1998, 25–26).

As Porter emphasises with regard to *Émile*, though Rousseau's focus was mainly on the question of how the innately good human individual could survive in a corrupt society, it also contained advice as to how to raise children. Interestingly, Rousseau utilised a novelistic style and constructed the fictitious characters Émile and Sophie; while the text celebrates the boy's upbringing as an "active, rational and assertive" individual, it applauds the girl's "yielding, loving and nurturing" character traits (Porter 2004, 262). For Rousseau, "it was for men to exercise their reason, [and] women to feel" (Porter 2004, 626). However, in Rousseau's unfinished sequel *Émile et Sophie*, Sophie commits adultery and is described by Rousseau as "the most odious of all monsters" (Rousseau [1783] 1969, 31).

In order to counter such "blatant sexism" with regard to the association of femininity with feeling as opposed to masculinity and rationality, women promoted John Locke's concept of the "mind as a *tabula rasa*" and his idea that the "mind had no sex" (Porter 2004, 262–263). In fact, there were many contradicting views as to the question on whether and how girls and young women should be raised and educated; what remained, though, was a notion of a "civilizing mission upon the sex" (Porter 2004, 263), similar to the British colonists' mission during this period. Fenwick's friend Mary Wollstonecraft also heavily criticised Rousseau's convictions in her proto-feminist work *A Vindication of the Rights of Woman* (1792) (Grundy 1998, 26).

Wollstonecraft advocated equality of the sexes and attacked Rousseau's depiction of women in *Émile*, especially the character construction of the beautiful and docile Sophie for being nothing but a product of male desire (Furniss 1992, 284; Speck 2016, 347). In particular, she rejected Rousseau's objectification of women that, in her view, could be prevented by (their) education (Furniss 1992, 285; Speck 2016, 347). Most importantly, Wollstonecraft challenged rigid associations between women and the body by making the 'radical' statement that women were equally capable of rationality (Gubar 1994, 454–455). In terms of *Secresy*, as Grundy contends, "[w]ether or not Fenwick was conscious of the fact, her heroines Caroline and Sibella, in following Wollstonecraft, take up an earlier feminist intellectual heritage," and she concludes: "Wollstonecraft's rebuttal of Rousseau in her *Vindication* is a major influence on *Secresy*" (Grundy 1998, 26).[2]

Yet, *Secresy* is not just a "critique of education, class and culture" or (secret) marriage but it especially deals with secret sexuality (Emsley 1999, 477). Sarah Emsley points out that Sibella, due to her "solitary life" as part of Mr Valmont's "tyrannical experiment in education," is convinced by the "contract between hearts" (their romance and sexual intercourse with Clement), to which she gives greater weight than the "economic contract of marriage in society" (Emsley 1999, 477). The "sexual union," as Emsley emphasises, is the novel's "central event" as it exposes the "flaws in Sibella's upbringing" and thus functions as a critique of patriarchal "social institutions" (Emsley 1999, 477). In other words, *Secresy* reveals the "tragedy of failed ideals in a system that necessitates secrecy about sexuality," while simultaneously failing to "offer any hope for change" by letting its heroine die (Emsley 1999, 478). The secret sex, however, eventually led to an initially secret and especially illegitimate pregnancy. In this context, the following subchapter discusses the meaning of 'hygienic motherhood' as well as the refusal of reproduction as a form of female agency.

2.4.3 Hygienic Motherhood & Mechanical Mothers

This section deals in more detail with *Secresy*'s negotiation of secret sexuality and female agency, while putting particular emphasis on reproductive bodies, (secret) pregnancies and (mechanical) motherhood. It mainly builds on two pivotal publications by Mercy Cannon (2008) and Meghan L. Burke (2009) and expands their core statements: Cannon argues that the novel's tragic end possesses the potential to subvert patriarchal norms by refusing reproduction, while simultaneously confirming stereotypical maternal norms by eliminating the "diseased 'other,'" the mother and the illegitimate child (Cannon 2008, 534). Burke's intriguing article, on the other hand, argues that *Secresy* is not just about secret sexuality and illegitimate offspring – it is also and especially about the power of women over reproduction which poses a threat to patriarchal authority that seeks to control childbirth.

Apart from this rather classic feminist reading, Burke's central argument is that Sibella's body literally embodies the new field of obstetrics, its discourses as well as its (material) technologies: In *Secresy*, Sibella represents the obstetrical machine, while her death can be interpreted as a prime example of the maternal body's erasure. Moreover, the secrets that saturate the novel render Sibella's reproductive body suspect, even monstrous. After offering a rendition of Cannon's and Burke's arguments, the concluding subchapter will go beyond a reading of *Secresy* as a (potential) critique of patriarchy and rethink, or think *through*, Sibella's material-discursive body by discussing its cyborgian potential.

Cannon's point of departure is William Buchan's *Domestic Medicine, Or: The Family Physician* ([1769] 2014), a "best-selling treatise" and home health guide. In this book, Buchan advocates for "hygienic motherhood," meaning that it is both the mother's power and responsibility to ensure her own health and that of her children (Cannon 2008, 535). The treatise, which Cannon largely mentions in passing and that shall be discussed here in more detail, is divided into two parts: Part I is about the causes of children's diseases and their prevention, and Part II deals with the distinction of diseases in general, ranging from fevers to smallpox to gout to melancholy and madness or hiccups.

The last three subchapters of Buchan's guide not only address surgery and, again, diseases of children but also devote roughly 20 pages to the "Diseases of Women" including pregnancy, childbirth and "barrenness" (Buchan [1769] 2014, vi). In this chapter, Buchan solely concentrates on the female's reproductive life phase, between about 15 and 50, and stresses the importance of her conduct during this period that requires the "greatest care" to ensure (future) "health and happiness" (Buchan 2014, 557). One of the main suggestions to women is to stay active, go outside and enjoy "exercise and free air" (Buchan 2014, 558):

> If a girl about this time of life be confined to the house, kept constantly sitting, and neither allowed to romp about, nor employed in some active business, which gives exercise to the whole body, she becomes weak, relaxed, and puny; [...] her health, spirits and vigour decline, and she sinks into a valetudinary for life.
>
> (Buchan 2014, 557)

Buchan hence clearly recommends an active lifestyle that exceeds the limits of the house. Furthermore, in the section "Of Pregnancy," he explicitly states that "PREGNANCY is not a disease"; however, he simultaneously emphasises that responsibility for preventing related 'fevers' lies with women (Buchan 2014, 566). Buchan continues with the "danger of abortion" that can equally be reduced by avoiding, for instance, "violent passions or affections of the mind, as fear, grief; &c.," thus again shifting responsibility to the mother (Buchan 2014, 567). The pregnant female should always "be kept cheerful and easy in her mind [because] [a]ll violent passions hurt the *foetus*, and endanger an abortion" (Buchan 2014, 568). Though Buchan advocates physical and mental stimulation to women during their reproductive years, he still holds mothers solely accountable for their pregnancy's 'product' – the foetus – and therefore attaches the greatest importance to female (moral) conduct.

Buchan's understanding of hygienic motherhood involves a "vigilant awareness" of one's child and own health that also includes an "acute attentiveness to mental and moral development" (Cannon 2008, 535). The latter is especially relevant as Buchan renders the (maternal) "power to shape the entire social realm" in fact the mothers' "duty as national [British] subjects" (Cannon 2008, 536). Yet, Cannon identifies a shift in "maternal virtue" in Buchan's *Domestic Medicine* that also manifests itself in Fenwick's *Secresy* (Cannon 2008, 536). By reference to Toni Bowers' *The Politics of Motherhood* ([1996] 2005) and Julie Kipp's *Romanticism, Maternity, and the Body Politic* ([2003] 2009), Cannon outlines how especially in the second half of the eighteenth century, maternal representations tended towards the "dangerously good" or the "naturally bad" mother who either cared too much or too little (Cannon 2008, 537). Bower, Kipp and Cannon all argue that the construction of (female) reproduction was an instrument for "expressing concerns over political and social power" (Cannon 2008, 537). Along these lines,

Secresy's character Sibella tends towards the 'naturally bad' mother who disregards her 'duty,' hygienic motherhood.

Health guides like those produced by Buchan were entangled with such material discourses and fed into the idea that women's bodies should be "safe spaces for unborn [British] children" to ensure a healthy (British) nation – a form of health care that "could only *materialize* through pregnant women's self-care" (emphasis added, Cannon 2008, 537). This maternal power, however, simultaneously meant "confinement within the maternal body"; it is this restriction within the female reproductive body that Sibella refuses in Fenwick's *Secresy* by seeking (secret) sex outside of (traditional) wedlock, becoming pregnant under such circumstances and thus "endanger[ing]" her (British) child and hence (symbolically) Britain's future (Cannon 2008, 537).

Fenwick's Sibella therefore refuses hygienic motherhood by actively promising herself to a morally questionable man. As a result, the novel entangles material (medical) maternal bodies, Sibella's literary "individual body" and the discursive "body politic" with one another (Cannon 2008, 538). As Cannon emphasises with reference to Buchan's health guide, "a clear connection exists between individual health and national health: medical manuals define the hygienic parent's relationship to the nation and her children" (Cannon 2008, 538). Following this logic, Sibella is "doomed by circumstance and choice to become the diseased 'other,'" the unhygienic mother, who "refuses to protect" her reproductive body (Cannon 2008, 539). Fenwick thus allows her main character agency as Sibella rejects the objectification of her reproductive body as a "healthy incubator" (Cannon 2008, 540). She recovers possession of her body while the text at the same time highlights women's reproductive bodies as prisons (Cannon 2008, 542).

Moreover, Sibella's character development is linked to the spaces she moves in: While Valmont Castle is associated with "disease – unhealthy, toxic, and even [the] deadly" and represents an "unhygienic environment" for the protagonist, she "thrives in the openness of the castle grounds" (Cannon 2008, 543–544). In a letter to her friend, Caroline describes the castle she remembers in a dream:

> [...] instead of smiling lawns and gay parterres, [...] I found moats, walls, and drawbridges, frowning battlements that looked as uninviting on the friend as threatening on the enemy, turrets all cheerless, all hostile, and discouraging to the wandering stranger. The castle's Gothic magnificence within reminded me of the Valmont race; the apartments received their guests without welcome; the domestics were obedient, but neither cheerful nor attentive.
>
> (*Secresy*, 52)

Sibella responds to Caroline by lamenting her situation at Castle Valmont in a similarly bleak manner:

> He [Mr. Valmont] demands my obedience [...]. I am held in the bondage of slavery. [...] Imprisoned, during so many years, within the narrow boundary of this castle and its parks, [...] my actions are confined to the mechanical

> operations of the body, that I am an imbecile creature, but a reptile of more graceful form, the half finished work of nature, [...] he would degrade me to the subordinate station he describes. He daringly asserts that I am born to the exercise of no will; to the exercise of no duties but submission; that wisdom owns me not, knows me not, could not find in me a resting place.
>
> (*Secresy*, 73–74)

Fenwick's text not only associates the castle's 'unhygienic' interior with (patriarchal) hostility, submission and the absence of free will but also seems to construct Sibella's (reproductive) body as both machine and animal, thus blurring the boundaries between the human and nonhuman. What is more, *Secresy* sets the interior – the castle – in stark contrast with its exterior – the woods – that is rendered a hygienic environment for Sibella in which she thrives as Caroline narrates to a group of ladies:

> A true child of nature, bold in innocence, day or night is equally propitious to her rambles; and always mentally alive, she has the glow of animation to her cheeks, the fire of vivacity in her eye, alone in a solitary wood at noon-day or at mid-night. [...] I spoke further, Sibella, of your favourite lonely haunt, the flying speed with which I have seen you bound there, the affectionate caresses of your little fawn and numberless other circumstances.
>
> (*Secresy*, 94–95)

The association of confinement with pathology and openness with health recalls Buchan's *Domestic Medicine* that explicitly advises against confining young women to the house and recommends an active lifestyle outside in the open air. The reason for Sibella's 'contagion' can clearly be found in her spatial confinement; Fenwick's text thus confirms Buchan's call for hygienic motherhood, while at the same time exposing this (material) medical discourse as a patriarchal product.

The novel's two central events are on the one hand Sibella's voluntary and deliberate secret sex with the morally degenerated Clement, and on the other hand, her illegitimate secret pregnancy that needs to be punished in the end: "With her pregnancy, the heroine becomes an infectious figure whose death is both tragic and necessary in the novel's domestic economy" (Cannon 2008, 546). In sum, the novel not only pathologises the female reproductive body but especially renders (female) secrecy an illness that threatens the wellbeing of the British nation. Despite Sibella's death, her body still owns agency by resisting its status as a birth machine. Yet, it is simultaneously constructed as a revolting, disturbing and monstrous body not only by the very man who impregnated her but also by other (male) characters such as Arthur. The latter feels particularly "unmanned" by Sibella's secret pregnancy and renders her a monster whose sight he can hardly stand (*Secresy*, 322):

> And so I am, Miss Ashburn. I think too, I should love revenge. I feel a rankling glow of satisfaction, as she [Sibella] walks past my chair, that I have so placed it I cannot look up and behold her. I recovered strength and courage

> while my horror remained unabated. [...] As she spoke, I turned my eyes from her now haggard and jaundiced face to my own, reflected in the mirror by which I was standing. "Moving corpses!" said I to myself – "Why encumber ye the fair earth?"
>
> (*Secresy*, 322)

Sibella is the 'monster' who, through her denial of hygienic motherhood, ultimately refuses reproduction and is thus equipped with female agency. Unfortunately, as Cannon concludes, Sibella's "radicalism dies with her and her child – the disturbing elements are no longer present" (Cannon 2008, 561).

Burke argues among similar lines and first reminds her readers that the novel's very title alludes to secret or "hidden maternity" (Burke 2009, 357). Sibella's "clandestine pregnancy," however, "both creates and destroys": On the one hand, her secret pregnancy is the "embodiment of [...] female agency" and "free female will," but on the other hand, her death signals the recapture of reproduction by "patriarchal authority" (Burke 2009, 357). Moreover, Sibella's secret pregnancy, which only Caroline knows of until it is revealed to everyone, correlates with very real material practices of (early) midwifery that was regarded as a female-only place and knowledge space from which "men were almost completely excluded" (Burke 2009, 358).

Sibella's reproductive body and her secret pregnancy therefore pose a threat to "male hegemony"; masculine authority loses not only "control over the facts of childbirth" but also over "social systems as a whole" (Burke 2009, 358–359). Burke draws a clear connection between Fenwick's *Secresy* and the shift from midwifery to obstetrics in the course of the eighteenth century during which male practitioners "physical[ly] penetrat[ed] [...] the secret world of the birthing room," hoping not only to investigate and (re)map the female reproductive body but ultimately to "reproduce other men without relying on the female sex" (Burke 2009, 359).

Burke goes even further and argues that the rise of "obstetric technolog[ies]" is "literalized" in Fenwick's novel not only by "render[ing] mothers obsolete agents in their own labour" but especially by constructing Sibella as the literary manifestation of the obstetrical machine, a "lifeless automaton" that feeds the "desire [of] masculine generative power" (Burke 2009, 360). Like Cannon, Burke identifies secrecy as both a form of agency and a "direct threat to masculine control" (Burke 2009, 364). As long as the female reproductive body cannot be controlled, it can only be othered as monstrous. This is exactly what happens in Fenwick's *Secresy*: Sibella is the 'monstrous,' 'unhygienic' and 'unnatural mother' whose secret pregnancy needs to be exposed in order to control reproduction (Burke 2009, 364).

Moreover, Sibella's death represents the prime example of the 'erased mother' – it points to the material-discursive suppression of the female subject, resulting in the objectification of the reproductive body that requires investigation by means of new obstetrics technologies (Burke 2009, 368). Ultimately, Sibella becomes a version of a passive, inert, mechanical mother, a mannequin, a machine, a "mock-woman" as Burke stresses by reference to the eighteenth-century midwife Elizabeth Nihell (Burke 2009, 370–371). In this context, Valmont can be read as an example of a man-midwife who seeks to control Sibella's reproductive body "according to his concept of the proper mechanized order of the world, as a perfect, passive, female object" (Burke 2009, 374).

Equally, Clement views Sibella's body as nothing more but a "passive, objectified, and utilitarian 'mechanical mother' through which he can (re)produce his fondest hopes for the future" (Burke 2009, 376–377). As Burke continues: "No one, then, is willing or able to recognize Sibella as an autonomous, living woman" except for her (female) friend Caroline (Burke 2009, 377). Both men's hopes, however, are "shattered by the sudden proof of her active, independent biological reproduction"; Sibella's "growing gravid body" is not a sign of frailty, but rather an "assertion of [female] agency" – as Burke concludes, "Sibella is literally pregnant with her own power and volition" (Burke 2009, 379). Sibella's 'monstrous' maternal body thus represents both her resistance to patriarchal authority as well as her downfall: Ultimately, her reproductive body confirms maternal as well as obstetrical norms.

2.4.4 (Re)Productive Monsters & Cyborgian Agency

The statement that Fenwick processed her dramatic life experiences in *Secresy* would certainly be too sweeping. Yet, it seems reasonable to assume that her difficult marriage and the close relationship with her children and grandchildren, her daughter in particular, of which many died tragically, had an impact on her writing. Furthermore, Fenwick might have also endured several traumatic birth experiences herself. While most of this can only be speculated, Grundy outlines how Fenwick gave birth to her daughter Eliza Anne "after a painful and dangerous labour," and though "[s]he had no more children till the (easier) birth of her son […] there may have been unrecorded miscarriages or still-births" (Grundy 1998, 8). This suggests that Fenwick' birth experiences could have influenced the character construction of Sibella who also "delivered […] a dead child" (*Secresy*, 347).

Of greater interest, however, is how the text links Sibella's reproductive body with that of the infant – both are associated with death and rendered lifeless: Sibella "insisted on having the corpse of her infant brought to her before its burial; and, while she pressed it to her burning bosom, she said":

> – Poor senseless earth [unconscious body]! In quitting life so soon, thou hast not lost but gained! What art thou? nothing! thy members will not swell into strength and proportion. Life will not inform them. Thy heart will never beat, and it shall not feel. – Babe, thou art gone for ever! None laments for thee. – Go, babe! go to thy cold shelter! soon will that shelter be mine. But I cannot afford thee warmth: for I shall be cold, senseless, dead, as thou art!.
>
> (*Secresy*, 353)

Read in light of early (radical) feminism, it is possible to argue that, although the text never reveals the infant's gender, Sibella is almost relieved about the death of her alleged daughter as she will not be born into a patriarchal system she cannot escape from. Read against the background of childbirth, medicine and the rise of obstetrics, however, the text seems to highlight the material-discursive entanglement of the (haptic) reproductive body on the dissection table, including its dead foetus, with its representations. Both mother and child are "cold, senseless, dead" and evoke images of reproductive bodies in the anatomy theatre, either in the form of human flesh or mechanical copies, as well as illustrations in Hunter's or Smellie's obstetrical atlases.

As a result, Fenwick's *Secresy* not only criticises the isolated education of women, as proposed by Rousseau in *Émile*, for instance, by allowing its main female characters Sibella and Caroline to resist through letter-writing and self-education – the novel also functions as a critique of the usurpation of childbirth my man-midwives or obstetricians. Sibella's fictional reproductive body, including its foetus, embodies the power shift from midwifery to obstetrics that reached its climax towards the turn of the century. The obstetrical machine materialises in, or rather through, Sibella's body and renders her both dead and alive, a moving but pathologised gravid body that needs to be regulated by patriarchal power. I would like to remind this book's readers, however, not to think about this form of materialisation in causal terms. Rather, both the material and the discursive reproductive body emerge simultaneously and are, in Barad's words, always already part of the world's becoming.

Obviously, secrecy plays a major role in Fenwick's eponymous novel and is its leitmotif, not only with regard to Sibella and Clement's secret sexual union that subverts patriarchal authority, but especially in terms of the resulting secret pregnancy that only Caroline and Sibella know of before it is revealed to everyone. It is this secret knowledge shared by female characters only that poses the largest threat not just to the field of obstetrics but, read along the lines of degeneration, to the British nation as a whole. Sibella resists the obligation to hygienic motherhood by actively choosing a morally degenerate man to reproduce with. Unfortunately, this radical feminist potential fizzles out when Sibella dies together with her illegitimate child.

Yet, I argue that the text still grants Sibella's reproductive body a degree of agency: Neither dead nor alive in the final chapters and int*ra*-linked with both the material, fleshy reproductive body on the dissection table as well as the mechanical obstetrical mock-woman, Sibella's body can easily be conceptualised as a productive monster, a cyborg body. Sibella's body has agency in that it 'speaks' (back) to the problematic pathologisation of the material reproductive body on the historically very real, material dissection table. It is therefore too simple to assume that Sibella's death is *only* to be read as an example of the erasure of motherhood. In fact, both interpretations are – simultaneously – possible: Fenwick's protagonist is dead as well as alive; Sibella is silenced but also speaks *through* her body.

As Burke emphasises, in the course of the eighteenth century and the rise of obstetrics, the "female reproductive body, then, became the foe for male midwives" – instead of acknowledging their patients as human, they regarded them as "potentially dangerous, oppositional objects" in need of constant surveillance and control (Burke 2009, 368). Part of this threat were secret knowledges that only women had access to and which threatened medical men's material-discursive power. Ironically, William Buchan directly addresses the notion of secrecy in his "Advertisement" to *Domestic Medicine* (Buchan 2014, vii–viii):[3]

> Had physicians been [...] less solicitous in hunting after wonderful medicines, and concealing their pretended virtues from the rest of mankind, the medical art would never have become an object of ridicule. [...] Every attempt to monopolize or conceal anything that relates to the preservation of health or the cure of diseases, must not only be injurious to the interests of society, but likewise detrimental to the medical art. [...] SECRECY in any art lays a foundation for imposition. Had physicians never affected mystery, quacks and quackery could never have existed. [...] Let us therefore act with candor, openness, and ingenuity, and mankind will soon learn to dread everything in medicine that has the smallest appearance of secrecy or disguise.
>
> (emphasis in the original, Buchan 2014, vii–viii)

Though it is quite clear that Buchan is also promoting his *domestic* health guide, the irony is that his critique seems to be directed towards male practitioners only since eighteenth-century "physicians" were largely male. Buchan's advertisement condemns a monopolisation of medical knowledge, as secrecy only leads to quackery or medical malpractice. He thus calls for "openness" for the benefit of *man*kind. In the section "Of Childbirth," however, Buchan seems to criticise traditional knowledge represented especially by women. Interestingly, there is no mention whatsoever of traditional midwives involved in the birth process, although Buchan does argue for as little medical invention as possible by letting nature take its course: "Nature, if left to herself, will seldom fail to expel the *foetus*" (Buchan 2014, 567–568).

As soon as the birth becomes difficult, however, Buchan strongly suggests to call a "skilful surgeon," while erasing the female midwives' existence by simply not mentioning them (Buchan 2014, 569). What Buchan finds most problematic during the birth process is the "greatest number of attendants in child-bed," whose presence would significantly hinder the mother's recovery (Buchan 2014, 568):

> These directions [minimal intervention] are sufficient in natural labours, and in all preternatural cases, a skilful surgeon, or man-midwife, ought to be called as soon as possible. [...] We cannot help taking notice of that ridiculous custom which still prevails in some country places, of collecting a number of women together on such occasions. These, instead of being useful, serve only to crowd the house, and obstruct the necessary attendants. Besides, they hurt the patient with their noise; and often by their untimely and impertinent advice, do much mischief.
>
> (Buchan 2014, 569)

It is quite clear that Buchan here alludes to traditional (female) midwives, whom he ignores or erases by referring only to a "ridiculous custom" that he never specifies but that involves a "number of women." Furthermore, his insistence on calling a man-midwife as soon as things become difficult recalls William Smellie's suggestion mentioned in PART I of this book: In his medical handbooks, Smellie offers kind but no less patronising advice to rely on male assistance during difficult births, while at the same time recommending to show understanding for the "weakness of the sex" by correcting their (the midwives') 'mistakes' (Woods/Galley 2014, 186). It is thus safe to say that in their medical texts, both Buchan and Smellie display a paternalistic if not derogatory attitude towards traditional female midwives who seem to cause 'mischief' and whose 'mistakes' male practitioners must correct.

Buchan also blames women for childbed fever that, according to his guide, can be avoided during pregnancy through proper diet and exercise (Buchan 2014, 572–573). Hence, the potential mother is made solely responsible for her own and her child's wellbeing. This regime as part of 'hygienic motherhood' shifts accountability to females who, ironically, also seem to require constant supervision due to their reproductive power. Surprisingly, though *Domestic Medicine* suggests that birthing women should rely on male assistance that can also involve the use of instruments during difficult births, Buchan also advocates minimal intervention during parturition: "When the labour is coming on, it is not to be hastened with forcing medicines, which inflame the humours, or put them into unnatural commotions" (Buchan 2014, 573). Like Fenwick's *Secrecy*, therefore, Buchan's health guide remains relatively ambiguous with regard to ('proper') childbirth practices. What both texts – the novel and the medical guide – confirm, however, is the gendered power struggle between traditional and institutionalised knowledges that both fought for (material-) discursive power during the eighteenth century in Britain.

This subchapter ends by revisiting the notion of secrecy a final time. Read from a feminist viewpoint, it was not Sibella's secret actions that led to her death, but rather Mr Valmont's attempt to secretly create a, what he regards, perfect human being, thus aligning this character with another literary megalomaniac – Victor Frankenstein (see Burke 2009, 374). Both characters ultimately seek to control reproduction, albeit in different ways. Yet, the main problem of both patriarchs is that their offspring develop a free will that backfires on the creators. This book discusses Mary Shelley's *Frankenstein* in more detail in the final analysis chapter, but what can safely be said about Fenwick's female characters is that they represent remarkable examples of female agency. Already during Filmar's abduction attempts, Sibella faces his attacker with strength and self-confidence by denying him access to both her mind and her body: "Mark, Sir, […] Mr. Valmont may bring you here; may make this castle my prison; but my will is free. I tell you, Sir, I am beyond your reach. Remember it, I am beyond your reach" (*Secresy*, 229). As discussed, the novel's end is, to use Grundy's words, reformist rather than revolutionary. Not only is the ('unhygienic') mother erased by death, but before Sibella dies, she ultimately blames herself, thus confirming maternal ideologies: "My uncle's secrets could have done me but a temporary harm, it was mine own secrets [that] destroyed me – Oh that fatal contract!" (*Secresy*, 358).

Like the cyborg figure, Fenwick's novel remains ambiguous in its meaning. This, I argue, is one of the text's main strengths as it dissolves the boundaries between medicine, the material and the literary reproductive body – Fenwick's novel allows the female body to 'speak' and thus grants it agency. Ultimately, the narrative criticises not female but rather male secrecy by letting Sibella's female friend function as her voice. Caroline confronts Mr Valmont and sends him all the letters written between the two women and between Sibella and Arthur to demonstrate whose secrecy is actually to blame:

> I send you, Sir, a pacquet [sic] containing all the letters [...] for I think they will serve to convince you [that] artifice and secrecy are dangerous vicious tools. Your secrets were the preparatory steps to the errors of Clement and Sibella. Had Sibella never departed from strict truth and sincerity, she had never formed her rash engagement with Clement. Had [Arthur] Murden never (with his dangerous refinements of fancy) longed secretly to view this rare child of seclusion, he had not bartered his life and happiness for a sigh. And lastly, had I not given way to the *fatal mistake that secrecy could repair the inability of reason*, I had, instead of availing myself of the *ruin on the rock*, ere now perhaps released Sibella by convincing you. And we had all been comparatively happy.
>
> (emphasis added, *Secresy*, 336)

Notes

1 Fenwick eventually became Wollstonecraft's nurse during her illness in 1797, attended her friend until her death and took care of her baby, Mary Shelley, for a couple of days before her father Godwin sent for his daughter (Grundy 1998, 10).

2 Furthermore, like *Vindication, Secresy* equally highlights the (negative) implications of "class privilege [,] gender dependence" and the problem of property in the form of "hereditary wealth" and criticises class-related vanity in the characters of Caroline's mother, Mrs Ashburn, and Mr Valmont (Grundy 1998, 27–28).

3 The quotes' orthography is adjusted to modern English for reasons of readability.

References

Bowers, Toni. 2005. *The Politics of Motherhood: British Writing and Culture, 1680–1760.* Cambridge: Cambridge University Press.

Buchan, William. 2014. *Domestic Medicine, Or: The Family Physician.* Cambridge Library Collection. Cambridge: Cambridge University Press.

Burke, Meghan L. 2009. "Making Mothers Obsolete: Eliza Fenwick's *Secresy* and the Masculine Appropriation of Maternity." *Eighteenth Century Fiction* 21 (3): 357–384.

Cannon, Mercy. 2008. "Hygienic Motherhood: Domestic Medicine and Eliza Fenwick's *Secresy*." *Eighteenth-Century Fiction* 20 (4): 535–561.

Close, Anne. 2004. "Into the Public: The Sexual Heroine in Eliza Fenwick's *Secresy* and Mary Robinson's *The Natural Daughter*." *Eighteenth-Century Fiction* 17 (1): 35–52.

Emsley, Sarah. 1999. "Radical Marriage." *Eighteenth-Century Fiction* 11 (4): 477–498.

Furniss, Tom. 1992. "Wollstonecraft, Mary (1759–97)." In *A Handbook to English Romanticism*, edited by Jean Raimond and John Richard Watson, 284–288. Basingstoke: Macmillan.

Fenwick, Eliza. 1998. *Secresy*. Edited with an introduction by Isobel Grundy. Peterborough, ON: Broadview Press.

Grundy, Isobel. 1998. "Introduction." In *Secresy, Or: The Ruin on the Rock*, 2nd ed., edited by Eliza Fenwick and Isobel Grundy, 7–36. Broadview.

Gubar, Susan. 1994. "Feminist Misogyny: Mary Wollstonecraft and the Paradox of 'It Takes One to Know One.'" *Feminist Studies* 20 (3): 452–473.

Isaac, Janice A. 1999. "*Secresy, or: The Ruin on the Rock*." Review of *Secresy*, by Eliza Fenwick. *ESC: English Studies in Canada* 25 (1): 114–116.

Kipp, Julie. 2009. *Romanticism, Maternity, and the Body Politic*. Cambridge: Cambridge University Press.

Paul, Lissa. 2019. *Eliza Fenwick: Early Modern Feminist*. Newark: University of Delaware Press.

Porter, Roy. 2004. *Flesh in the Age of Reason*. London: Penguin.

Rousseau, Jean Jacques. [1789] 1969. *Oeuvres Completes*. Vol. 4. Ed. Pierre Burgelin. Paris: Gallimard.

Speck, William Arthur. 2016. "Social Structure, Class and Gender: 1770–1832." In *The Oxford Handbook of the Eighteenth-Century Novel*, edited by Alan Downie, 339–354. Oxford: Oxford University Press.

Todd, Janet. 1989. "Introduction." In *Secresy, Or: The Ruin on the Rock*, by Eliza Fenwick, vii-x. Norfolk/UK: Pandora.

Wollstonecraft, Mary. 2008. *A Vindication of the Rights of Men*. Edited with an introduction by Janet Todd. Oxford: Oxford University Press.

Wollstonecraft, Mary. 2009. *A Vindication of the Rights of Woman: An Authoritative Text, Backgrounds, and Contexts, Criticism*. Edited by Deidre S. Lynch. New York: Norton.

Wollstonecraft, Mary. 2009. *Mary, A Fiction*. Edited by Gary Kelly. Reissued. Oxford: Oxford University Press.

2.5 Mary Wollstonecraft's *Maria, Or: The Wrongs of Woman* (1798)

2.5.1 Introduction

Like *Secresy*, Mary Wollstonecraft's *Maria, Or: The Wrongs of Woman* (1798) can be regarded as a highly ambiguous novel. It touches on reproduction and female embodiment insofar as it criticises the 'horrors' of pregnancy and motherhood. It is this eighteenth-century text in particular that constructs reproduction as 'women's wrongs.' This chapter first offers a short introduction to the text (Kaplan 2002; Kelly 2009; Bergès 2013) before it continues with its context including selected aspects of Wollstonecraft's life, works and the world she was part of (Furniss 1992; Gubar 1994; Mellor 1996; Jones 1997; Kaplan 2009; Poovey 2009; Guralnick 2009; Bergès 2013; Sill 2016; Speck 2016; Benedict 2016; Schabert 2017). The final two sections proceed with a discussion of maternal metaphors and instances of female agency (Lanser 1992; Homans 1994; Conboy et al. 1997; Johnson 2002; Cooper 2004; Dolan 2008; Tegan 2011). This analysis chapter ends with the question of how the text int*ra*-links especially Jemima's (discursive) body with the (material) body on the eighteenth-century dissection table.[1]

Wollstonecraft is mostly known for her pivotal proto-feminist essay *A Vindication of the Rights of Woman* (1792), following her political pamphlet *A Vindication of the Rights of Men* (1790). What some readers do not know is that she also wrote reviews, conduct literature and novels. Others might remember her eventful life including her romantic relationships with the Swiss painter and writer Henry Fuseli, the US-American writer and officer Gilbert Imlay and their illegitimate child as well as her marriage with the British writer and political philosopher William Godwin. Most people recall her tragic death shortly after giving birth to her prominent daughter and later author of the Gothic masterpiece *Frankenstei*n, Mary Shelley. One of the reasons for the emphasis on her life experiences is the scholarly neglect of her work until the second half of the twentieth century. Until then, authors had predominantly focussed on her personal biography[2] at the expense of her oeuvre, including her fiction. It was not until the second-wave women's movement that Wollstonecraft was celebrated as a feminist "foremother" (Kaplan 2002, 253).

In fact, Wollstonecraft wrote two novels in addition to her political pieces, her first a quasi-autobiographical text titled *Mary, A Fiction* (1788), published shortly

DOI: 10.4324/9781003467977-10

before the French Revolution began in 1789, and her second purely fictional text *Maria, Or: The Wrongs of Woman* (1798), released towards the end of this revolutionary moment. *Wrongs* was also Wollstonecraft's final work as she died before the novel was finished. Her husband William published it posthumously. Both novels bear similarities in that they feature a female protagonist who is trapped in an unhappy marriage, engages in an affair and ends up either depressed, suicidal or dead. Yet, the two texts differ immensely in terms of their politics, which can be partly explained by their publication dates: They were written ten years apart and document Wollstonecraft's development from a governess, journalist and writer of fiction to a novelist, political philosopher and radical proto-feminist.

Wollstonecraft's *Wrongs* starts *in medias res* and revolves around the life story of the middle-class mother Maria Venables. Maria is married to an abusive husband who first abducts their only child and then imprisons her in a mental asylum. Maria thinks her daughter is dead and befriends a female ward, Jemima, to whom she tells her story. Later, Maria begins an affair with the inmate Henry Darnford and mainly communicates with him through letters. As the story progresses, the working-class Jemima also narrates her life stories to both Maria and Henry. These include her mother's early death, her experiences with starvation, violence, rape, an unwanted pregnancy, abortion, poverty, homelessness and prostitution. Maria then starts to write her memoirs for her presumed dead daughter addressing the subordinate status of women in society. *Wrongs'* final chapter remains incomplete and consists of two different endings, one describing Maria's escape from the asylum, followed by a miscarriage, Henry's unfaithfulness and her suicide, and the other allowing the distraught pregnant protagonist to be united with her child by the help of Jemima who imagines an alternative female family unit together.

The novel's structure is noteworthy for a variety of reasons. *Wrongs* begins with a "Preface," signed by William Godwin, that comments on the text's unfinished and fragmented nature, its many revisions and the announcement of the subsequent and equally unfinished preface. What follows are the "Author's Preface," 17 chapters of varying length as well as a short "Conclusion" consisting of two versions, the first divided into numbered sentences or even keywords only, and the second into paragraphs, all signed by William Godwin. The notion of fragmentation pervades the whole novel: Not only does the text start in the midst of things, but its characters frequently interrupt one another and the perspectives change repeatedly. Moreover, sentences remain unfinished and the narrator's relation to the protagonist is often antithetic (Kelly 2009, xxiii–xxv, xxix). Some modern readers might also be irritated by embodied (female) horrors the novel establishes from the beginning, only to then resort to overtly sentimental language, especially with regard to Maria and Henry's romantic relationship. Nevertheless, these interruptions enable a productive feminist discussion.

Contrary to Wollstonecraft's *Vindications*, *Wrongs*' reception was mixed, which was partly due to her husband. William published her final and unfinished novel in his *Posthumous Works of the Author of 'A Vindication of the Rights of Woman'* (1798) together with *Memoirs of the Author of A Vindication of the Rights of Woman* (1798), a biography of his late wife that rather concentrated on

Wollstonecraft's previous relationships with other men, her illegitimate child and her suicide attempts, thus contributing to her reputation as a tragic and "loose woman" that lasted until the twentieth century (Bergès 2013, 12–13). Scholarship did not accelerate until the 1980s and was equally mixed: While some authors criticised Wollstonecraft's emphasis on motherhood, her supposed "assault on female sexuality" and a dismissal of feminine desire in *Vindication of the Rights of Woman*, others recognised her work's significant impact on feminist movements (Poovey 1984, 74; Kaplan 2002, 258–259). Since the millennium, scholars like Janet Todd (2000), Ashley Tauchert (2002), Claudia L. Johnson (2002), Barbara Taylor (2003), Lyndall Gordon (2005) or Jane Moore (2012) have revisited Wollstonecraft's biography and rehabilitated this historically significant proto-feminist.

Today, scholarship has shifted its attention to newer concepts such as embodiment in conjunction with female sexuality, pregnancy and motherhood. Yet, Wollstonecraft's *Wrongs* remains under-analysed. The manageable amount of research on this novel so far has mainly focussed on questions of narration, genre, as well as (a critique of) *Wrongs*' overtly sentimental tone that counteracts the revolutionary ideas expressed in *A Vindication of the Rights of Woman*. Other established authors, however, have praised the novel for its ambiguity with regard to the displayed 'wrongs' that are done not only to women by men but also to women by women. The subsequent sections move beyond a discussion of *Wrongs*' aesthetic strategies and sharpen the focus on questions of womanhood by putting particular emphasis on reproduction and female embodiment. What follows is a discussion of *Wrongs'* body politics, pregnancy, the figure of the prostitute and abortion as female agency. The aim is to demonstrate how the material-discursive, fragmented female reproductive body not only manifests in but is rather entangled with the novel.

2.5.2 Wollstonecraft's Revolutions & Womanhood

In contrast to authors like Cleland or Fenwick, a significant amount of information is available about Mary Wollstonecraft's life and works. Though a concentration on her turbulent life had been the main reason for the neglect of her oeuvre until the twentieth century, it nevertheless makes sense to shed light on selected aspects of her biography in order to fully grasp her work's significance and her attitudes to gender issues, especially with regard to sexuality, pregnancy and motherhood. The following sections therefore focus on some of her challenging personal relationships, her 'unusual' profession, her often misunderstood stance on female sexuality, and most importantly, her revolutionary and radical body politics.

Though Wollstonecraft grew up in a middle-class family and did not experience the hardships of a working-class upbringing, she struggled with the burdens of living with a father addicted to alcohol and gambling. Edward John Wollstonecraft also abused her mother, Elizabeth Dixon, which is why Mary avoided marriage for a long time (Bergès 2013, 2–4). The first 'revolutionary' act she performed was to enter employment, first as a governess, then as a founder of a girls-only boarding school, and later as a journalist and writer of fiction for the well-known bookseller and publisher Joseph Johnson (Furniss 1992, 285). Wollstonecraft's 'revolution' was to fend for herself financially; she worked in positions that had hitherto been unprecedented for women due to their essentially non-existent citizenship. As W. A. Speck explains, women were legally not granted personhood but instead passed on as property, including potential wages, from their fathers to their husbands: Once married, pregnancy usually followed, and with motherhood came full financial dependency (Speck 2016, 347). Ina Schabert adds that the denial of women's legal status was paired with social anxieties about unrestrained female sexuality; these, however, must be read in light of major revolutions that occurred during this period, ranging from the French to the scientific to the commercial to the print revolution (Laqueur 2012, 808; Schabert 2017, 51).

While opponents of the revolution in France associated the country with uncontrolled female desire, monstrosity and prostitution, medicine equally contributed to the idea of dangerous female sexuality. As outlined in PART I of this book, by the end of the eighteenth century, science, anatomy and medicine had firmly established a clear hierarchical division between people's sex in terms of their biology that was, of course, entangled with their gender. Given that, according to medicine, the female orgasm was rendered unnecessary for reproduction, women were held fully responsible for their pregnancies, both in terms of their prevention and outcome. This, in combination with the increased access to reading materials due to the print revolution, enhanced the fear of unbridled female sexuality that could only be controlled through marriage. This book goes a step further by arguing that it was also medicine that sought to control reproduction by containing female sexuality, which resulted in an indivisible entanglement of matter, meaning, bodies and discourses.

Wollstonecraft's own life experiences and the fact that women were denied citizenship and thus personhood, while at the same time being 'imprisoned' in the domestic sphere through pregnancy and motherhood, all influenced her protofeminist work. Her first political pamphlet *A Vindication of the Rights of Men* (1790) was a radical response to Edmund Burke's defence of the British aristocracy and class system as well as his critique of the French Revolution. She later complemented this publication with her manifesto *A Vindication of the Rights of Woman* (1792): This essay argued for the equality of women who had been ignored by proponents of the revolution in France (Bergès 2013, xi, 4). As outlined in the previous chapter, Wollstonecraft also criticised Jean-Jacques Rousseau, whom she both admired for his general politics but disagreed with in terms of his depiction of women in *Émile* (1726).

Wollstonecraft especially challenged the gendered distinction between the (sexualised female) body and the (rational male) mind by arguing that women were equally capable of rational thinking (Gubar 1994, 454–455). In *Wrongs*, Wollstonecraft attempted to fictionalise the political statements she made in *A Vindications of the Rights of Woman* by focussing on the embodied plights of women, poor women in particular, that accompanied "[s]equential pregnancies, exhausting child care in the grimmest conditions," and the "double yoke of waged and unpaid domestic labour" (Kaplan 2009, 347). Both her *A Vindication of the Rights of Woman* and her unfinished novel *Wrongs* are therefore to be regarded as a call for a "complete transformation of society and the body politic" (Guralnick 2009, 316).

Unfortunately, many of Wollstonecraft's contemporaries were not able (or willing) to fully understand her statements about women and reduced her work to a demand for female education only. What she actually wanted to say, however, was not just that women should enjoy the same education as men, but that they should also reject their status as "insignificant object[s] of desire and as [essentially] desiring object[s]" that some misunderstood as an attack on or even condemnation of female sexuality (Kaplan 2009, 338). Unless proponents of a patriarchal society understood her main critique, women and their reproductive bodies would remain hostage to "sexuality, pregnancy, birth and motherhood," the roots of women's wrongs in her view (Poovey 2009, 357).

Wollstonecraft's works were influenced not only by her personal life experiences, (body) politics, changes in anatomy, medicine and the events of the French Revolution but also by eighteenth-century developments in literature and culture. As mentioned above, due to the print revolution those women who could read had access to an increasing number of literary products. For instance, the novel was regarded as a symptom of the French Revolution as it brought the autonomous individual to the fore. In this context, one particular literary mode reflected a gendered fear with regard to female sexuality and reproduction: sentimentalism (Benedict 2016, 356). Sentimental literature primarily celebrated strong feelings that led to emotional states of sentimentality and sensibility (Kaplan 2002, 248; see also Neumann/Schmidt-Haberkamp 2015, 140–141, 147). One has to consider, however, that the eighteenth-century term 'sentimentalism' did not imply the same negative connotations that it does today; rather, it was used to display a "longing after an imagined world [...] in which sympathy, benevolence and goodness are the predominant virtues" (Sill 2016, 426). Furthermore, als Neumann and Schmidt-Haberkamp emphasise, the new 'culture of sentimentalism' did not exclude rational thinking altogether – both modes completed each other and melded into a new definition of 'man,' including contemporary gender relations (Neumann/Schmidt-Haberkamp 2015, 141).

In this context, as older scholarship argues, early sentimental fiction's goal was also to control female sexuality by reinforcing the idea of proper female conduct as becomes clear by examples such as Samuel Richardson's *Pamela, Or: Virtue Rewarded* (1740). In this sentimental novel, the eponymous heroine's 'virtuous' (meaning chaste) behaviour – or rather successful resistance against her 'Master,' Mr B., and his attempted rape – is 'rewarded' in the end with marriage to said male character. This form of testing a young woman's virtue was a common characteristic of sentimental literature. Other topoi could also include the protagonists' abduction or the redemption of a poor prostitute who functioned as an "object of sentimental pity" (Jones 1997, 201, 202).

In *Wrongs*, Wollstonecraft utilised the sentimental mode to challenge the patriarchal idea that women's sexuality must be controlled either through reward or redemption (Mellor 1996, 418). In her unfinished novel, it is Jemima who literally and literarily embodies the figure of the poor prostitute who is forced to resort to this profession in order to survive. Wollstonecraft uses her main character as a means to comment on eighteenth-century contradicting discourses regarding female desire, reproduction (and the control thereof), sentimentalism and the general plights of womanhood of the time with the aim to evoke "actual social change" (Sill 2016, 438).

The following sections shift the focus from sentimentalism to reproduction and fragmentation that, I argue, are *Wrongs*' leitmotifs. In Wollstonecraft's novel, the 'wrongs of woman' manifest themselves in the female character's reproductive bodies: Maria is tormented by her husband and her daughter's assumed death, and Jemima is not only raped but also forced to perform an abortion. Moreover, Jemima's body is treated like a machine in the laundry or an object to be studied at the hospital. This form of dehumanisation recalls the fragmented female reproductive body on the eighteenth-century dissection table. Interestingly, the novel's narrative structure is entangled with this fragmentation as it is dismembered from the beginning: Not only is Maria's story narrated retrospectively but the other characters repeatedly interrupt one another, resulting in a constant change of perspectives.

The novel's tragic irony is that Jemima seeks to escape the physical threat of rape by resorting to prostitution. Wollstonecraft's prostitute figure can thus be read as the incarnated version of the mechanical woman who is sexualised, controlled and gazed at by (medical) men. As a result, *Wrongs* criticises not only women's social status in general, but in particular it demonstrates how social roles are entangled with the material conditions of women's bodily existence. Women seem to be primarily defined by their ability – or responsibility – to (re)produce (healthy) offspring. The next subchapter discusses in more detail the question of how the text int*ra*-links discourses of reproduction with contemporary medical bodies of knowledge. Though at first glance Wollstonecraft's novel seems quite futile in terms of female agency, at a second it does allow Jemima's body to 'act.' In fact, the novel suggests a way out of the lived bodily fate of pregnancy: Through abortion, Jemima not only refuses reproduction but reappropriates her body.

2.5.3 Maternal Metaphors & Embodied Horrors

While research on *Wrongs* still remains relatively scarce, those scholarly texts that deal with this novel predominantly focus on its aesthetic and narrative strategies, the meaning of its shifting perspectives or on Wollstonecraft's critique of sentimentalism (see Lanser 1992; Homans 1994; Tegan 2011). Mary B. Tegan, however, draws attention to how the text both challenges concepts of "conventional femininity" and also relentlessly unmasks the horrors of motherhood by utilising "too many maternal metaphors" (Tegan 2011, 358–361). The subsequent sections hence shift the focus to Wollstonecraft's use of maternal metaphors as well as the horrors of female embodiment that manifest themselves in the reproductive body. As Katie Conboy already argued in the late 1990s, in *Wrongs,* especially pregnancy, birth and motherhood define the female characters' "road to ruin" (Conboy et al. 1997, 15). It is (the power of) reproduction in particular that reinforces women's status as (embodied) property lacking personhood or citizenship (Conboy et al. 1997, 12).

Wollstonecraft's extensive use of maternal metaphors becomes apparent in the very first chapter. From the beginning, the text renders women's 'wrongs' a body problem in particular. Chapter I directly associates maternity with horror by using Gothic descriptions of motherhood. The heterodiegetic narrator starts *in medias res* to reconstruct Maria's story by situating her in the hostile environment of the asylum. Maria's prison is described as "ABODES OF HORROR" and a "mansion of despair" that 'scatters' the protagonist's (maternal) thoughts from the outset (spelling in the original, *Wrongs*, 69):

> [...] waking by degrees to a keen sense of anguish, a whirlwind of rage and indignation roused her torpid pulse. One recollection with frightful velocity following another, threatened to fire her brain, and make her a fit companion for the terrific inhabitants, whose groans and shrieks were no unsubstantial sound of whistling winds [...] but such tones of misery as carry a dreadful certainty directly to the heart. What effect must they then have produced on one, true to the touch of sympathy, and tortured by maternal apprehension.
>
> (*Wrongs*, 69)

Maria's "maternal apprehension" pertains to her daughter who, torn away by her husband when abducting and imprisoning his wife, she thinks is dead. The severity of her maternal anguish tortures Maria's mind to the extent that it materialises in, or *through*, her in her reproductive body:

> Her infant's image was continually floating on Maria's sight, and the first smile of intelligence remembered, as none but a mother, an unhappy mother, can conceive. She [...] felt the little twinkling fingers on her burning bosom– a bosom bursting with the nutriment for which this cherished child might now be pining in vain.
>
> (*Wrongs*, 69)

Maria's grief about the alleged death of her child is not only entangled with her aching maternal body, her "burning bosom" in particular, but – like Fenwick's Sibella – she at the same time also bemoans her infant's sex: "Still she mourned for her child, lamented she was a daughter, and anticipated the aggravated ills of life that her sex rendered almost inevitable, even while dreading she was no more" (*Wrongs*, 69). Later in the chapter, Maria is described as a "wretched mother" who asks herself if "not the world [was] a vast prison, and women born slaves?" (*Wrongs*, 73). By utilising a significant number of maternal metaphors, Wollstonecraft's text highlights not just the ill fate of mothers but of women in general who are doomed to exist in the prisons of their own reproductive bodies.

Chapter IX further illustrates the plight of female embodiment. Maria here reconstructs the unhappy marriage to George in her memoirs addressed to her daughter. She describes how she deeply regretted marrying her "tyrant," while outlining that it was especially her pregnancy that had led her to the realisation she was "caged for life" (*Wrongs*, 70, 127):

> Fatal error! How quickly is the so much vaunted milkiness of nature turned into gall, by an intercourse with the world [...]! One trait in my character was extreme credulity; but, when my eyes were once opened, I saw but too clearly all I had before overlooked. [...] While circumstances were ripening my faculties, [...] I could not sometimes help regretting my early marriage; and that, in my haste to escape from a temporary dependence, and expand my newly fledged wings, [...] I had been caught in a trap, and caged for life.
>
> (*Wrongs*, 127–128)

During her progressing pregnancy, Maria's husband not only drank and displayed inappropriate affection for other women, but she also describes humiliating sexual encounters she had to endure with George that further stress the horrors of female embodiment in *Wrongs*:

> He now seldom dined at home, and continually returned at a late hour, drunk, to bed. [...] I was glad [...] to escape from his; for personal intimacy without affection, seemed, to me the most degrading, as well as the most painful state in which a woman of any taste [...] could be placed. But my husband's fondness for women was of the grossest kind, and imagination was so wholly out of the question, as to render his indulgences of this sort entirely promiscuous, and of the most brutal nature. My health suffered, [...] but as a victim to the prejudices of mankind, who have made women the property of their husbands?
>
> (*Wrongs*, 129–130)

Shortly after these recollections, Maria realises that men of this sort tend to degrade women out of male anxiety: "Men who are inferior to their fellow men, are always anxious to establish their superiority over women" (*Wrongs*, 130). Furthermore, Maria's lived bodily experiences bear similarities with Jemima's later accounts of her work as a prostitute on the streets and in the brothel in chapter V:

> [...] taught to put on my rags to the best advantage, I was accosted from different motives, and yielded to the desire of the brutes I met, with the same detestation that I had felt for my still more brutal master. I had still read in novels of the blandishments of seduction, but I had not even the pleasure of being into vice. "I shall not," interrupted Jemima, "lead your imagination into all the scenes of wretchedness and depravity, which I was condemned to view; or mark the different stages of my debasing misery. Fate dragged me through the very kennels of society: I was still a slave, a bastard, a common property.
>
> (*Wrongs*, 98)

Both Maria and Jemima had to endure rape, both had to bear brutal and humiliating sexual encounters, and both characters are constructed as male property. By drawing these connections, the text merges marriage with prostitution (and slavery, though this comparison is rather misleading as outlined earlier), a link that *A Vindication of the Rights of Woman* equally establishes. In both novels and essays, women's reproductive bodies are rendered objects to be owned and controlled.

Wrongs is, in fact, saturated with examples of the appropriated female body. Not only is female sexuality contained through marriage, but Maria also recalls how George tried to sell her body to a male friend to whom he owned money. Yet, the text allows Maria to defend herself against the attempt and reconstructs how she spoke up to her husband:

> 'I continued, with solemnity, "I have borne with your tyranny and infidelities. I disdain to utter what I have borne with. [...] Neglected by you, I have resolutely stifled the enticing emotions, and respected the plighted faith you outraged. And you dare now to insult me, by selling me to prostitution! – Yes – equally lost to delicacy and principle – you dared sacrilegiously to barter the honour of the mother of your child."
>
> (quotation marks in the original, *Wrongs*, 143)

The text thus grants Maria a degree of agency by letting her use her voice to resist George's attempts to further appropriate her body. However, after she had escaped the marriage, she was chased down "like a felon" and came to the conclusion that "men would be men while the world stands" (*Wrongs*, 152). During her flight, Maria hid at her uncle's place where she gave birth to her child and recalls how she, "after the pains of child-bed," mourned the absence of a "respectable father," while trying to prevent her daughter's purity from being "sullied" by showering her with "maternal fondness" (*Wrongs*, 159). Maria continues to narrate how her despair increased after her uncle's death and further laments the plights of female embodiment:

> But, born a woman – and born to suffer, in endeavouring to repress my own emotions, I feel more acutely the various ills my sex are fated to bear – I feel that the evils they are subject to endure, degrade them so far below their oppressors, as almost to justify their tyranny; leading at the same time superficial reasoners to term that weakness the cause, which is only the consequence of short-sighted despotism.
>
> (*Wrongs*, 159–160)

The oppression of women is clearly entangled with female embodiment here. Maria further explains the "maternal anxiety" she experienced while, as a mother without protection of any sort, worrying that George would track them down and wrest her daughter from her (*Wrongs*, 160). Wollstonecraft's novel thus renders embodied motherhood a particularly traumatic experience. Yet, Maria finds comfort in

Jemima, who is deeply moved by her friend's "tears of maternal tenderness" and "sufferings" as a "wretched mother" (*Wrongs*, 73). Due to her own life stories, Jemima can relate to the status of an "outcast from society" who is "hunted from hole to hole" like a "beast of prey, or infected with a moral plague" (*Wrongs*, 73). As a result, both characters merge into one body – they simultaneously represent the figure of the prostitute, whose material-discursive body is objectified and controlled by male society.

After listening to Maria's life story, Jemima begins to narrate her own and starts with the "misfortune of her birth," being born into a family that neglected her from the outset:

> An insulated being, [...] she despised and preyed on the society by which she had been oppressed, and loved not her fellow-creatures, because she had never been beloved. No mother had ever fondled her, not father or brother had protected her from outrage; and the man who had plunged her into infamy, and deserted her when she stood in greatest need of support, deigned not to smooth with kindness the road to ruin. Thus degraded, she was let loose on the world; and virtue, never nurtured by affection, assumed the stern aspect of selfish independence.
>
> (*Wrongs*, 75)

Again, Maria and Jemima share the fate of finding themselves in emotionally and physically degrading relationships that lead them to their own particular "road to ruin." Especially Jemima bears similarities with another well-known literary character who is born into a problematic family constellation, experiences substantial parental neglect in a moment of "greatest need of support" and is "let loose on the world" without ever having learnt how to love or be loved – Victor Frankenstein's progeny, the Creature.

Moreover, Mary Shelley's Creature represents the embodiment of a fragmented identity. The motif of fragmentation in *Wrongs*, however, mainly manifests itself on the level of narration: While the two female characters share their life stories, they constantly interrupt one another to express their compassion and thus fragment the plot line: "for she [Jemima] would listen to her with earnestness, and then suddenly interrupt the conversation, as if afraid of resigning, by giving way to her sympathy, her dear-brought knowledge of the world" (*Wrong*s, 75). Though this narrative strategy is part of the sentimental mode, it changes into a kind if *un*sentimentalism due to the (embodied) horrors the narrative revolves around (Dolan 2008, 201). Wollstonecraft's strategy is therefore not to simply trigger sympathy in the reader who shall be moved by the women's life stories and their empathy for one another – her aim is rather to demonstrate the embodied plight of female embodiment by illustrating the horrors of marriage and prostitution that culminate in pregnancy and motherhood.

Despite the novel's horror stories and its radical feminist potential, it has been criticised by both feminist scholars and readers for the representation of Maria's naïve romance with the inmate Henry Darnford. Regardless of her previous experiences, Maria blindly trusts Henry and expresses her love for him in overtly sentimental language. Henry, on the other hand, openly reflects on the inferiority of those women he met during his many travels abroad. Some of them bored him to the extent that he was forced to make "downright love to them" to avoid falling asleep (*Wrongs*, 87). Surprisingly, Maria's affection is not impaired by Henry's "fancy for prostitutes" he writes to her about (Johnson 2002, 204):

> I will not disgust you with a recital of the vices of my youth, which can scarcely be comprehended by female delicacy. I was taught to love by a creature I am ashamed to mention, and the other women with whom I afterwards became intimate, were of a class of which you can have no knowledge. I formed my acquaintance with them at the theatres; and, when vivacity danced in their eyes, I was not easily disgusted by the vulgarity which flowed from their lips.
>
> (*Wrongs*, 85–86)

One might argue in this case that Henry only values these women for their bodies since he expresses a degree of disgust regarding their (verbal) vulgarity and especially class that, however, does not keep him from becoming "intimate" with them. Henry appropriates these women's bodies in a way that bears resemblance to the general appropriation of wives by their husbands who disregard their minds and 'domesticate' their bodies. Henry therefore echoes the character George, Maria's first husband, who likewise sought to control her (reproductive) body.

Wrongs' tragic irony is Maria's inability to recognise Henry's true character until she escapes. Yet, the fact that her new spouse tends to be equally misogynist does not reduce her wish to marry him:

> With Darnford she did not taste uninterrupted felicity; there was a volatility in his manner which often distressed her; but love gladdened the scene; besides, he was the most tender, sympathizing creature in the world. [...] Marriage, as at present constituted, she considered as leading to immorality – yet, [...] she wished to avow her affection to Darnford, by becoming his wife [...].
>
> (*Wrongs*, 169)

Nevertheless, the text grants Maria a degree of agency when she later insists in court, to which she has to defend herself against committing adultery, that she freely entered into a relationship with Henry:

> I voluntarily gave myself, [...] While no command of a husband can prevent a woman from suffering for certain crimes, she must be allowed to consult her conscience, and regulate her conduct, in some degree, by her own sense of right.
>
> (*Wrongs*, 172)

Though the novel allows Maria to claim her right as an individual by choosing her romantic partner, which enables her to refuse the status of embodied property, her newfound autonomy is soon thwarted by the (male) judge. He laments the "fallacy of letting women plead their feelings" that he regards as an "excuse for the violation of the marriage-vow" (*Wrongs*, 174):

> We did not want French principles in public or private life – and, if women were allowed to plead their feelings, as an excuse or palliation of infidelity, it was opening a flood-gate for immorality. What virtuous woman thought of her feelings? – It was her duty to love and obey the man chosen by her parents and relations, who were qualified by their experience to judge better for her, than she could for herself.
>
> (*Wrongs*, 174)

Obviously, the judge's worldview evokes cynicism since it was George's inhumane and especially promiscuous behaviour that drove Maria away. The same holds true for Jemima whose 'road to ruin' was caused by the men who exploited, raped, impoverished and drove her into prostitution. The novel's first 'conclusion' ends in a similarly bleak manner. Yet, though the end implies there is no way out of the horrors of female embodiment, it does leave room for female agency by suggesting a particularly drastic measure to escape the plights of pregnancy and motherhood – abortion.

2.5.4 Gender, Class & Abortion as Agency

Wollstonecraft's *Wrongs* not only addresses the burden of female embodiment in general – it also intersects questions of gender and reproduction with those of class. Poverty plays a major role in this text. Jemima is not just a woman but also belongs to the poor working class. This is important to note as her social background significantly influences her bodily fate. In chapter V, Jemima narrates her own life story and begins with her mother who, as a young servant, was seduced by her master who had promised to marry her. Shortly after the affair began, Jemima's mother "perceived the dreaded consequence [...] that she was ruined" (*Wrongs*, 92). Due to her immense fear of shame with regard to her pregnancy, her mother pressured Jemima's father to fulfil his promise by marrying her. He refused and developed a strong antipathy towards his servant and her unborn child: "he [thereupon] began to hate, as well as despise me [Jemima], before I was born" (*Wrongs*, 92).

In response, Jemima's mother attempted suicide by starving herself to death. The attempt failed and she continued her hard work as a maid in her master's house until she died in the attic during "pangs of labour," while the father and his wife "felt no sympathy for the poor wretch" (*Wrongs*, 92). After her mother's death, Jemima was given to "the cheapest nurse" her father could find (*Wrongs*, 92). The nurse housed as many foster children as possible but focussed on the wellbeing of her own child, thus neglecting her and the others (*Wrongs*, 92). The narrator makes

Jemima's class-based life experiences particularly responsible for her character development:

> 'Poverty, and the habit of seeing children die off her hands, has so hardened her heart, that the office of a mother did not awake the tenderness of a woman; nor were the feminine caresses which seem a part of the rearing of a child, ever bestowed on me. […] Left in dirt, to cry with cold and hunger till I was weary, […] could I be expected to become any thing but a weak and ricket babe? Still, in spite of neglect, I continued to exist, to learn to curse existence' […].
>
> (quotation marks in the original, *Wrongs*, 92–93)

Wrongs not only blames class and poverty for Jemima's fate but this example also points to Wollstonecraft's critique of female solidarity or rather the lack thereof that is repeated in the course of the text. Tragically, her mother's life experiences recurred when Jemima, also working as a housemaid at the age of 16, was raped by her employer, leaving her pregnant or, in other words, imprisoned in her reproductive body: "I discovered, with horror – ah! what horror! that I was with child" (*Wrongs*, 96). However, the female reproductive body in *Wrongs* poses a threat not only to Jemima's existence but also to that of male characters, albeit to a different extent.

When Jemima's master, who was also an alcoholic, discovered her unwanted pregnancy, he only "feared his wife and public censure," while he continued to rape the girl (*Wrongs*, 96). After a few weeks, he gave her some "medicine in a phial" to abort the pregnancy, but Jemima refused at first:

> He cursed me for a fool, and left me to my own reflections. I could not resolve to take this infernal potion; but I wrapped it up in an old gown, and hid it in a corner of my box.
>
> (*Wrongs*, 96)

The text also criticises the lack of female solidarity when her master's wife, after catching her husband raping Jemima, threw her out of the house, leaving her penny- and homeless.

Jemima, however, is allowed bodily agency when she, after confronting her master who offered "to get a nurse for the brat [she] laid to him," decided to eventually terminate the pregnancy by swallowing the medicine he had previously given to her:

> I hurried back to my hole, and, rage giving place to despair, sought for the potion that was to procure abortion, and swallowed it, with a wish that it might destroy me, at the same time that it stopped the sensations of new-born life, which I felt with indescribable emotion. My head turned round, my heart grew sick, and in the horrors of approaching dissolution, mental anguish was swallowed up. The effect of the medicine was violent and I was confined to

> my bed several days; but, youth and a strong constitution prevailing, I once more crawled out, to ask myself the cruel question, "Whither should I go?"
>
> (*Wrongs*, 98)

Though this scene constructs pregnancy as a plight, especially for poor women, it nevertheless proposes a way out of the prison of motherhood many eighteenth-century women had to face. By aborting her pregnancy, Jemima refused reproduction and thus reappropriated her body, which lent her a certain degree of agency. As she continues to tell her friend Maria, she remained confronted with poverty and homelessness. In order to survive she was forced to first wander the streets as a prostitute, "[d]etesting her occupation," and then "accept[ed] a place in a house of ill fame" to escape the brutal "watchmen" who hunted down women engaged in this profession, harassed and treated them like "outlaws of society" (*Wrongs*, 98–99). The 'fall' from one desolate state into the next is the novel's real tragedy and resonates with the very real material living conditions of many poor eighteenth-century women.

Wollstonecraft's *Wrongs* further entangles class with medicine. Jemima continues her story and tells Maria about the time she worked as a washerwoman for a family that "cast [her] aside as the filth of society" (*Wrongs*, 103). The text describes how Jemima, "[c]ondemned to labour," was forced to work "like a machine, only to earn bread, and scarcely that" (*Wrongs*, 103–104). When she seriously injured her shin one day and needed to be admitted to hospital, she struggled to pay the required admittance fee, including a "security for burying" her (*Wrongs*, 105). With the help of her poor landlady and the family that hired her, she finally gained access to this space usually reserved for the "rich and respectable" (*Wrongs*, 105). She describes the way she was treated in this medical environment as follows:

> I cannot give you an adequate idea of the wretchedness of an hospital; every thing is left to the care of people intent on gain. The attendants seem to have lost all feeling of compassion in the bustling discharge of their offices; death is so familiar to them, that they are not anxious to ward it off. Every thing appeared to be conducted for the accommodation of the medical men and their pupils, who came to make experiments on the poor, for the benefit of the rich. […] After my dismission, I was more at a loss than ever […], I began to consider the rich and poor as natural enemies, and became a thief from principle.
>
> (*Wrongs*, 105)

This scene demonstrates the entanglement of gender, class, medicine and the body. The hospital's interior is as wretched as Jemima's treatment by the attendants as well as the "medical men and their pupils"; they use the bodies of the poor for their experiments, not for the benefit of humankind but for the "benefit of the rich." Wollstonecraft also allows her character to give an explanation for becoming a thief, which in this case is a result of her treatment as a poor working-class patient in the hospital who learns to despise the rich as well as the poor. Ultimately, Jemima is rendered an object to be investigated by (unsympathetic) 'rational' physicians, this scene representing a prime example of the Foucauldian medical gaze. This recalls the examination of the female reproductive body by obstetricians, either on the dissection table or in the birth room. In conclusion, when discussing material-discursive entanglements of the female reproductive body in terms of general medical treatment but also prostitution or pregnancy, one has to consider other categories as well. The goal should be an intersectional analysis that int*ra*-links gender with class, for example. In the case of Jemima, it is especially her status as a poor working-class woman that eventually forces her to abort her pregnancy.

In fact, as Christine Cooper explains, the abortion motif is *Wrongs'* driving force: As a synonym for 'failure,' it refers not only to aborted pregnancies but also to institutional miscarriages, for "reproductive failure acts as evidence of larger institutional and ideological failures" (Cooper 2004, 739). Put another way, Wollstonecraft's text utilises the abortion motif to criticise the oppressive reproductive logic of her time. This critique also manifests itself on the level of narration as most of the novel's (maternal) acts and narrative processes are either interrupted or misunderstood (Cooper 2004, 739). In this context, Maria's memoirs represent the novel's greatest failure. Though addressed to her daughter, Henry reads everything the novel's readers have also read about Maria's life stories and the 'wrongs of woman' – but he learns nothing. As Cooper concludes, Henry eventually morphs into the "replication of Maria's husband" by cheating on and forsaking her while pregnant (Cooper 2004, 774). The abortion motif takes particular effect in the novel's unfinished and fragmented ending. Here, it not only serves as a final challenge towards patriarchal ideology, but it can also be read as a critique of medicine's attempt to erase the mother. This, in turn, leaves room for bodily agency.

Both versions of the novel's fragmented "Conclusion" that were written "by the editor" William Godwin are characterised by notions of reproduction, abortion, death and birth (*Wrongs*, 175, 178). In the first short version, Maria is "[o]nce more pregnant," separates from Henry, and "[f]inds herself again with child" (*Wrongs*, 176). This version ends with the entry "Divorced by her husband – Her lover unfaithful – Pregnancy – Miscarriage – Suicide" (*Wrongs*, 176). The second, slightly longer version commences with the information that Maria had "swallowed the laudanum [...] to escape from this hell of disappointment" but to no avail:

> 'Still her eyes closed not – one remembrance with frightful velocity followed another – All the incidents of her life were in arms, embodied to assail her, and prevent her sinking into the sleep of death. – Her murdered child again appeared to her, mourning for the babe of which she was the tomb. [...] "this cannot last long; and what is a little bodily pain to the pangs I have endured?"
> (quotation marks in the original, *Wrongs*, 176)

Maria attempts suicide because she still thinks her daughter is dead, but the horrific memories of her experiences keep her from succeeding – they are literally "embodied" to the extent that the text renders Maria's womb a "tomb" for her assumed dead child, thus adhering to the Gothic mode by merging life with death.

In terms of reproduction, Cooper calls Wollstonecraft's *Wrongs* a "fetus-text" as it also refers to the eighteenth-century novel that was "still gestating" at the time (Cooper 2004, 760, 778). I wish to go one step further and argue that especially the novel's fragmented ending, consisting of two versions, not only amalgamates birth, death and the female reproductive body but can equally be read as an example of cyborgian agency.

Following this interpretation, it is possible to conceptualise Maria's body as a cyborg body since she is, from the narrative's very beginning, metaphorically speaking neither alive nor dead in the 'abodes of horror' she finds herself in. In chapter IV, Maria describes the asylum as a "tomb of living death," thus rendering her own body a 'living dead' one, blurring the boundaries between life and death, health and pathology (*Wrongs*, 91). Furthermore, the novel begins and ends with Maria's 'maternal apprehensions' that frame the narrative. The two endings, however, simultaneously render Maria dead and alive: She succeeds and does not succeed in committing suicide. Her body both 'aborts' a foetus ("miscarriage"), and she learns from Jemima that her presumed dead daughter is alive. In the second version, Maria is literally "restored to life," while her child, saved by Jemima, is equally "alive again" (*Wrongs*, 177). The second version's final sentence belongs to Maria who exclaims: "The conflict is over! – I will live for my child!" (*Wrongs*, 177).

Not only does this ending display female solidarity by positioning Jemima as Maria's saviour, but taken together, the two different versions also allow for a reconceptualisation of Maria's body as a cyborg body that blurs the boundaries between life and death, pregnancy and abortion. In fact, both Maria's and Jemima's bodies bear cyborgian potential – Maria's body through the entanglement of womb and tomb, and Jemima's body through her othered status as a poor working-class woman who is forced to work 'like a machine' to survive. Both female reproductive bodies in Wollstonecraft's *Wrongs* succumb to objectified and sexualised machines controlled by material-discursive patriarchal power structures from domestic work to medicine to prostitution. Apart from abortion as a possible way out of the bodily prison of motherhood, the text also proposes another option – female solidarity. When Jemima returns Maria's long-lost child and asks "would you leave her alone in the world, to endure what I have endured," she eventually replies that she will continue to live for her daughter's sake (*Wrongs*, 177).

To conclude, with *Wrongs*, Wollstonecraft sought to fictionalise the radical proto-feminist politics she had expressed in *A Vindication of the Rights of Woman* to reach a broader (female) audience. The unfinished novel criticises the patriarchal concept of sentimentalism that also aimed at controlling female sexuality and thus reproduction through reward or redemption. The text's fragmented structure as well as the many interrupted, failed or 'aborted' life stories, however, fulfil various functions: On the one hand, the abortion motif offers a way out of the bodily plights of motherhood and also renders the body 'active,' and on the other hand, the novel's fragmentation points to the incomplete identity of women during the eighteenth century who were, legally speaking, not granted personhood. On a metaphorical level, women therefore represented both persons and non-persons, humans and non-humans, the living and the non-living, just like the maternal body on the physician's dissection table. The novel's two endings, however, both erase and do not erase the mother. It is this ambiguity that poses the greatest feminist potential against the backdrop of reproduction.

Last but not least, Jemima's accounts in *Wrongs* emphasise the particular and very real bodily fates of many poor eighteenth-century women who could often only escape physical harassment by sexualising and objectifying their own bodies as a means of survival. In Jemima's case, the text makes both poverty and women's lack of citizenship responsible for this dilemma. Hence, the prostitute Jemima represents the incarnation of the mechanical woman as sexualised object who works 'like a machine' and is controlled by men. While *Wrongs* constructs motherhood as the ultimate imprisonment, it also leaves room for hope. Both Maria and Jemima can be conceptualised as mechanical beings, as cyborgs that blur boundaries between life and death, pregnancy and abortion but also between classes. Especially their female solidarity towards one another merges their bodies into one productive monster that has the power to disrupt divisions between gender, class, medicine and reproduction and thus criticise the very material-discursive structures they are themselves entangled with.

Notes

1 Parts of this chapter are based on results I also discuss in a corresponding handbook contribution (see Henke 2022).

2 See, for instance, Margaret George's *One Woman's "Situation": A Study of Mary Wollstonecraft* (1970) and Claire Tomalin's *The Life and Death of Mary Wollstonecraft* (1974) or Lyndall Gordon's *Vindication* (2005).

References

Benedict, Barbara M. 2016. "'Male' and 'Female' Novels? Gendered Fictions and the Reading Public, 1770–1832." In *The Oxford Handbook of the Eighteenth-Century Novel*, edited by James Alan Downie, 355–371. Oxford: Oxford University Press.

Bergès, Sandrine. 2013. *The Routledge Guidebook to Wollstonecraft's A Vindication of the Rights of Woman*. London: Routledge.

Conboy, Katie, Nadia Medina, and Sarah Stanbury, eds. 1997. *Writing on the Body: Female Embodiment and Feminist Theory*. New York: Columbia University Press.

Cooper, Christine M. 2004. "Reading the Politics of Abortion: Mary Wollstonecraft Revisited." *Eighteenth-Century Fiction* 16 (4): 735–782.

Dolan, Elizabeth A. 2008. *Seeing Suffering in Women's Literature of the Romantic Era*. Aldershot; Burlington, VT: Ashgate.

Furniss, Tom. 1992. "Wollstonecraft, Mary (1759–97)." In *A Handbook to English Romanticism*, edited by Jean Raimond and John Richard Watson, 284–288. Basingstoke: Macmillan.

Gordon, Lyndall. 2005. *Vindication: A Life of Mary Wollstonecraft*. New York: Harper.

Gubar, Susan. 1994. "Feminist Misogyny: Mary Wollstonecraft and the Paradox of 'It Takes One to Know One.'" *Feminist Studies* 20 (3): 452–473.

Guralnick, Elissa S. 2009. "Radical Politics in Mary Wollstonecraft's A Vindication of the Rights of Woman." In Mary Wollstonecraft, *A Vindication of the Rights of Woman: An Authoritative Text, Backgrounds, and Contexts, Criticism*, edited by Deidre S. Lynch, 309–319. New York: Norton.

Henke, Jennifer S. 2022. "Mary Wollstonecraft, *Maria: or, The Wrongs of Woman* (1798)." In *Handbook of the British Novel in the Long Eighteenth Century*, edited by Katrin Berndt and Alessa Johns, 449–466. Berlin; Boston, MA: De Gruyter.

Homans, Margaret. 1994. "Feminist Fictions and Feminist Theories of Narrative." *Narrative* 2 (1): 3–16.

Johnson, Claudia L., ed. 2002. *The Cambridge Companion to Mary Wollstonecraft*. Cambridge: Cambridge University Press.

Jones, Vivien. 1997. "Placing Jemima: Women Writers of the 1790s and the Eighteenth-Century Prostitution Narrative." *Women's Writing* 4 (2): 201–220.

Kaplan, Cora. 2002. "Mary Wollstonecraft's Reception and Legacies." In *The Cambridge Companion to Mary Wollstonecraft*, edited by Claudia L. Johnson, 246–270. Cambridge: Cambridge University Press.

Kaplan, Cora. 2009. "From *Wild Nights: Pleasure/Sexuality/Feminism*." In Mary Wollstonecraft. *A Vindication of the Rights of Woman: An Authoritative Text, Backgrounds, and Contexts, Criticism*, edited by Deidre S. Lynch, 335–349. New York: Norton.

Kelly, Gary. 2009. "Introduction." In *Mary and The Wrongs of Woman*, by Mary Wollstonecraft. Oxford World's Classics. Oxford: Oxford University Press.

Laqueur, Thomas W. 2012. "The Rise of Sex in the Eighteenth Century: Historical Context and Historiographical Implications." *Signs: Journal of Women in Culture and Society* 37 (4): 802–813.

Lanser, Susan S. 1992. *Fictions of Authority: Women Writers and Narrative Voice*. Ithaca, NY: Cornell University Press.

Mellor, Anne K. 1996. "Righting the Wrongs of Woman: Mary Wollstonecraft's *Maria*." *Nineteenth-Century Contexts* 19: 413–424.

Moore, Jane. 2012. *Mary Wollstonecraft*. Farnham: Ashgate.

Neumann, Birgit and Barbara Schmidt-Haberkamp, eds. 2015. *Emotionen, Wissen und Aufklärung: Gefühlskulturen im Großbritannien des 18. Jahrhunderts/Emotions, Knowledge and Enlightenment: Cultures of Emotion in 18th-Century Britain*. Ed. by Carsten Zelle. Special Issue *Das 18. Jahrhundert* 39 (2).

Poovey, Mary. 2009. "*A Vindication of the Rights of Woman* and Female Sexuality." In Mary Wollstonecraft. *A Vindication of the Rights of Woman*, edited by Deidre S. Lynch, 349–363. New York: Norton.

Richardson, Samuel. [1740] 2008. *Pamela: Or, Virtue Rewarded*. Edited by Thomas Keymer and Alice Wakely. Oxford World's Classics. Oxford: Oxford University Press.

Schabert, Ina. 2017. "Gender and Class." In *Handbook of British Romanticism*, edited by Ralf Haekel, 49–66. Berlin; Boston, MA: De Gruyter.

Sill, Geoffrey. 2016. "Developments in Sentimental Fiction." In *The Oxford Handbook of the Eighteenth-Century Novel*, edited by Alan Downie, 426–439. Oxford: Oxford University Press.

Speck, William Arthur. 2016. "Social Structure, Class and Gender: 1770–1832." In *The Oxford Handbook of the Eighteenth-Century Novel*, edited by Alan Downie, 339–354. Oxford: Oxford University Press.

Tauchert, Ashley. 2002. *Mary Wollstonecraft and the Accent of the Feminine*. Basingstoke; New York: Palgrave.

Taylor, Barbara. 2003. *Mary Wollstonecraft and the Feminine Imagination*. Cambridge: Cambridge University Press.

Tegan, Mary Beth. 2011. "Mocking the Mothers of the Novel: Mary Wollstonecraft, Maternal Metaphor, and the Reproduction of Sympathy." *Studies in the Novel* 42 (4): 357–376.

Tomalin, Claire. 2012. *The Life and Death of Mary Wollstonecraft*. London: Penguin.

Todd, Janet. 1989. "Introduction." In *Secresy, Or: The Ruin on the Rock*, by Eliza Fenwick, vii-x. Pandora.

Todd, Janet. 2000. *Mary Wollstonecraft: A Revolutionary Life*. London: Phoenix Press.

Wollstonecraft, Mary. [1790] 2008. *A Vindication of the Rights of Men*. Edited with an introduction by Janet Todd. Oxford: Oxford University Press.

Wollstonecraft, Mary. 2009. *A Vindication of the Rights of Woman: An Authoritative Text, Backgrounds, and Contexts, Criticism*. Edited by Deidre S. Lynch. New York: Norton.

Wollstonecraft, Mary. [1792] 2009. *Mary and the Wrongs of Woman*. Edited with an introduction by Gary Kelly. Oxford: Oxford University Press.

2.6 Mary Shelley's *Frankenstein, Or: The Modern Prometheus* (1818)

2.6.1 Introduction

Mary Shelley's *Frankenstein, Or: The Modern Prometheus* (1818) concludes the analysis section and represents both the initial spark of this book as well as the place where almost all of the above-mentioned aspects come together, from science to secrets to the reproductive body to obstetrics to cyborgism. This chapter not only revisits both traditional as well as selected newer scholarship on this literary masterpiece (Bewell 1988; Rauch 1995; Cody 2008; Francus 2012; Gilbert/Gubar [1979] 2012; Hunter 2012, 2022; Lieske 2012; Moers [1974] 2012, [1974] 2022; Mangham/Depledge 2012; Sommers 2012; Buchan 2014; Buckley 2017; Kitson 2017; Cook 2022) – it also turns to an extended in-depth (re)reading of the text. The following sections first introduce the novel and discuss its entanglement with the material-discursive culture of obstetrics and end with the conclusion that the greatest threat to both Victor Frankenstein and the field of obstetrics is the loss of power over reproduction. In *Frankenstein*, the Creature's fragmented, half-dead body functions as a critique of contemporary obstetric practices. Last but not least, the novel dismembers the female reproductive body by tearing the Creature's companion into pieces, thus int*ra*-linking it with the eighteenth-century maternal body on the anatomist's dissection table.[1]

As the English scholar Alan Rauch already acknowledged in the 1990s: "New perspectives on *Frankenstein* are hard to come by" (Rauch 1995, 1). J. Paul Hunter added in the 2010s that Mary Shelley's *Frankenstein, Or: The Modern Prometheus* has become an integral part of the canon as one of the most studied texts in literary and cultural studies (Hunter 2012, ix). In the 2020s, Daniel Cook stated that *Frankenstein* still "takes a prominent place in the upper echelons of the European canon" (Cook 2022, 539). In the newest Norton edition of 2022, Hunter confirms that *Frankenstein* is still "one of the world's most popular, widely read, thoroughly studied, and celebrated novel" (Hunter 2022, vii). Nevertheless, the narrative's persistent popularity is quite surprising given its difficult 'birth' and reception: "*Frankenstein* was not an immediate hit" and had to overcome some hurdles with regard to its publication as both publishers and booksellers initially rejected it (Cook 2022, 551).

DOI: 10.4324/9781003467977-11

The novel's reception was equally mixed; while some reviewers celebrated it, others criticised the narrative for its blasphemy and lack of morals (Cook 2022, 551). Eventually, *Frankenstein* gained broad popularity due to its first adaptation to the stage, Richard B. Peake's *Presumption, Or: The Fate of Frankenstein* (1823). This highly successful production resulted in a second, though "heavily revised," edition of *Frankenstein* in 1831 that was sold multiple times with several reprints until the late 1840s and cemented the novel's popularity (Cook 2022, 551). "By 1831, Frankenstein had become a household name" that further inspired countless adaptations, ranging from James Whale's *Bride of Frankenstein* (1935) to Haifaa al-Mansour's *Mary Shelley* (2017), to name only a few (Cook 2022, 551–552).

Despite or rather because of its pronounced canonicity, the novel is superbly suited for a critical reading of the history of childbirth, obstetrics and reproduction. Needless to say, most readers associate the novel's title with monstrosity, either with regard to the 'monstrous' Creature Victor Frankenstein stitched together from dead body parts, or in terms of the megalomaniac scientist himself, who does not anticipate his action's consequences. Frankenstein engages in 'monstrous science' and attempts to make a human being, only to cruelly reject his 'monstrous' progeny, which thereupon turns on its ambitious and obsessed creator. As J. Paul Hunter sums up, the name Frankenstein has become an "all-purpose watchword for creativity gone wrong and monstrosity gone wild" (Hunter 2012, xi, 2022, ix). But what role exactly does monstrosity play in Shelley's Gothic narrative against the backdrop of science and reproduction? How are medicine, maternity and the monstrous int*ra*-linked through this text?

To begin with, it is entirely possible to read Shelley's *Frankenstein* as a birth narrative. Ellen Moers is one of the first scholars to interpret the narrative as a "birth myth" or "trauma of the *after*birth" (emphasis in the original, Moers 2012, 319, 321; see also Moers 2022, 462–463). In her pivotal essay on the female Gothic, she argues that *Frankenstein* not only serves as a, in Cook's words, "sublimated confession of the author's perceived failure of giving birth," but also as a critique of medicine; Shelley blamed the obstetricians for not treating her mother correctly who died only a few days later after giving birth to her daughter (Cook 2022, 552; see also Moers 2012, 325, 2022, 468).

Against this background, Alan Bewell even regards *Frankenstein* as a "cautionary obstetric tale" since the novel extensively draws on this scientific discourse (Bewell 1988, 8). The cruel neglect of the Creature's body on the dissection table by the scientist Victor can therefore be read as an analogy to the treatment of the pregnant body by the field of obstetrics, which viewed the female patient not as a living and feeling subject but rather as a conglomerate of inert body parts. In addition, Sandra M. Gilbert and Susan Gubar agree that the language Shelley uses to describe, for instance, the Creature's animation during the doctor's "midnight labours" in his "workshop of filthy creation" also evokes images of Victor's metaphorical pregnancy and (painful) parturition (Gilbert/Gubar 2012, 336; *Frankenstein*, 36).

Reproduction, or rather the control thereof, is thus central to the narrative and entangles a multitude of material-discursive bodies of knowledge, from pregnancy to childbirth to obstetrics to Shelley's own biography. Regarding the latter, connections "between authorship and gender" prompted further feminist scholars such as Barbara Johnson (1982), Mary Poovey (1984) or Anne Mellor (1988) to explore this link (Cook 2022, 552). In general, Shelley's *Frankenstein* has been and still is a popular research object for a variety of scholarly fields, ranging from postcolonial studies (Spivak 1985), psychoanalysis (e.g. Mulvey-Roberts 2000), posthumanism (e.g. Mossmann 2001), queer studies (e.g. Rigby 2009) to ecocriticism (e.g. Morton 2016) (Cook 2022, 552).

This book, however, is situated in the fields of the critical medical humanities and feminist new materialism with a focus on childbirth, medicine and the reproductive body. It reads Victor's secret laboratory in which he dissects and reanimates dead body parts as a metaphor for the eighteenth-century anatomy theatre or dissection room. Moreover, the whole narrative can be conceptualised as a manifestation of the material-discursive reproductive body, of (man-)midwifery practices, obstetrical atlases as well as medical illustrations, and, last but not least, of obstetric machines. After all, Victor is, among other things, an anatomist and, like the historical obstetricians Smellie and Hunter before him, dissects and dismembers his 'patient(s).' Finally, Victor brings his experiment to 'life,' like the medical illustrations or obstetrical machines '(re)animate' the (inert) fragmented reproductive body, without considering the consequences. Yet, both the material-discursive reproductive body and the literary Creature are alive but not alive, whole but fragmented, fresh but decaying, fleshy but machine-like, human but non-human. This form of bodily ambiguity opens up the possibility for cyborgian agency as the following subchapters demonstrate.

In conclusion, it is safe to say that Frankenstein's Creature literally embodies the fragmented mechanical mother who is denied subjectivity and whose reproductive powers need to be controlled by male-connoted science. This becomes especially clear in the scene in which Victor follows the Creature's demand to create a companion only to then tear it apart, fearing they would independently reproduce. Shelley's *Frankenstein* is thus not only about pregnancy and birth (trauma) as such, but especially about the control of reproduction by male-dominated science and medicine. In order to fully grasp how lived birth experiences, scientific discourses, obstetrical practices and ideas of monstrosity are entangled *through* the literary bodies in *Frankenstein*, it is first necessary to discuss selected aspects of Shelley's life and the novel's conception.

2.6.2 Shelley & The Conception of *Frankenstein*

Reading *Frankenstein* as a birth narrative makes sense if one considers Mary Shelley's biography and traumatic birth (and death) experiences. These started with her mother, the radical philosopher and proto-feminist Mary Wollstonecraft, who died shortly after giving birth to her daughter (Gilbert/Gubar 2012, 330; Hunter 2012, xiii, 2022, xiii, xv; Moers 2012, 325, 2022, 468). Hence, Shelley's mother–daughter relationship "would only be textual" (Cook 2022, 539). Based on previous scholarship by Moers, Bewell, Gilbert/Gubar and others it can therefore be speculated that Shelley used her novel as a vehicle to criticise the practice of obstetrics that was not able to save her mother during her difficult birth. As Alan Rauch explains, Wollstonecraft's body was partially dismembered by doctors who had unsuccessfully tried to remove her placenta piece by piece (Rauch 1995, 3, 4, 11). This led to her death from puerperal fever roughly two weeks later (Cook 2022, 539).

Shelley's traumatic birth experiences continued during and after her own pregnancies. Not only had she been almost constantly pregnant from age 16 to 21, but she was also with child when she wrote *Frankenstein* at the age of 18 (Gilbert/Gubar 2012, 331; Moers 2012, 319). In addition, most of her children did not survive (Hunter 2012, xv, 2022, xv; Moers 2012, 325, 2022, 462). After her first child had died only a few weeks postpartum, her second followed in 1818 and her third in 1819, leaving her with one surviving child, Percy Florence Shelley, while she experienced further miscarriages throughout the 1820s (Cook 2022, 541). In general, Shelley's biography was "overshadowed by [...] untimely deaths" (Cook 2022, 541). Having grown up in what we would today call a patchwork family, consisting of two stepsisters and her half-sister Frances 'Fanny' Imlay, the latter Wollstonecraft's "illegitimate daughter" from her relationship with Gilbert Imlay, she witnessed Fanny's suicide as well as her later husband's death who drowned in Italy during an accident (Hunter 2012, xiii, 2022, xv; Cook 2022, 541). Unsurprisingly, the themes of birth and death also play a major role in *Frankenstein*.

Mary Shelley's upbringing equally influenced her work. Born into a family of writers and political philosophers, she received a formal education, enabled by her father William Godwin, the well-known English journalist, novelist and author of political tracts such as *Enquiry Concerning Political Justice and its Influence on Morals and Happiness* (1793). This book argued for Enlightenment thought and criticised institutions like the monarchy, the government and marriage that "kept personal responsibility in check" (Cook 2022, 539). Four years after Wollstonecraft's death, Godwin remarried, and together with his new wife Mary Jane Clairmont, he acquainted his daughter with their intellectual circle (Cook 2022, 540). In 1812, the teenaged Mary first met the aspiring – and still married – Romantic poet Percy Bysshe Shelley, whom she married in 1816 after Percy's wife committed suicide (Cook 2022, 540–541). During a visit to Villa Diodati at Lake Geneva that same year, "ideas for the novel took shape" (Kitson 2017, 347).

Frankenstein was 'conceived' during a ghost story writing competition in said villa between Mary Shelley, Percy Shelley and the famous poet Lord Byron, the latter accompanied by his "personal physician" Dr John William Polidori, who subsequently also became the author of the short story *The Vampyre* (1819) and thus the literary precursor of the fantasy genre (Hunter 2012, x, 2022, xv; Cook 2022, 540). The year 1816 further came to be known as the "year without summer" due to a volcanic eruption a few months earlier in Southeast Asia that darkened the sky for a long period afterwards (Hunter 2012, x–xi, 2022, x). It was in this atmosphere that the contestants read and conversed about "ancient classics, [...] scientific discovery [as well as] British and European social politics" (Hunter 2012, x; see also Hunter 2022, xi).

Though it is impossible to determine what exactly this group discussed day after day, it is safe to say that their conversations and the geographical surroundings substantially influenced Mary Shelley's masterpiece (Hunter 2012, x, 2022, xi). The contest as such, however, failed because Percy Shelley and Byron soon "lost interest," while Polidori's "ludicrous" attempt did not convince any of the participants (Hunter 2012, xi). The main result of the writing competition was Mary Shelley's *Frankenstein*, "published nineteenth months later anonymously," and "reviewers [first] *assumed* that it was written by a man" (emphasis in the original, Hunter 2012, xi, 2022, xi).

Turning to selected aspects of Mary Shelley's biography is necessary to emphasise two aspects that significantly informed her work; first, her unstable family, and second, the insatiable reading influenced by her upbringing in a household of intellectuals (Hunter 2012, xii, 2022, xii; Cook 2022, 539). Both circumstances help to better understand *Frankenstein*'s themes that revolve around "creativity, ambition, responsibility, duty, family, friendship, authority, education, and social integrity" (Hunter 2012, xii, 2022, xii). Further, Shelley's parents, both radical political philosophers and novelists, had themselves experienced difficult domestic relationships; Wollstonecraft in particular had to endure family abuse in a household "where girls hardly mattered" (Hunter 2012, xii; see also Hunter 2022, xii). As a result of these experiences, Godwin and Wollstonecraft had strong views on issues such as the French Revolution, political justice and women's education, and their companionship was characterised by a mutual understanding (Hunter 2012, xii–xiii, 2022, xii–xiii; Cook 2022, 539). Though critical of the institution of marriage, they married shortly before Mary Shelley was born, but unfortunately, as mentioned above, Mary was never able to meet her mother who "died of childbirth complications" (Hunter 2012, xiii, 2022, xiii).

As Hunter claims, given Shelley's traumatic experiences with birth and death, it does not surprise that "vitality and its opposites preyed on Mary's thinking" (Hunter 2012, xv, 2022, xv). But that is not all – considering Shelley's own reading matter in more detail significantly adds to an interpretation of *Frankenstein*. She was not only familiar with Romantic poetry produced by Samuel Taylor Coleridge as well as that of her own husband Percy but also with well-known literary pieces such as John Milton's seventeenth-century epic poem *Paradise Lost* (1667), a reworking of the biblical story of the book of Genesis and the expulsion of Adam and Eve from paradise (Hunter 2012, xvi). Moreover, Shelley's *Frankenstein* evokes "classical [...] myths of creativity and destruction" by referencing the Greek myth of Prometheus in her subtitle (Hunter 2012, xvi, 2022, xvi).[2] Shelley further alludes to images of paradise when she sends Walton out to sea in search for a "perfect climate and utopian world," thus also addressing the wanderlust and manifold (colonial) explorations of her time (Hunter 2012, xvii; see also *Frankenstein*, 9–10).

Moreover, *Frankenstein* is not only considered as one of the first examples of science fiction published in the English language, but it is also seen as a prime example of Gothic fiction. Yet, as opposed to other representatives of this genre like Horace Walpole's *Castle of Otranto* (1764) or Matthew Gregory Lewis's *The Monk* (1796), it exhibits a "nearly contemporary setting" and also deals with "recent developments in scientific thought" (Kitson 2017, 346). Because the novel does not, in the traditional sense, contain Gothic elements such as ghosts or castles, to name but a few, it can indeed be categorised as an "early work of science fiction" (Kitson 2017, 346; Cook 2022, 539). In essence, as Peter Kitson states, Shelley's *Frankenstein* "avoids much of the cliché of Gothic writing" and tackles aspects like "education, environment, crime and responsibility" (Kitson 2017, 347). In particular, the novel negotiates questions of medical responsibility towards the (female) reproductive body.

Reading *Frankenstein* as a birth narrative is not a new endeavour. As mentioned above, Moers understands *Frankenstein* as a "drama of guilt, dread, and flight surrounding birth and its consequences" (Moers 2012, 320; Moers 2022, 463). Bewell, however, emphasises that the novel's leitmotif of childbirth is not simply rooted in Shelley's biography, but moreover has to be regarded as a "discursive event, which made her [Shelley] familiar [...] with the language of obstetrics" (Bewell 1988, 2). To use Barad's words, the novel is therefore int*ra*-linked or entangled with material-discursive phenomena surrounding pregnancy, childbirth and medicine. In fact, for Bewell, obstetrics is the "master-code" of Shelley's aesthetics by which she criticises the scientific culture of her time. He goes so far as to call *Frankenstein* a "cautionary obstetrical tale" that "draws extensively on this discourse" (Bewell 1988, 8). These critical reflections on the material-discursive culture of obstetrics constitute this book's core. Hence, the words 'monster' and 'body' have manifold meanings: The 'monstrous' is not only limited to Frankenstein's fictional Creature but further refers to both the 'monstrous' theory and practice of obstetrics that together form material-discursive 'bodies' of knowledge.

Scholars like Moers, Rauch and Bewell produced their publications of reasonable length on birth myths and obstetrics in *Frankenstein* more than three decades ago. What new insights have been gained since then? Is it really so hard to come by new perspectives on Shelley's novel? What can be said for sure is that research on *Frankenstein* and reproduction, including the history of obstetrics and/in literature and culture, still remains surprisingly scarce. Lisa F. Cody states in *Birthing the Nation* ([2005] 2008), a book on the revolutionary and uniquely British shift from midwives to man-midwives in the eighteenth century, that the rise of man-midwifery is still clearly under-analysed (Cody 2008, 3, 8). Cody's work, however, predominantly focuses on the history of medicine and only superficially addresses cultural artefacts such as literature that negotiates obstetrics. Furthermore, Christa Knellwolf and Jane Goodall's anthology *Frankenstein's Science* ([2008] 2016), released in the same year as Cody's study, also features only a short chapter by Melinda Cooper on the teratological tradition in science and literature against the backdrop of Shelley's novel, while largely ignoring the theme of reproduction (Knellwolf/Goodall 2016, 87).[3]

Knellwolf and Goodall's collection for the most part neglects the implications of obstetric theory and practice for *Frankenstein* and other cultural artefacts of the time. Furthermore, Andrew Mangham and Greta Depledge claim that their 2012 anthology *The Female Body in Medicine and Literature* is one of the few works that investigates the "impact of women's surgery, gynaecology, and obstetrics on literary production" (Mangham/Depledge 2012, 1). Strangely enough, neither the editors nor their authors mention Shelley's *Frankenstein* in their contributions. To my knowledge, only Jenifer Buckley's 2017 monograph *Gender, Pregnancy and Power in Eighteenth-Century Literature* deals explicitly with questions of reproduction and/in *Frankenstein*. Yet Buckley mainly focuses on how the novel "draws on the language, conventions, and legacy of the discourse of maternal imagination" in particular without placing the body at centre stage (Buckley 2017, 242). Another recent book worth mentioning is Diana Peréz Edelman's *Embryology and the Rise of the Gothic Novel* (2021). This is an extraordinary study that reads the Gothic novel, including Shelley's *Frankenstein*, through the lens of embryology by the examples of authors such as Horace Walpole and Ann Radcliffe and asks how embryology is related to genre theory. Its focus on this particular field of science and literary genre is, however, not the centre of my book that rather seeks to entangle meaning and matter against the backdrop of reproduction in the eighteenth century.

It is this gap this book seeks to close. It not only aims at continuing the still ongoing debate surrounding science, medicine, reproduction and the body; its goal is also to offer appropriate terms and concepts to talk about material-discursive entanglements of matter and meaning, body and mind, physicality and fiction. Current scholarship has indeed shifted attention away from the question of how Shelley's biography, her reading habits and the period she wrote in influenced her writing towards an investigation of the "history of science" (Hunter 2012, xviii). Today, research is more interested in how scientific and medical ideas shaped – or rather int*ra*-linked with – the novel *Frankenstein*. I wish to continue this endeavour and extend beyond a mere historical reading of childbirth, obstetrics and the reproductive body in *Frankenstein* by making matter matter again. In particular, I argue that Shelley's masterpiece functions as the embodiment of a material discourse that sought to control reproduction.

2.6.3 Science, Secrecy & The Control of Reproduction

Shelley's *Frankenstein* is predominantly about bodies: bodies of knowledge, monstrous bodies, reproductive bodies and secret/ive bodies. It is a novel in which contradicting bodies of knowledge clash and in which secrecy is (mis)used to control reproduction. The leitmotif of fragmentation dominates this narrative more than any other of this book's fictional texts: It manifests itself not only in the novel's form, namely its epistolary mode, but especially in the Creature's fragmented physicality that consists of dead body parts and thus functions as a critique of contemporary obstetrics. The novel's context, form and content are therefore inextricably int*ra*-linked *through* the material-discursive body that takes centre stage in the novel. Though this subchapter does discuss the novel's form, the focus lies on science, secrecy and the fragmented reproductive body.

Certainly, one of *Frankenstein*'s distinguishing features is its extraordinary and fragmented narrative form. Like Wollstonecraft's *Wrongs*, Shelley's novel consists of several inset tales. These mainly revolve around the stories of Robert Walton, the seafarer, Victor Frankenstein, the megalomanic scientist, and the Creature, Victor's abandoned progeny, who share their thoughts and memories. However, readers are left in the dark as to what "moral values" the text wishes to transport due to the lack of a heterodiegetic narrator (Kitson 2017, 347).[4] At the same time, *Frankenstein*'s high degree of ambiguity facilitates a multitude of interpretations, especially with regard to questions of embodiment and reproduction.

What follows first, however, is a discussion of how the text negotiates two contradicting bodies of knowledge, namely that of traditional or proto- and modern science. The aim is to shed light on the (negative) effects of secrecy for science by the example of obstetrics. This chapter argues that Victor can be read as the obstetrician who not only disregards his patient's subjectivity by (literally) treating the Creature as an object, but he also hoards his knowledge, including his medical instruments. This aligns the fictional character Victor Frankenstein with real historical obstetricians, some of which equally kept their new tools such as forceps – that sometimes did more harm than good – a secret.

To begin with, the novel's core text is preceded by a 'Preface' added to the 1831 edition, which is also included in the 2012 reprint of the 1818 version. The preface starts by reassuring the readers that what will follow is not simply a ghost story with supernatural elements. It rather situates the narrative "in the context of natural philosophy," the archaic term for science (Kitson 2017, 347):

> I have not considered myself as merely weaving a series of supernatural terrors. The event on which the interest of the story depends is exempt from the disadvantages of a mere tale of spectres or enchantment. […] I have thus endeavoured to preserve the truth of the elementary principles of human nature […] I am by no means indifferent to the manner in which whatever moral tendencies exist in the sentiments or characters it contains shall affect the reader; yet my chief concern in this respect has been limited to the avoiding the enervating effects of the novels of the present day, and to the exhibition of the amiableness of domestic affection, and the excellence of universal virtue.
>
> (*Frankenstein*, 7–8)

The preface here outlines the novel's main purpose: It is not supposed to merely display a "series of supernational terrors" or "tale[s] of spectres or enchantment," but instead aims to shed light on the "truth of […] human nature" and emphasises the "amiableness of domestic affection." In other words, according to the preface, *Frankenstein*'s aim is not to judge a man playing God, but rather to highlight the "excellence of universal virtue." One has to factor in, however, that the preface is not a product of Shelley's mind – it was actually written by Percy anonymously (*Frankenstein*, 7, fn 1). It is therefore necessary to treat the preface with caution and accept the possibility that the novel *Frankenstein*, conversely, criticises exactly what Percy seemed to have tried to relativise in the preface – a megalomaniac male scientist playing God. Against the backdrop of this book, Victor does so at the expense of the (female) reproductive body.

After the preface, the narrative commences with its frame story of Captain Robert Walton and his letters to his sister Margaret Saville who "shares the same initials" as Mary Shelley (Kitson 2017, 348). In the novel's first paragraph, Walton tries to soothe his sister by informing her he is safe. He also attempts to convince Margaret of his "enterprise" that she had viewed "with such evil forebodings" (*Frankenstein*, 9). The text thus entangles the author Shelley with the female character Saville who both caution their readers. As Walton continues in his first letter to his sister, with whom he shares a close relationship, he describes how he is "already far north of London" on his way to the north pole and hopes to discover a "country of eternal light," a "land never before imprinted by the foot of man," to "satiate" his "ardent curiosity" (*Frankenstein*, 7). He is inspired by a "wind of promise" and the hope to "conquer all fear of danger" by "discovering a passage near the pole" and unlocking the "secret of the magnet" that makes his heart "glow with enthusiasm" – all for the "benefit [...] on all mankind" (*Frankenstein*, 10). On the very first pages, therefore, Shelley's text constructs an over-ambitious adventurer who, like Victor, claims to embark on his mission for the benefit of humankind only. Robert is driven not only by an insatiable desire for knowledge but also fame since he believes "to deserve to accomplish some great purpose" in compensation for his difficult upbringing (*Frankenstein*, 10).

Furthermore, Robert's first letter is saturated with contrasts of "frost and desolation [...] beauty and delight [...] agitation [and] enthusiasm" (*Frankenstein*, 9–10). These point to this character's dual nature that he shares with both Victor and the Creature who are each other's Gothic doppelgangers. Robert then continues to reflect on his neglected education, his contact with the works of great poets and his problematic relationship with his father who opposed his "embark[ment] in a sea-faring life" (*Frankenstein*, 10). He calls himself both a poet and a "naval adventurer" who "devoted [his] nights to the study of mathematics, the theory of medicine, and those branches of physical science," thus further aligning him not only with the scientist Victor Frankenstein but also with Shelley herself who was surrounded by philosophers and physicians alike (*Frankenstein*, 10–11).

The following epistolary chapters of the novel consist of Victor's intradiegetic narrative about his life – his birthplace, upbringing, family relations, his future wife Elizabeth and the "birth of that passion" – natural philosophy or science – "which afterwards ruled [his] destiny" (*Frankenstein*, 24). However, it is not 'modern' science Victor first came into contact with as he tells Walton:

> Natural philosophy is the genius that has regulated my fate; I desire therefore, in this narration, to state those facts which led to my predilection for that science. When I was thirteen years of age, we all went on a party of pleasure to the baths near Thonon: the inclemency of the weather obliged us to remain a day confined to the inn. In this house I chanced to find a volume of the works of Cornelius Agrippa. I opened it with apathy; the theory which

> he attempts to demonstrate, and the wonderful facts which he relates, soon changed this feeling into enthusiasm. A new light seemed to dawn upon my mind; and, bounding with joy, I communicated my discovery to my father. I cannot help remarking here the many opportunities instructors possess of directing the attention of their pupils to useful knowledge, which they utterly neglect. My father looked carelessly at the title-page of my book, and said, "Ah! Cornelius Agrippa! My dear Victor, do not waste your time upon this; it is sad trash."
>
> (*Frankenstein*, 24)

At first glance, Victor tells his new friend Robert how his interest for science was sparked during his childhood. However, he conflates occultism with natural science: Heinrich Cornelius Agrippa was not a representative of modern science but a "German physician, author of *De Occulta Philosophia* (1531)" and known as a "magician" (*Frankenstein*, 24, fn 6). The novel thus addresses a clash between esoterism and science early on. It is this form of 'alternative science' that triggers Victor's "enthusiasm" for what he thinks is "useful knowledge." Though Victor's father had cautioned him about the "entirely exploded [...] principles of Agrippa," he had ignored his warning and "continued to read with the greatest avidity" (*Frankenstein*, 24). The character therefore distanced himself from the responsibility required for his later practice of science and medicine (*Frankenstein*, 24).

Victor continued to study the "wild fancies" in the works of "Paracelsus and Albertus Magnus," thirteen- and fifteenth-century scientists who concerned themselves with "natural sciences [...] chemistry, medicine" but also alchemy, again blurring the lines between ancient, proto-scientific traditions and modern science (*Frankenstein*, 25; fn 8). Victor read "with delight" these "secret stores of knowledge" (*Frankenstein*, 25). He decided not to share these 'secrets' with his father, who would have advised against these questionable works, and also orders his fiancée Elizabeth to "strict secrecy" (*Frankenstein*, 25). This form of (scientific) secrecy is, in fact, one of the main problems Shelley seems to criticise in her novel. Against the backdrop of reproduction, one could further interpret the text's contrasts between outdated theories and modern science as an allusion to the still circulating orthodox ideas and concepts during the eighteenth century such as the myth of maternal imagination.

Furthermore, Victor conducts experiments with electricity later in the novel, which alludes to the debate on vitalism and the practice of galvanism. In fact, Victor came into contact with electricity during his teenage years and was fascinated by his father's experiments with kites and "small electrical machine[s]" that could not hinder him from becoming "disgusted with the science of natural philosophy" (*Frankenstein*, 26). Mary Shelley and the members of the ghost-writing context were "well aware" of the discussions surrounding the 'old' and 'new' sciences that heavily influenced the novel (Kitson 2017, 349).

Frankenstein's subsequent chapters consist of the Creature's embedded autodiegetic accounts, who tells about its "abandonment and the adventures it has experienced since its 'birth'" (Kitson 2017, 349). It recollects, among other things, how its own violent deeds – especially the murder of Victor's younger brother William – were the "result of his treatment by society" (Kitson 2017, 349). Towards the end of the novel, the narrative shifts back to Victor's narrative about how he refused to create a female companion for his progeny and the latter's "revengeful murder of his [Victor's] wife Elizabeth on their wedding night" (Kitson 2017, 349). The novel ends with Robert's report of Victor's death whose last words are directed towards him: "Farewell, Walton! Seek happiness in tranquillity, and avoid ambition, even if it be only the apparently innocent one of distinguishing yourself in science and discoveries" (*Frankenstein*, 163–164).

Victor's hubris is that he "fails to take responsibility" for his actions (Kitson 2017, 352). He conceals his (pseudo-scientific) experiments and isolates himself from his family. What is more, as feminist scholars have argued, Victor does not only function as a "negligent parent" towards his 'child,' the Creature, but also "usurps the female role of giving birth" (Kitson 2017, 351; see also Moers [1974] 2012, 2022). Along the lines of this argument, Shelley's novel criticises representatives of the male-connoted field of science who attempt to violently 'penetrate' and thus appropriate a female-coded sphere – childbirth. Read in this context, Victor functions as the male surgeon, the obstetrician, who intrudes into the field of midwifery with disastrous results. In fact, the way in which Victor brings his progeny into the world creates the impression that he himself is pregnant and thus has control over reproduction:

> I began the creation of a human being. […] the moon gazed on my midnight labours, with unrelaxed and breathless eagerness, I pursued nature to her hiding places. […] My limbs now tremble […] but then a resistless, and almost frantic impulse, urged me forward; […] It was indeed but a passing trance […] In a solitary chamber […] I kept my workshop of filthy creation […] It was on a dreary night of November, that I beheld the accomplishments of my toils. With an anxiety that almost amounted to agony, I collected the instruments of life around me […] How can I describe my emotions at this catastrophe, or how delineate the wretch whom with such infinite pains and care I had endeavored to form? […] the beauty of the dream vanished, and breathless horror and disgust filled my heart […] I rushed out of the room […] I passed the night wretchedly […] Mingled with this horror, I felt the bitterness of disappointment […].
>
> (*Frankenstein*, 35–39)

As mentioned above, Gilbert and Gubar largely agree with Moers and argue that the language of this scene evidently describes Victor's metaphorical pregnancy and (painful) childbirth (Gilbert/Gubar [1979] 2012, 336). Indeed, words like "midnight labours," "limbs now tremble," "frantic impulse," "passing trance," "anxiety," "agony," "infinite pains" and "breathless horror" do recall images of a birthing mother. Furthermore, Victor's strongest efforts leading up to the Creature's 'birth' took approximately nine months, adding to the reading that he is metaphorically pregnant.[5] What needs to be stressed in particular, however, are the mentioned "instruments of life." These can clearly be associated with the obstetrician's forceps that aimed at saving the life of both mother and child. Unfortunately, the outcome of Victor's 'medical intervention' is not what he had wished for: His progeny is not only already 'dead,' but eventually turns on him. As a result, Victor's "workshop of filthy creation" can be conceptualised as a metaphor for the eighteenth-century dissection room. It is the leitmotif of bodily dismemberment that looms large in this novel: Victor is the anatomist who, like the historical obstetrician, dissects his 'patients' and regards them not as a subject but as a collection of inert body parts.

The novel *Frankenstein* can therefore be understood as a prime example of the (masculine) attempt to control (female) reproduction. Such a reading repeatedly aligns the fictional Victor with the historical obstetrician who seeks control over female sexuality and thus reproduction. One scene particularly demonstrates Victor's greatest fear – that he might not be the only one to create a human being without the help of a female reproductive body. In volume II, chapter IX, the Creature demands the following from his creator:

> I am alone, and miserable; man will not associate with me; but one as deformed and horrible as myself would not deny herself to me. My companion must be of the same species, and have the same defects. This being you must create. […] You must create a female for me, with whom I can live in the interchange of those sympathies necessary for my being.
>
> (*Frankenstein*, 105–106)

At first, Victor agrees for reasons of his own safety as the Creature had promised to end its revengeful pursuit in exchange for a female companion. However, once Victor (finally) anticipates his actions' results, he fears the worst – free will, female in particular:

> I was now about to form another being, of whose dispositions I was alike ignorant; she might become ten thousand times more malignant that her mate, and delight, for its own sake, in murder and wretchedness. He [the Creature] had sworn to quit the neighbourhood of man, and hide himself in deserts; but she had not; and she, who in all probability was to become a thinking and reasoning animal, might refuse to comply with a compact made before her creation.
>
> (*Frankenstein*, 124–125)

Much worse, however, is the idea that the Creature and his companion could reproduce without his help as Victor outlines:

> Even if they were to leave Europe, and inhabit the deserts of the new world, yet one of the first results of those sympathies for which the daemon thirsted would be children, and a race of devils would be propagated upon the earth, who might make the very existence of the species of man a condition precarious and full of terror. Had I a right, for my own benefit, to inflict this curse

> upon everlasting generations? [...] now, for the first time, the wickedness of my promise burst upon me [...].
>
> (*Frankenstein*, 125)

Victor goes so far as to argue that uncontrolled reproduction would endanger the whole human race. This idea evokes so much horror and terror that the anatomist Frankenstein eventually tears his second child's body apart in a violent scene of madness and passion:

> As I looked on him [the Creature] [...] I thought with a sensation of madness on my promise of creating another like to him, and, trembling with passion, tore to pieces the thing on which I was engaged. [...] The remains of the half-finished creature, whom I had destroyed, lay scattered on the floor, and I almost felt as if I had *mangled the living flesh of a human being.*
>
> (emphasis added, *Frankenstein*, 125, 128)

To conclude, it is safe to say that Mary Shelley's Gothic narrative *Frankenstein* not only tackles questions of reproduction in general but also negotiates the control thereof. In this light, the anatomist Victor Frankenstein can be conceptualised as the man-midwife or obstetrician who not only dreams of 'birthing' a human being without the help of a female body, exemplified by his metaphorical pregnancy – once he realises he might lose this control by complying to the Creature's demand to create a companion, he literally erases the female reproductive body through dismemberment.

2.6.4 Monstrous Bodies & Monstrous Medicine

Shelley's Gothic narrative is not only about (reproductive) bodies (of knowledge) but especially about monstrosity. A reading of Victor as the novel's actual monster who fails to take responsibility for his actions has long since established itself.[6] Newer studies such as those by Jenifer Buckley (2017) have revisited the narrative against the backdrop of reproduction and medicine. Buckley moves beyond biographical readings of the novel; she draws a connection between Shelley's description of Victor's 'new-born' and previous reports of children being born with birth defects, which implicitly blamed the mother's maternal imagination for the outcome.

Indeed, *Frankenstein*'s text bears similarities with such reports as outlined in PART I with regard to Paré's accounts of 'monsters and marvels.' In addition to the already mentioned exemplary cases of monstrous births as a result of the mother's maternal imagination, Paré chronicles a particular incidence in Turin in 1578. He describes the birth of a child in much detail that, despite its "well-proportioned" face, had multiple 'monstrous' horns attached to its head and pieces of flesh hanging down its back:

> In Piedmont, [...] a good woman gave birth to a monster on the seventeenth day of January [...], the face being well-proportioned in all its parts. It was found to be monstrous on the rest of the head [....]. It had around its neck a

> flap of double-layered flesh like a shirt collar of all one piece, the extremities of the fingers resembling the talons of some bird of prey, its knees like hams. The foot and right leg were an intense color. The remainder of the body was a smoky gray color. It is said that at the birth of this monster it uttered a great bellow which so astonished the midwife and the whole crowd [gathered there] that the fright they had caused them to leave the building.
>
> (Paré 1982, 10–11)

Though otherwise "well-proportioned," Paré stresses the child's monstrous extremities as well as the unnatural colour of its skin that, together with its own "bellow" during parturition, caused such a "fright" that all those present fled the building. Paré then continues with further reports of monstrous births, while especially focusing on the children's hair that resembled little live snakes (Paré 1982, 12–13). In general, his accounts are very detailed, verbally fragmenting the child's body into pieces. Such accounts do bear an eerie resemblance to Shelley's construction of Victor's 'afterbirth':

> It was a dreary night of November, that I beheld the accomplishments of my toils. […] His limbs were in proportion, and I had selected his features as beautiful. Beautiful! – Great God! His yellow skin scarcely covered the work of muscles and arteries beneath; his hair was of a lustrous black, and flowing; his teeth of a pearly whiteness, but these luxuriances only formed a more horrid contrast with his watery eyes, that seemed almost of the same colour as the dun white sockets in which they were set, his shrivelled complexion, and straight black lips. […] now that I had finished, the beauty of the dream vanished, and breathless horror and disgust filled my heart. Unable to endure the aspect of the being I had created, I rushed out of the room […].
>
> (*Frankenstein*, 37–38)

The similarities are striking – the mentioning of the month of birth, the child's proportions, their unusual skin colour, their flowing hair that (might) resemble living snakes and the horror that follows. Though we can only speculate whether Shelley was familiar with accounts of monstrous births such as those described by Paré, it is safe to say that she at least knew about the "doctrine of maternal imagination" that could, as the myth has it, result in birth defects (Buckley 2017, 243). By reference to Marie-Hélène Huet's classic study *Monstrous Imagination* (1993) as well as Bewell's pivotal research mentioned earlier, Buckley argues that Shelley's text, by constructing Victor as a 'mother' whose monstrous imagination eventually results in his "self-blame," functions as a critique of a "culture of guilt" attached to the "discourse of maternal imagination" (Buckley 2017, 242–244). I, however, want to extend beyond a mere discourse analysis and shift attention towards matter, in this case, the (material) maternal body.

Against this background, Victor can not only be understood as the man-midwife or obstetrician who seeks control over reproduction – it is especially the bodily fragmentation of the Creature and its female companion that entangles literature with medicine or meaning with matter. It is *through* the material-discursive entanglement of the reproductive body in fiction, medical handbooks, obstetrical atlases, as well as on the actual dissection table and in the medical theatre that the novel achieves its critique. Fragmentation plays a major role in this entanglement as it further complicates the distinction between meaning and matter: Not only is the eighteenth-century female reproductive body actually dismembered in order to keep it fresh as long as possible so it can be re-presented on the pages of the obstetrical atlas, but it is also entangled with Shelley's own biography and the Creature she gives birth to in her novel.

Both bodies – Victor's progeny and the maternal body on the dissection table – are dismembered and thus rid of subjectivity. What is more, they are both dead and alive, the Creature a "demoniacal corpse [...] given life" and the pathologised female reproductive body in midwifery manuals a "female corpse [...] giving birth" (*Frankenstein*, 39; Nichols 2013, 114). Beyond that, Victor's destruction of the companion's body before even bringing it to life not only links this violent act with actual obstetrical practices that could result in the unborn child's death, but the frantic dismemberment by Victor, "trembling with passion", is at the same time eroticised (Frankenstein, 125). As a result, the female companion's body is both violated and sexualised; it becomes the "deadly erotic" represented in many midwifery handbooks and through (haptic) obstetric machines, thus further entangling meaning with matter (Nichols 2013, 110).

Shelley wrote and published her literary masterpiece in the late 1810s, only a few years after the power shift from (female-dominated) midwifery to (male-connoted) obstetrics was completed. As mentioned in PART I by reference to Cody, from a political viewpoint the "revolutionary nature of this shift cannot be overstated" (Cody 2008, 3). It is thus highly likely that she also drew her inspiration from this material discourse. Despite the Enlightenment's emphasis on reason and rationality, wondrous stories about sex and birth remained popular and continued to circulate well into the nineteenth century. Moreover, these tales and myths helped to reinforce binary hierarchical gender formations among the British population, which in turn affected the self-image not only of the sexes but also of the nation state (Cody 2008, 7, 8, 11).

As outlined in this book, childbirth was initially a "site of strength for women," the maternal body, in particular, a "site of power" (Burke 2009, 1, 4). The knowledge of female midwives was based on experience, manual labour, and especially on subjective feeling and sympathy towards the delivering person (Cody 2008, 36). Their domain largely excluded men; the man-midwife was only called in rare cases of difficult births. Shelley's text entangles (material) dissection as well as midwifery and obstetrical practices with literature by constructing the character Victor as the unsympathetic doctor who prefers his 'instruments of life' over manual labour and sympathy for his patient. In this context, Sommers claims that the eighteenth-century obstetrician indeed treated his female patients rather as "bodies or body parts," as "silent object[s], composed of dismembered parts [...] lacking subjectivity" (Sommers 2012, 100).

Lieske adds that this material-discursive practice of objectifying the maternal subject became especially apparent in the use of obstetrical machines which, as discussed above, were "life-sized models of pregnant female women and fetuses" that further contributed to the displacement of midwives (Lieske 2012, 71). As Cody repeatedly stresses, by the end of the eighteenth century, female midwives were almost entirely replaced by man-midwives or obstetricians who had successfully "enter[ed] British birth rooms" (Cody 2008, 43; see also Francus 2012, 41). It is very likely that Shelly's novel criticises this power shift from childbirth based on hands and feeling in an almost all-female lying-in chamber to a more mechanical birth in a male-dominated 'workshop of filthy creation' full of instruments.[7]

Moreover, it is no coincidence that Victor's lab and instruments are secret. As scholars like Williams have pointed out, male obstetricians not only objectified female reproductive bodies but were also known for their radical secretiveness. In order to preserve their monopoly and advance their careers, male practitioners hoarded their knowledge and kept it secret from the public. This manner is best exemplified in the Chamberlens, a family of man-midwives, who assisted childbirth from the sixteenth to the eighteenth century, used instruments such as forceps but kept these devices under strict secrecy for reasons of profit among others (Williams 2012, 26). By the time Shelley began to write her novel, male obstetricians had almost entirely replaced female midwives. This cultural change in combination with the high degree of secretiveness on the side of the obstetricians meant the "end of maternity as a site of female agency" (Burke 2009, 6).

The fictional Frankenstein, like his fellow eighteenth-century historical obstetricians, hoards his knowledge and thus works against the aim of science that should, ideally, as Buchan also mentions in *Domestic Medicine*, not be monopolised. Rather, knowledge should be made accessible to everyone in order to avert damage to both the profession and society (Buchan 2014, vii-viii). In other words, had obstetricians such as the Chamberlen family shared their knowledge with female midwives as well as the broader public, it might have saved some mothers and children from damage or death during or after birth. Shelley's criticism is thus directed not only towards Victor Frankenstein's scientific egotism and "lack of sensitivity" towards his patient, but she moreover attacks his (social and spatial) isolation and radical secretiveness (Rauch 1995, 8). Frankenstein's hubris, as Rauch concludes, is therefore primarily a social hubris (Rauch 1995, 13). The novel as a whole, however, can be understood as a negotiation of the (material) discourse of obstetrics "on a literary level" (Cooper 2004, 93).

This subchapter ends with a reflection on embodiment. For Ursa, Shelley's *Frankenstein* – the novel about a man playing God with the help of dead body parts as well as old and new technologies such as "galvanism, mesmerism and electricity" – not only addresses the, here masculine connoted, dream of controlling reproduction (Ursa 2014, 133); the narrative also grapples with Enlightenment's "fear of disembodiment" due to possible consequences of emerging new technologies, especially those involved in "creating an artificial being" (Ursa 2014, 134). Ironically, this simultaneous fascination with and fear of creating a 'human' with the help of technology complicates the Cartesian dualism that renders the mind superior to the body. Humanity, as Ursa stresses, was (or is) viewed as "going beyond the material body, if not escaping embodiment altogether on the ground of rationality alone" (Ursa 2014, 134). However, Victor's Creature is both human (rational) and non-human (animal-like) and thus blurs the boundaries between body and mind – it fascinates and threatens at the same time.

However, Ursa criticises the "amnesia" or "erasure" of the maternal body in narratives such as Shelley's Gothic novel (Ursa 2014, 136). In this context, *Frankenstein* can be understood as a prime example of a story of "mothering father[s]," in which the womb is substituted for the "container of rationality (the head [...]), announcing the final demise of the pregnant body" (Ursa 2014, 137). Actually, in many science-fiction narratives, the "biological mother" is employed as a negative opposite of the "technological mother who, in most cases, is actually a father" (Ursa 2014, 137).

To clarify her point, Ursa turns to a modern example, the science-fiction film series *Alien* (1979–2017) that constructs birth as a "messy, horrific and bloody event," while simultaneously excluding other normal physiological processes such as "[b]leeding, excreting, eating, [or] coughing" from human life (Ursa 2014, 137–138). In this context, she adds one more aspect that contributes to the othering of birth and motherhood in *Alien* and similar narratives – monstrosity: "when representing monsters or monstrous births [...], animal organics is introduced in the narrative in order to underline the monstrosity establishing a direct connection between mother and bestiality" (Ursa 2014, 138). This makes sense if we think of the best-known scene from *Alien* (1979), in which the male character Kane, previously impregnated by one of the 'facehuggers' with a parasite, gives birth to an alien through his upper abdomen in a horrific scene of blood, fear and terror.

Such representations of birth processes have had two material-discursive consequences; first, the erasure of 'natural' pregnant bodies throughout the centuries in favour of grotesque and monstrous ones that has surely contributed to the worldwide fear of childbirth; second, the pathologisation of the female reproductive body that enabled control over the "fruit of her [the mother's] bearing" and culminated in the "cultural lack of trust in the mother's body" (Ursa 2014, 139). Ursa claims that technologised fictional beings have "major implications upon imagining a corporeal birth" (Ursa 2014, 140). The effect of the female reproductive body's erasure – with all its material bodily aspects – is the rejection of the "idea of natural maternity," meaning a non-pathologised process of gestation without unnecessary medical supervision and intervention (Ursa 2014, 140).

To conclude, Shelley's *Frankenstein* does, in fact, offer new perspectives on reproduction if subjected to a material-discursive analysis. Though I agree that the narrative functions as a cautionary obstetric tale that criticises the practice of man-midwifery, I argue that the Creature's bodily ambiguity also bears cyborgian potential. Not only can it be read as the embodiment of the mechanical mother who is denied subjectivity, but its fragmented nature also questions the superiority of science over nature and blurs the boundaries between mind and body or meaning over matter. One of the greatest threats, however, manifests itself in the Creature's attempt to reproduce with a female companion, thus ridding Victor of his power of creation. This loss of control is the reason why the scientist literally dismembers the female reproductive body – just like the verbal, visual and haptic practices and representations fragmented and thus erased the maternal body on the (discursive) page of the obstetric atlas, and the (material) dissection table of the medical theatre.

Notes

1 Parts of this chapter are based on some results already discussed in another book chapter of mine that was submitted in 2019 and published in an anthology titled *Contradiction Studies* (2023).
2 In this myth, the titan Prometheus fabricates humans from soil, steals fire and hands it over to humanity, thus enabling civilisation. The immortal Prometheus is then punished by the gods for his theft by binding him to a rock while an eagle devours his liver over and over again.
3 The scientific theory of teratology refers to the study of the monstrous, i.e., of deformed or disabled human beings and babies with birth defects in particular (see Knellwolf/Goodall 2016, 87).
4 Morrissey stresses the importance of the narrator's attempt to "persuade their auditors to act in a certain way" – since there is no extradiegetic narrator, the readers are only confronted with the "perspective of other characters whose own moral judgements may be suspected or biased" (Morrissey 2017, 349).
5 "Winter, spring, and summer, passed away during *my labours*" (emphasis added, *Frankenstein*, 37).
6 See Mellor's "Making a 'Monster': An Introduction to *Frankenstein*" (2003).
7 The presumption that this shift occurred as a male backlash resulting from men's fears of female knowledge and thus power which needs to be controlled is obvious, but far too simple. Jane Sharp's seventeenth-century work on the art of midwifery still belonged to the most widely read handbooks throughout the eighteenth century and beyond. What especially loomed large in her publication is the belief that mother's minds were capable of affecting the unborn child, which, as far as the baby showed severe deformities or died postpartum, could even result in the accusation of infanticide (Cody 2008, 33).

References

Bewell, Alan. 1988. "An Issue of Monstrous Desire: 'Frankenstein' and Obstetrics." *The Yale Journal of Criticism* 2 (1): 105–125.

Buckley, Jenifer. 2017. *Gender, Pregnancy and Power in Eighteenth-Century Literature: The Maternal Imagination*. Basingstoke: Palgrave Macmillan.

Buchan, William. 2014. *Domestic Medicine, Or: The Family Physician*. Cambridge Library Collection. Cambridge: Cambridge University Press.

Burke, Meghan L. 2009. "Making Mothers Obsolete: Eliza Fenwick's Secresy and the Masculine Appropriation of Maternity." *Eighteenth Century Fiction* 21 (3): 357–384.

Cody, Lisa Forman. 2008. *Birthing the Nation: Sex, Science, and the Conception of Eighteenth-Century Britons*. Oxford: Oxford University Press.

Cook, Daniel. 2022. "Mary Shelley, Frankenstein, or the Modern Prometheus (1818)." In *Handbook of the British Novel in the Long Eighteenth Century*, edited by Katrin Berndt and Alessa Johns, 231–249. Berlin; Boston, MA: De Gruyter.

Edelman, Diana Pérez. 2021. *Embryology and the Rise of the Gothic Novel*. London; New York: Palgrave Macmillan.

Francus, Marilyn. 2012. *Monstrous Motherhood: Eighteenth-Century Culture and the Ideology of Domesticity*. Baltimore, MD: Johns Hopkins University Press.

Gilbert, Sandra M., and Susan Gubar. [1979] 2012. "Mary Shelley's Monstrous Eve." In Mary Shelley. *Frankenstein*, edited by J. Paul Hunter, 328–344. New York: Norton.

Godwin, William. [1793] 2013. *Enquiry Concerning Political Justice*. Edited by Mark Philp. Oxford: Oxford University Press.

Henke, Jennifer S. 2023. "Contesting Spaces of Knowledge: Reproduction, Medicine and Literature." In *Contradiction Studies: Mapping the Field/Inaugural Conference on Concepts of Contradiction in the Humanities*, edited by Kerstin Knopf, Gisela Febel, and Martin Nonhoff, 233–256. Heidelberg: Springer.

Huet, Marie Hélène. 1993. *Monstrous Imagination*. Cambridge, MA: Harvard University Press.

Hunter, Paul. 2012. "Introduction." In *Frankenstein: The 1818 Text, Contexts, Criticism*, 2nd ed., edited by Mary Shelley and J. Paul Hunter, ix–xviii. New York: Norton.

Hunter, Paul. 2022. "Introduction." In Frankenstein*: The 1818 Text, Contexts, Criticism*, 3rd ed., edited by Mary Shelley and J. Paul Hunter, vii–xix. New York: Norton.

Johnson, Barbara. 1982. "My Monster/My Self." *Diacritics* 12 (2): 2–10.

Kitson, Peter. 2017. "The Romantic Period, 1780–1832." In *English Literature in Context*, 2nd ed., edited by Paul Poplawski, 406–420. Cambridge; New York: Cambridge University Press.

Knellwolf, Christa, and Jane Goodall, eds. 2016. *Frankenstein's Science: Experimentation and Discovery in Romantic Culture, 1780–1830*. London; New York: Routledge.

Lewis, Matthew G. 2016. *The Monk*. Oxford: Oxford University Press.

Lieske, Pam. 2012. "'Made in Imitation of Real Women and Children': Obstetrical Machines in Eighteenth-Century Britain." In *The Female Body in Medicine and Literature*, edited by Andrew Mangham and Greta Depledge, 16–33. Liverpool: Liverpool University Press.

Mangham, Andrew, and Greta Depledge, eds. 2012. *The Female Body in Medicine and Literature*. Liverpool: Liverpool University Press.

Mellor, Anne K. 1988. *Mary Shelley: Her Life, Her Fiction, Her Monsters*. New York: Routledge.

Mellor, Anne K. 2003. "Making a 'Monster': An Introduction to Frankenstein." In *The Cambridge Companion to Mary Shelley*, edited by Esther Schor, 9–25. Cambridge: Cambridge University Press.

Milton, John. 2014. *Paradise Lost*. London: Penguin.

Moers, Ellen. 2012. "Female Gothic: The Monster's Mother." In *Frankenstein: The 1818 Text, Contexts, Criticism*, edited by Mary Shelley and J. Paul Hunter, 213–218. New York: Norton.

Moers, Ellen. 2022. "From Female Gothic: The Monster's Mother." In *Frankenstein: The 1818 Text, Contexts, Criticism*, 3rd ed., edited by Mary Shelley and J. Paul Hunter, 214–219. New York: Norton.

Morton, Timothy. 2016. "Frankenstein and Ecocriticism." In *The Cambridge Companion to Frankenstein*, edited by Andrew Smith, 143–157. Cambridge: Cambridge University Press.

Mossmann, Mark. 2001. "Acts of Becoming: Autobiography, Frankenstein, and the Postmodern Body." *Postmodern Culture* 11(3).

Mulvey-Roberts, Marie. 2000. "The Corpse in the Corpus: Frankenstein, Rewriting Wollstonecraft and the Abject." In *Mary Shelley's Fictions: From 'Frankenstein' to 'Falkner'*, edited by Michael Eberle-Sinatra, 197–210. New York: Macmillan.

Nichols, Marcia D. 2013. "Venus Dissected: The Visual Blazon of Mid-Eighteenth-Century Medical Atlases." In *Sex and Death in Eighteenth-Century Literature*, edited by Jolene Zigarovich, 119–138. New York; London: Routledge.

Poovey, Mary. 1984. *The Proper Lady and the Woman Writer: Ideology as Style in the Works of Mary Wollstonecraft, Mary Shelley, and Jane Austen*. Chicago, IL: University of Chicago Press.

Rauch, Alan. 1995. "The Monstrous Body of Knowledge in Mary Shelley's 'Frankenstein'." *Studies in Romanticism* 34 (2): 227–253.

Rigby, Mair. 2009. "'Do you Share my Madness?' Frankenstein's Queer Gothic." In *Queering the Gothic*, edited by William Hughes and Andrew Smith, 36–54. Manchester: Manchester University Press.

Shelley, Mary. 2022. *Frankenstein*. Edited with an introduction by J. Paul Hunter. New York: Norton.

Sommers, Sheena. 2012. "Transcending the Sexed Body: Reason, Sympathy, and 'Thinking Machines' in the Debates over Male Midwifery." In *The Female Body in Medicine and Literature*, edited by Andrew Mangham and Greta Depledge, 89–106. Liverpool: Liverpool University Press.

Spivak, Gayatri Chakravorty. 1985. "Three Women's Texts and a Critique of Imperialism." *Critical Inquiry* 12 (1): 235–261.

Ursa, Mihaela. 2014. "Giving Birth the Posthuman Way: Technology, Disembodiment and Cyber-Progenies." *Ekphrasis: Images, Cinema, Theatre, Media* 12 (2): 131–140.

Walpole, Horace. 2014. *The Castle of Otranto*. Oxford: Oxford University Press.

Williams, Carolyn. 2012. "Difficulties, at Present in No Degree Clear'd Up: The Controversial Mother, 1600–1800." In *The Female Body in Medicine and Literature*, edited by Andrew Mangham and Greta Depledge, 16–33. Liverpool: Liverpool University Press.

Part III

Stitching the Pieces Together

3.1 Stitching

3.1.1 The British Enlightenment & The Rise of New Knowledges

Needless to say, the Enlightenment in Britain was a period that witnessed manifold revolutions, some of which persist until today, from the rise of reason and a culture of debate, new concepts of freedom and individualism, the rise of the middle class, urbanisation and industrialisation, the scientific and industrial revolution, early capitalism, colonialism, the rise of science to the print revolution – and last but not least the 'birth' of the novel as a distinct genre. As a respected colleague and expert in Anglophone eighteenth-century studies recently pointed out, this era can only be likened to the digital revolution of the twentieth and twenty-first centuries, also known as the third industrial revolution (Schmidt-Haberkamp 2022, n.p.).[1] The final subchapters of this book, however, single out three particular emergences that, I claim, are entangled with one another in a manner that does suggest progress in terms of human rights, however at the cost of the maternal body and in consequence the female subject. These include (1) the *rise of science*, (2) the *rise of the novel* and (3) the *rise of the individual*. I argue that these three changes in fact led to a rise in 'knowledge' and elevated individual (human) rights, however mainly those of *male* individuals at the cost of female embodiment as will be summarised in the following.

While PART I of this book aimed at an extensive history of the body and practices of reproduction, it further set the scene for the subsequent exemplary analyses of selected texts not only by problematising representation but also by proposing a material-discursive approach to pregnancy and childbirth. As demonstrated, medical as well as literary and cultural representations of the female reproductive body cannot be separated from actual, material practices of (man-)midwifery and obstetrics, including dissection. Both the verbal or visual (i.e., novels or illustrations) and the haptic (i.e., wax models or machines) examples thus interlink – or intr*a*-link – the reproductive body with the dissection table. One of the main points of criticism formulated in PART I is not just the simultaneous pathologisation and eroticisation of the pregnant body through material-discursive practices, but especially the elevation of the (male) foetus to a *homunculus*, literally meaning 'little *man*,' that, however, occurred at the cost of the mother's individuality.

DOI: 10.4324/9781003467977-13

It is the maternal body's *fragmentation* in particular that contributed to the mother's *erasure,* while at the same time granting medical men more discursive power. At the same time, however, the fragmented pregnant body can be conceptualised, from our present perspective, as a cyborg body that equally allows for a certain degree of agency; the cyborg's ambiguous and dismembered body actively criticises the male-dominated sphere of science and medicine during the eighteenth century. Cultural artefacts of this period work well for a critical analysis of medicine and reproduction as this time frame is associated with the *Enlightenment* or *Age of Reason*, as mentioned above a period that witnessed not only manifold and rapid developments in the field of science but also the challenge of old beliefs, the reformation of societal norms and the much-invoked 'rise of the novel.'[2] Though the term 'Enlightenment' emerged in retrospect and was not coined until the nineteenth century, it vividly illustrates the emergence of (new) knowledges by the use of reason (Robertson 2015, 2, 7).

It is safe to say that the Enlightenment was predominantly characterised by the rise of science; it particularly defended "reasoned debate," "open critique" and can thus be considered as an "age of criticism" in its own right (Morrissey 2017, 234–235). As Kitson emphasises, however, the last couple of decades of the twenty-first century have seen "wide-ranging" discussions about the Enlightenment's achievements. Due to the "recent 'rise of religion,' [and] the return of new enthusiasm and scepticism towards science," some scholars express concerns about an "undoing of the Enlightenment's legacy" (Kitson 2017, 235). Revisiting the Enlightenment therefore helps to understand our present; eighteenth-century literature and culture "can make an important contribution to the discussion" (Morrissey 2017, 235).

In addition to new knowledges that emerged in the fields of science, medicine and technology, the eighteenth century also saw an explosion of literary and cultural art forms. As most readers of this book know, the period is especially known for witnessing the rise (or birth) of the novel, a phrase popularised by the literary critic and historian Ian Watt in his eponymous classic *The Rise of the Novel* (1957).[3] As opposed to the nineteenth-century novel, however, that rather centres on the domestic and is usually "set in great country houses" or the "British countryside," the eighteenth-century novel is "often engaged globally, rather than domestically" (Morrissey 2017, 228). Many eighteenth-century narratives such as Daniel Defoe's *Robinson Crusoe* (1719) or Jonathan Swift's *Gulliver's Travels* (1726) revolve around travellers undertaking voyages or trips around the world and deal with the "*'terra incognita'* of colonial locations" or the 'New World' that was explored and colonised by the British Empire (Morrissey 2017, 228). The notion of exploration is certainly also characteristic of the Enlightenment, and the Scientific Revolution as the '(con)quest' for/of new knowledges dominated the period. This also included the 'colonisation' or 're-mapping' of the female reproductive body that was still largely regarded as a *terra incognita* by both laypeople and (medical) experts.

A final characteristic of the eighteenth century that is also entangled with both the rise of science and the birth of the novel is that of modern individualism. As John Richetti argues, Enlightenment readers experienced a "hunger for actuality" and predominantly asked whether a narrative they encountered was "'true history' or a 'romance'"; they began to regard genres like the epic as "preposterous and irrelevant in their unreality" (Richetti 1998, 2–3, 4). The reason for this increased demand for 'true' stories can be partly explained by the rise of individualism that occurred in conjunction with Enlightenment thought and its focus on reason. In this context, the eighteenth-century novel "tends in these preferences to validate the perspective of the newly conceptualized modern individual, whose particularized and personalized view of the world is explored" (Richetti 1998, 5). As Richetti recalls, "notions of autonomy, agency, and self-consciousness" were anything but natural for the eighteenth-century reader – what we take "for granted" today was actually

> only emerging as new and controversial [...] for European thought [...] when the modern individual is, in effect, invented and naturalized, that is to say, presented as an inevitable feature of the order of the world rather than as an entity constructed in a cultural moment, conceptualized and in that sense produced by modern historical circumstances.
>
> (Richetti 1998, 5)

Yet, the notion of modern individualism that merged with a new literary genre occurred only slowly – "over a long century and a half" – and existed alongside "older forms" (Richetti 1998, 6). Moreover, it is impossible to determine the exact time and place in which the novel emerged; what can be said for sure is that readers longed for "new 'realistic' fictions that featured ordinary people in familiar, everyday, contemporary circumstances" with a special focus on the "individual, local, and the particular" (Hunter 1998, 9–10).[4] This has been confirmed by Katrin Berndt and Alessa Johns in their impressive *Handbook of the British Novel in the Long Eighteenth Century* (2022); with reference to Christoph Bode (2011) and Sandra Macpherson (2010), Berndt and Johns emphasise the new literary form's "predilection to tell stories that invited identification rather than representing elevated exemplification" as one of the main characteristics of modernity (Berndt/Johns 2022, 2). Furthermore, the eighteenth-century novel was driven by a "reconciliation of individual agency" and an "unprecedented notion of citizenship" (Berndt/Johns 2022, 2). Yet, the rise of individualism, as outlined previously by reference to Newman (1996) and Porter (2004), occurred at the cost of the body, female in particular, while simultaneously elevating that of the (mostly) male foetus.

Last but not least, Hunter stresses the danger of talking about 'the' eighteenth-century novel and urges us not to think of either the period, the genre or the culture, including science, in strictly "synchronic and generic terms as if all [...] were more or less alike" – rather, as he stresses, "cultures change as rivers do" (Hunter 1998, 28). In a way, Hunter here already engages in a Baradian non-linear way of thinking. In addition, shifts in the era's novel "roughly trace the changes in eighteenth-century social and cultural history, but *only* roughly" (emphasis in the original, Hunter 1998, 29). It is therefore necessary to avoid simply drawing "large conclusions about cultural characteristics" from eighteenth-century artefacts such as novels: "all novels select ruthlessly; they do not try to characterize a century or a culture" (Hunter 1998, 29). Berndt and Johns argue along similar lines when they emphasise how the eighteenth-century novel "did not necessarily suggest challenging society in general, but encountered a critical recognition of how customs, beliefs, and institutions were translated into action" (Berndt/Johns 2022, 7). One aspect Hunter adds is especially relevant: Novels do not simply select, "they are themselves [...] part of the mechanism of development and change [...] – novels are also players within the culture, *agents* as well as portrayers [...]; they *embody* rhetoric as well as representation" (emphasis added, Hunter 1998, 30). Again, in Barad's words, it is possible to argue that novels certainly are also always part of the world's becoming.

In sum, already 20 years ago, Hunter criticised the long-outdated idea that texts "reflect" or "mirror" the world and thus "suggest accuracy and exactitude" (Hunter 1998, 30). Though he prefers the term 'representation,' he also stresses that both the novel and the writer are "active agent[s] *within* history as well as [...] scribe[s] of it" and thus complicates the notion of 'accuracy' (emphasis in the original, Hunter 1998, 30). The term 'within,' however, still suggests two separate entities – the writer (or novel) situated in a pre-existing world that is then artistically processed, despite the fact that they are in turn influenced by their culture and also influence it themselves within a seemingly never-ending feedback loop. Hunter does acknowledge the "cultural condition of the writer as part of an ongoing process" (Hunter 1998, 30). However, he lacks the appropriate language to describe how the world (including its matter), the writer and the text are *entangled* with one another. They are, simply speaking, inseparable and *simultaneously* participate in the world's becoming. The same holds true for the body – both its materiality and representation function as *active agents*.

To conclude, this book's aim is to discuss how the female reproductive body is entangled with the world. Reproduction is, in fact, at the core of eighteenth-century culture. Not only is this period characterised by a general inequality between the sexes (and classes), but Paul Goring describes it as a "fiercely patriarchal society" involving women's "secondary status both through prevailing attitudes and through the law" (Goring 2009, 29):

> Financial independence was denied to most women due to restrictions on their rights to own property: a married women's property came under control of her husband, and property would be passed on through sons before it could be inherited by a daughter. And many areas of public life were closed to women: for example, they could not vote, and were debarred any direct role in politics. A few women were in a position to influence politicians or the monarch, but they were excluded from direct power.
>
> (Goring 2009, 29)

Goring also mentions the maintenance of a "firm double standard" with regard to "sexual practice" and the "nuclear family" as a "basic building-block of British society": "Clear chains of ownership and the unity of a family were seen to depend upon the preservation of female chastity until marriage, and of monogamy after marriage" (Goring 2009, 29). To be unmarried and become pregnant was regarded as a "great shame" and met with "hostility" towards both the mother and the illegitimate child (Goring 2009, 30). Most importantly, this "inequality of the sexes" was viewed as the "natural order of the world"; according to Goring, the eighteenth century largely "saw nothing that could really be described as a feminist 'movement'" (Goring 2009, 30). Only in the last decades of the century, proto-feminists like Mary Wollstonecraft began to slowly establish a "feminist agenda," while the majority of society was still convinced that "inequality on earth was inherent to human existence [...] that men and women were positioned within a [godly] 'chain of being'" (Goring 2009, 30). Yet, some scholars have recently argued that both historical and textual reproductive bodies and/of women were not completely without agency as the following sections discuss.

3.1.2 (Re)Productive Agency

This subchapter turns to possibilities of female agency during conception, pregnancy, and childbirth both by the example of actual, material practices during the eighteenth century as well as their literary representations. The order of discussion, i.e. – history first, literature second – is entirely arbitrary. I wish to emphasise that neither takes priority over the other nor is the order to be thought in causal terms. Rather, both material practices and discursive representations are to be understood as always already entangled with each other in a non-linear manner. The following chronology has therefore been chosen for reasons of structure only – the practices and representations could just as well be discussed in reverse order.

This section first concerns itself with what the shift from midwifery to obstetrics might have meant for women's agency during (actual) pregnancy and childbirth and builds on older and newer studies in the history of medicine and reproduction (Wilson 1995; Murphey-Lawless 1998; Waddington 2011; Williams 2012; Buckley 2017). In particular, this chapter outlines contradicting views on female reproductive agency: While some scholars take a more radical stance on the (alleged) loss of agency during childbirth as a result of the shift from midwifery to obstetrics, others offer a more nuanced reading of this development. They argue that this change was more gradual than previously assumed and award the female birthing subject more agency. Recent studies have also begun to carve out the complexity of the myth of maternal imagination by rethinking it rather as evidence of female agency, at least to a certain degree. What these studies lack, however, is a discussion of the entanglement of matter and meaning, of the material pregnant female body and its representations.

The sociologist and feminist Jo Murphey-Lawless is one of the scholars who paints a more radical picture of reproduction and medicine in *Reading Birth and Death – A History of Obstetrics Thinking* (1998). Murphey-Lawless chooses the late twentieth century as a vantage point. She addresses the "problem of agency" in today's Western world and criticises women's "incapacity to judge and take action"; for her, this lack of bodily agency during the birthing process is linked to the status of "obstetrics medicine [...] as the principal authority" (Murphey-Lawless 1998, 4). Murphey-Lawless concerns herself less with the reasons for the shift from midwifery to obstetrics and instead emphasises the impact this change has had on pregnant women until the present. She particularly questions biomedicine's "remarkable exercise of power" and states that the rise of obstetrics has made alternative ways of birth care nearly impossible (Murphey-Lawless 1998, 4). The reasons for the lack of female agency, she explains, can be found in the history of medical practices that actually "predate obstetric science" (Murphey-Lawless 1998, 5).[5]

Murphey-Lawless' core argument is that "obstetrics science" has led to the widespread assumption that "no birth is normal except in retrospect," which renders childbirth a risky or dangerous medical condition (Murphey-Lawless 1998, 8). As opposed to traditional midwifery that allowed the woman enough time for delivery by simply assisting and not managing or forcing the birth process, obstetrical practices like the C-section started to "override the woman's body," depriving her of agency (Murphey-Lawless 1998, 9–10).[6] For Murphey-Lawless, the practice of obstetrics can be "dehumanizing"; women are usually advised not to give birth at home due to potential risks and should agree to severe medical interventions such as the C-section, if necessary, although the "risks to the mother of Caesarean section will not be discussed" (Murphey-Lawless 1998, 14).

Murphey-Lawless' radical stance is that obstetrics deliberately obscures the relatively low risks of the birth process and mainly intervenes "with the ambition of exercising power over life which is so characteristic of science" (Murphey-Lawless 1998, 15). As a result, obstetrics "maximis[es] its control of [the reproductive] body" (Murphey-Lawless 1998, 15). Murphey-Lawless hence calls for "taking [back] control of and re-forming the knowledges of these [...] bodies" (Murphey-Lawless 1998, 61). Since the turn of the millennium, however, scholars have moved away from such radical stances towards a more nuanced historiography of reproduction.

In his impressive guide *An Introduction to the Social History of Medicine* (2011), the medical historian Keir Waddington draws on previous scholarship by Foucault, Laqueur, Wilson and others. In his section on women, health and medicine, he stresses that the shift from midwifery to obstetrics was actually gradual, while "[t]raditional practices and cultures of childbirth continued" (Waddington 2011, 74). Waddington explicitly emphasises the importance of women's agency in childbirth: "[W]omen had choices. Experiences varied, but women also welcomed medical intervention" (Waddington 2011, 74). One factor, however, that shaped the rise of obstetrics was the "creation of the lying-in hospital" that contributed to the "trend [...] from home to hospital births" and resulted in the medicalisation, pathologisation and institutionalisation of reproduction: "childbearing women became patients" (Waddington 2011, 74–75).

What strikes the eye in Waddington's account is the amount of self-determination he attributes to both birthing women and hospitalised patients in general. As opposed to more radical feminist voices like Murphey-Lawless' that lament women's relatively abrupt loss of agency regarding practices of childbirth, Waddington states:

> Rather than a [sudden] shift from female cultures to male medical intervention [...] a different process can be detected. It is one that points to gradual changes and growing institutionalization in which women had agency and were often willing partners.
>
> (Waddington 2011, 77)

In addition to this rather positive perspective, Waddington also stresses that "[t]he sick have never been passive" and always engaged in "self-diagnosis": This practice of (medical) "self-help" has rendered "patients [...] active agents" with "agency and choice" (Waddington 2011, 79). He emphasises how "popular medicine, vernacular medicine and folk medicine" merged with "formal medicine," thus establishing "networks of information, power and authority" (Waddington 2011, 80–81, 83).

Certainly, class and wealth also played a role in the shift from midwifery to obstetrics, but Carolyn D. Williams underscores that there "is no single obvious reason for this important social change" (Williams 2012, 25). What she is certain of, however, is that this shift was not a medical necessity but rather a reaction to cultural developments like (mostly wealthy) women's own preference for fashionable new instruments such as forceps, thus arguing along similar lines as Waddington (Williams 2012, 26; see also Cody 2008, 197). In fact, the role of new medical or mechanical tools and instruments produced by male practitioners and introduced into the sphere of childbirth should not be underestimated. Like Williams, Wilson, too, attributes a certain bodily autonomy to women and argues that early-modern English expectant mothers "were not passive victims either of their bodies or of men, but active agents who made their own history" (Wilson 1995, 7).

As outlined earlier, one of the most recent studies on the history of reproduction by the literary critic Jenifer Buckley turns to a discourse that not only seems to have been largely neglected by historians of medicine but also opens up new possibilities for female agency. In her 2017 book, Buckley offers a remarkable study of the medical, literary and cultural history of pregnancy and mainly focusses on the discourse of maternal imagination in literature and culture of the (long) eighteenth century.[7] She stresses not only (common) prejudices towards women's minds but also "a degree of agency" simultaneously ascribed to them; some myths tell stories about pregnant women deliberately exposing themselves to situations that would put them in emotional states of anger or passion (Buckley 2017, 3).

Buckley's aim is to investigate the phenomenon of maternal imagination as a complex discourse in relation to female agency and how it "penetrates different genres, shapes experience, and regulates discursive practice" (Buckley 2017, 3–4). She argues that the myth of maternal imagination was controlled through "discrete, localized and period-specific discursive practices" including both "specialist" and "speculative" knowledge of pregnant women's capabilities (Buckley 2017, 4). In this context, she points to "new modes of writing" that emerged in the eighteenth century, such as the "medical treatise, midwifery guide, [...] novel [...] or satire," that showed a "persistent fascination" with the pregnant body's ability to endanger the foetus (Buckley 2017, 5). Buckley draws on Foucault's discourse theory and makes this approach central to her study (Buckley 2017, 5). Her goal is to demonstrate how "female agency" by the example of maternal imagination renders "woman's mind[s]" active rather than passive (Buckley 2017, 6).[8]

Buckley's study makes an important contribution to the cultural and medical historiography of reproduction. However, her investigation largely disregards an analysis of material-discursive practices of reproduction; her case studies, for the most part, consist of literary examples like novels and poetry as well as myths. What is more, Buckley focusses on the mind and what it can 'do' to the body, thus confirming a linear and causal perspective. The notion of materiality is not mentioned in her study – material practices of representing the body are not yet considered. These, however, need to be questioned in order to literally grasp a more extensive picture of how the (material) body is entangled with (its) representation. This omission is all the more surprising given the fact that earlier studies have already addressed this problem. This book thus aims to contribute to a closing of this gap by making matter matter again.

After establishing a historical and methodological basis for questions of reproduction in literature and culture of the eighteenth century in PART I, PART II of this book attempted to discuss these issues by the example of selected well-known and lesser-known texts. As mentioned earlier, one of the main criticisms with regard to reproduction in eighteenth-century literature revolves around the erasure of (maternal) embodiment either through fragmentation or the avoidance of the maternal body altogether. This form of literary erasure is in turn entangled with both the (material) female body on the dissection table and the historical lack of women's individuality and personhood. In addition to the rise of individualism, new knowledges, and the usurpation of midwifery by obstetrics during the eighteenth century, some of the material-discursive textual analyses also confirm the simultaneous pathologisation and eroticisation of the female reproductive body, the pregnant body in particular.

Yet, these (ambiguous) bodies enable a certain degree of (cyborgian) agency, which is at least two-fold. On the one hand, the bodies' fragmentation criticises the dispersal or, in Barad's terms, *diffraction* of traditional midwifery knowledges as well as the (mal)treatment of very real material reproductive bodies by obstetricians during the eighteenth century. On the other hand, some of the literary bodies demonstrate agency by resisting the control of reproduction – they simply refuse to reproduce. Last but not least, in conclusion some of the verbal and visual analyses also indicate the entanglement of the *Venus vulgaris* – a material-discursive symbol for the total possession of the sexualised female reproductive body – with the way the very real female reproductive body and its haptic representations were 'used.'

In Jonathan Swift's *Gulliver's Travels* (1726), actual pregnancy and childbirth do not play a role. However, the reproductive body certainly does; *Travels* is not only saturated with giant bodies, tiny bodies and general questions of the flesh – the protagonist struggles with both female and his own reproductive embodiment. During Gulliver's encounters with giant female bodies or rather parts thereof, the text fragments and therefore objectifies female physicality. This dismemberment, however, also enables a certain degree of agency: It entangles the discursive reproductive body on the page with the material maternal body on the dissection table. The fragmented female body thus bears the potential to actively criticise the pathologisation of pregnancy and childbirth.

Moreover, Gulliver's own body can be conceptualised as an agential cyborg body, especially during the scenes in which he is gazed at by giant scholars; these render him monstrous and even draw connections to (failed) reproduction by calling him "an Embrio, or abortive Birth" (*Travels*, 86). Gulliver, the surgeon, is here himself looked at, his body visually fragmented or dissected and objectified by the male medical gaze.[9] Especially the maids' bodies are of particular importance in terms of reproduction. Not only is their physicality equally objectified through fragmentation, but Gulliver finds them both revolting and sexually appealing. This form of eroticising the 'monstrous' female reproductive body int*ra*-links the way the maternal body is displayed both on the dissection table and the pages of the obstetrical atlas. As Nichols has argued, such bodies that merge the erotic with violence represent the *Venus vulgaris*, whereby female sexuality is rendered profane, not divine. In this light, Swift's text can be read as a mockery of material-discursive practices of medicine and reproduction – the novel satirises the pathologisation and simultaneous eroticisation of the female reproductive body by the (male) surgeon.

Ironically, Gulliver's own body is sexualised and objectified by the maids' use of it as a human 'plaything.' Not only does this female sexual act emasculate the male surgeon, a representative of rational and powerful science, but it is equally entangled with material discourses of science, sexuality and microscopy. The pocket microscope, also commodified and used as a fashion item, posed a threat to both science and the concept of masculinity as it could either enable women to enter the scientific sphere or (allegedly) be used as a false penis, thus making the male body redundant. Swift therefore mocks the masculine sphere of science through Gulliver's body. He also expresses his scepticism towards tactile empiricism advocated by microscopists like Robert Hooke, who argued for the union of vision and touch that created an odd intimacy between observer and observed. However, this reduced distance, I argue, is in fact the very potential of both Swift's and Hooke's work as it mingles meaning with matter.[10]

John Cleland's *Fanny Hill* (1749) equally evades direct representations of pregnancy and birth. Instead, it centres strongly on sexuality and sexual reproduction. Though some scholars have claimed that Cleland's erotic novel is in fact characterised by a total lack of vulgarity, I argue that, although this might be the case on the level of register, female reproductive bodies are nevertheless rendered both sexually inviting and repulsive. While the text uses mechanical metaphors associated with technology, knowledge and power to describe male reproductive body parts, the botanical metaphors applied to female bodies tend towards the grotesque and revolting. Vulvas in *Fanny Hill* resemble "greasy landskip[s]" or "grizzly bush[es]" in contrast to penises that enjoy the status of a "wonderful machine" or "plenipotentiary instrument," the latter additionally evoking images of technology and science as opposed to those of feminised or 'monstrous' nature (*Memoirs*, 24, 25, 113). It is thus safe to say that, although the text lacks explicit vulgar language, the botanical metaphors allow for a reading of some female reproductive bodies as an example of the *Venus vulgaris*, a grotesque leaky vessel, whose sexuality cannot be constrained.

Furthermore, Cleland's othered female bodies are closely int*ra*-linked with the historical body of the eighteenth-century prostitute. Female sexuality as well as prostitution posed a threat to male authority as it not only endangered the individual due to its divisibility but also embodied a feminised marketplace. In order to control the unrestrained female sexual body, it had to be rendered monstrous, both in medical as well as literary terms as is also apparent in, for instance, Swift's poems. Cleland equally dissects his literary bodies in great detail, just like the surgeon on the dissection table. In this context, the discursive prostitute's body in *Fanny Hill* functions as an embodiment of the material and dismembered female reproductive body in the medical theatre. It can therefore equally be conceptualised as a cyborg body whose fragmentation functions as a critique of male connoted scientific power over the female body.

In this context, erotic literature serves as a useful arena to conduct such criticism: Through the conventional use of botanical and mechanical metaphors the narrative mocks emerging scientific terminology that drew on the binary, heteronormative and sexualised language of reproduction. In sum, Cleland's satire entangles prostitution not only with eighteenth-century early capitalism and the remapping of the body but also with (emerging) scientific and medical material discourses. Fanny's sexuality and reproductive power, however, are not controlled, at least not until she marries Charles. What is more, the text allows her to refuse reproduction; when pregnant, she – or rather her body – miscarries and is able to continue her activities as a more or less independent prostitute. For most parts of the novel, her body is not erased – she retains her individuality until entering marriage. As a result, the text does grant Fanny's body a certain degree of agency.

Not just birth but especially conception dominate Laurence Sterne's *Tristram Shandy* (1759). Fragmentation is the anti-novel's leitmotif both in terms of form and content. The narrative largely revolves around the (initial) inability of Tristram to birth himself until a sloppy obstetrician assists during childbirth but harms Tristram's nose, a symbol for his phallus. In fact, *Tristram Shandy* can be read as a story about bodily impotence that manifests itself especially in Sterne's male bodies. The novel's first half centres on the (male) *homunculus*/protagonist/narrator (Tristram) who rather unsuccessfully reconstructs his own conception, discusses foetuses' rights to personhood, reflects on the subject of birth and (male) 'opinions' on the latter, thereby reducing material discourses of reproduction and obstetrics to absurdity. Tristram's birth is disastrous precisely *because* Walter calls the obstetrician against the will of his wife Elizabeth who prefers the midwife. The novel can therefore be understood as a critique of the usurpation of female-connoted midwifery by male-dominated medicine.

Bodies in *Tristram Shandy* are equally fragmented either through descriptions in almost clinical detail or injuries to (male) noses, foreskins, hands or groins. Women's bodies are mostly rendered suspect. Walter blames Elizabeth for interrupting intercourse and his maid Susannah for verbally 'circumcising' his son's name from Trismegistus to Tristram. In Sterne's novel, female bodies symbolically castrate male bodies by interrupting both their material and discursive reproduction: They are therefore equally constructed as a threat to male authority. By rendering Elizabeth's body particularly untrustworthy, the novel also mocks the myth of maternal imagination and draws connections to spectacular 'monstrous' births such as that of Mary Toft.

At the same time, the text satirises eighteenth-century anatomists' mechanical approach to the body when Elizabeth asks whether her husband had 'wound up the clock.' In fact, both male and female bodies can be conceptualised as cyborgs in Sterne's novel. They are fragmented and/or rendered human-machine-like, thus further contributing to a critique of eighteenth-century myths and medical discourses. In conclusion, *Tristram Shandy* cleverly entangles material discourses of science, medicine and reproduction with the body. It satirises reproductive myths from *animalculism* to *homunculism* to the maternal imagination. In Sterne's narrative world, male bodies are impotent and obstetricians are quacks. The text therefore int*ra*-links itself with the historical power struggle between the female-dominated field of midwifery and the masculine-connoted sphere of science.

More than three decades later and in the midst of the wars in France, Eliza Fenwick published the ambiguous novel *Secresy, Or: The Ruin on the Rock* (1795). Though this text equally avoids graphic descriptions of pregnancy and childbirth, female sexuality, the reproductive body and motherhood play a central role. *Secresy*'s critique is two-fold: On the one hand, it contradicts Rousseau's postulate of the (sexually) submissive woman in *Émile*, and on the other hand, it criticises the medical treatment of the female reproductive body as an obstetric machine that largely erased the maternal subject. The text, however, allows for a certain degree of agency – not only do Caroline and Sibella refuse isolation by remaining in conversation with one another, but especially Sibella independently acts out her own sexuality. It is her secret sexual union with Clement that forms the central act of resistance towards patriarchal authority. Moreover, this sexual act leads to pregnancy, which allows the female character to escape her father's attempt to control (her) reproduction. However, Sibella also represents the *Venus vulgaris*, a symbol for unrestrained female sexuality.

Yet, female reproductive agency is rendered questionable in the novel's second half. After giving birth to her illegitimate and dead child, Sibella also dies. Though the text allows this character to refuse reproduction, it at the same time confirms patriarchal notions of reproduction that were based on the concept of hygienic motherhood to the benefit of the British nation. Since Sibella reproduced with a degenerate man, she must die. As a result, bodily agency remains highly ambiguous in Fenwick's *Secresy*: It resists masculine control over reproduction while at the same time affirming the material discourse of hygienic motherhood.

In the novel's end, Sibella is reduced to an inert obstetric machine, deadened and held responsible for her independent sexual act and illegitimate offspring. Yet, her mechanically dead or non-human body bears the potential to function as a cyborg body that criticises precisely what it confirms: the (material) treatment of the female reproductive body on the obstetrician's dissection table and its (discursive) representation on the pages of medical handbooks and atlases, thus merging meaning with matter. Ultimately, the erasure of the maternal body at the end of the novel also criticises the subordination of the female subject in favour of the rise of (masculine) individuality during the eighteenth century.

The lack of female personhood is particularly highlighted in Mary Wollstonecraft's *Maria, Or: The Wrongs of Woman* (1798). Reproduction plays a role insofar as the text constructs pregnancy and motherhood as the main plight of womanhood. Wollstonecraft's fragmented Gothic novel revolves around the horrors of female embodiment, from domestic violence, poverty, rape to prostitution. As outlined, towards the end of the eighteenth century, women did not enjoy British citizenship; instead, they were regarded and treated as property passed on from fathers to husbands, while marriage and especially motherhood cemented their sexual and economic dependency. At the same time, anxieties regarding unrestrained female sexuality circulated within British society that, when performed outside of wedlock, could lead to illegitimate offspring. As a result, female reproduction needed to be controlled by patriarchal authority including medical practices that (ironically) both sexualised and pathologised the maternal body.

One of Wollstonecraft's aims was to transform eighteenth-century unequal body politics by constructing sexuality and reproduction as the 'wrongs of woman.' Yet, she does not condemn female sexuality altogether – rather, the novel, a fictionalised version of her *Vindication*, criticises the idea of woman as an *essentially* desiring and desired object lacking any sense of rationality. I argue that the text utilises especially Jemima's objectified body as a mouthpiece for criticising the lack of female personhood to which medical material discourses equally contributed. Jemima's body can be read as a materialisation of the sexualised and dehumanised obstetric machine on the dissection table. However, the text also lends this female character a certain degree of agency: Jemima's way out of the plight of pregnancy and motherhood, especially as a working-class woman, is abortion.[11] She thus refuses reproduction and lives on to exhibit female solidarity towards Maria and her child, with whom she envisions a new form of family life. In sum, Wollstonecraft's *Wrongs* equally entangles meaning with matter by merging (material) motherhood with (discursive) questions of female personhood.

Frankenstein, Or: The Modern Prometheus (1818), written by Wollstonecraft's daughter Mary Shelley, forms the final analysis chapter and allows this book to come full circle. Shelley's Gothic narrative combines all of the previously discussed aspects: fragmentation and material-discursive dismemberment, monstrosity and machines, science and secrecy as well as reproduction and responsibility. Though finding new perspectives on this extraordinarily canonised literary masterpiece was indeed challenging, I hope to have contributed to a reframing of this text that heavily draws on the language of obstetrics. My aim was not just to rethink reproduction by the example of *Frankenstein*, but rather to think *through* the female reproductive body by carving out its entanglement with both material medical practices and discursive visual and verbal representations.

Indeed, as previous scholarship has already noted, *Frankenstein* serves as a cautionary obstetric tale that criticises medicine's objectification and pathologisation of pregnancy and childbirth. The text achieves its entanglement of meaning and matter by int*ra*-linking Victor's secret lab with the historical dissection room that exhibited dismembered female corpses but also human-like obstetric machines. In this context, the Creature can be conceptualised as a materialisation of the mechanical mother, lacking subjectivity, whose reproduction needs to be controlled by (seemingly) rational male science. Like *Tristram Shandy* negotiates two contradicting bodies of knowledge – that of midwifery and obstetrics – *Frankenstein* equally discusses the dangers of pseudo-science such as alchemy that ultimately leads to Victor's downfall. In this light, the novel is also very much about the gullibility – a term that is also played with in *Gulliver's Travels* – of a megalomanic male scientist who keeps his 'alternative' scientific procedures and instruments secret for reasons of fame. He only considers the importance of responsibility when threatened to lose control over reproduction.

In conclusion, it is safe to say that what Shelley's novel particularly negotiates is not only Victor's failed responsibility as a doctor or man-midwife who seeks to usurp reproduction – the text especially renders female free will in combination with uncontrolled reproduction the main threat. It is for these reasons that Victor dismembers the female reproductive body of the Creature's companion by literally tearing it to pieces in a scene that also resembles sexual violence, an act strongly associated with power. With regard to agency, I argue that it is precisely the Creature's fragmented body and identity that function as a critique of women's lack of subjectivity during the eighteenth century, as well as the treatment of the female reproductive body by masculine-connoted medicine: Both are entangled with one another. It is essential to note that medical discourses and material practices significantly contributed to women's status by reducing the maternal body to a fragmented object or birth machine. However, one could equally argue that women's inferior legal status influenced medical practices and representations. This 'chicken or the egg' question cannot be answered. The only way out of this impasse is to think *through* the material-discursive body and acknowledge its non-linear, non-causal entanglement with the world's becoming.

3.1.3 Towards a Material History of Reproduction

This book's final chapter returns to the introduction and revisits the question of to what extent the shift from midwifery to obstetrics actually improved pregnancy and childbirth. Points of criticism do not only refer to the resulting erasure of maternal embodiment, pathologisation of childbirth, and global 'fear of childbirth' (FOC), but also to recent reports of obstetric violence, a form of abuse during childbirth that is still in dire need of investigation.[12] Before concluding, this section discusses problematic and (possibly) progressive modern material-discursive representations of reproduction; these include iconic photographs produced in the second half of the twentieth century that are still investigated and, in some cases, referenced publicly today. This final subchapter ends with a renewed call for a material approach to history. As I hope to have demonstrated with this book, studying the history of reproduction is as topical as ever as it enables to draw connections between or rather entangle past and present, body and meaning. In order to grasp the full picture – a metaphor that already merges tactility with vision – we need to make matter matter more again.

That said, the question remains what impact eighteenth century's 'new obstetrics' actually had on the birthing process, especially with regard to maternal and infant mortality. The demographers Woods and Galley conclude that their documented notes confirm "positive advances" in both midwifery and obstetrical practices throughout the period (Woods/Galley 2014, 307). Yet, they also admit that due to the "absence of long-run data" there is no satisfactory answer to this question (Woods/Galley 2014, 307). Moreover, the "overall impact" of both fields was "accompanied by epidemiological changes"; certain infections during pregnancy such as those with smallpox triggered "antepartum stillbirths," which makes it even harder to come to a reliable conclusion (Woods/Galley 2014, 307). What the majority of scholars agree on, however, is that births were largely uncomplicated. As Woods and Galley state, it is very likely that even the most "ignorant midwives" were "able to ensure a successful outcome, there being little to do other than to receive the child, cut and tie the cord and then deal with the placenta" (Woods/Galley 2014, 308).

In line with Woods and Galley but also historians like Wilson, Sprang equally states that "maternal mortality was lower than usually presumed" (Sprang 2013, 139). He argues that in reality, "most women survived childbirth without complications" and continues to emphasise by reference to the historian David Cressy that "early modern childbirth was not so dangerous as was feared" (Cressy in Sprang 2013, 139). This optimistic view, however, stands in stark contradiction with the rise of maternal mortality in the scope of the "experimental phase in obstetrics" that took place in hospitals and was "often five or even ten times as high as it was in home deliveries in the worst of slums" (Louden in Sprang 2013, 139–140). This high rate of maternal mortality was mainly due to bad hygiene and still developing germ theories that did not reach their climax until the mid-nineteenth century.

Certainly, hygienic conditions in today's hospitals have significantly improved. Generally speaking, in the twenty-first century, maternal death is very rare in most industrialised countries. Yet, anxieties surrounding pregnancy and childbirth continue to circulate. This fear of childbirth (FOC) is still very much alive and can have serious implications according to healthcare scholars and practitioners:

> [FOC] is a common problem affecting women's health and wellbeing before and during pregnancy, as well as after childbirth. [...] [It] has consequences

> for women's relationships with their baby, partner and family [...], and often leads to requests for caesarean section (CS) by women striving for control in an exposed situation [...].
>
> (Nilsson et al. 2018, 1)

As a result, insisting on a C-section out of fear renders agency relative. In addition, recent reports of as well as scholarly articles on obstetric violence such as bullying during childbirth by both midwives and obstetricians, unnecessary episiotomies, C-sections, or the horrific 'husband stitch,' only to name a few, have contributed to FOC even within the hospital environment (see Abrams 2022; Smith-Oka 2022; Mena-Tudela et al. 2023). Still, 99% of birthing people prefer the hospital over the home, for instance – it seems as if childbirth continues to be regarded as a highly dangerous bodily process in constant need of medical supervision and intervention.

Against the backdrop of this book, the question arises as to how these problems – FOC as well as obstetric violence – can be tackled from the perspective of the medical humanities. I argue that part of the solution is to turn to the (cultural) history of childbirth and medicine. As this study has demonstrated, the history of (man-)midwifery is more complex than generally assumed. Focussing on the eighteenth century makes much sense as it was this period in particular that witnessed the more gradual than abrupt shift from the female-connoted traditional sphere of midwifery to the male-dominated institutionalised medical field of obstetrics. Ever since the rise of obstetric discourses and material practices, pregnancy and childbirth have been pathologised and regarded as bodily processes in need of control.

I claim that studying the history of material-discursive practices of reproduction can significantly contribute to a better understanding of the current situation surrounding childbirth and the fear thereof. Most importantly, we need a way to acknowledge the non-linear and non-causal entanglement of past and present, meaning and matter, body and representation, in short: We need appropriate ways to talk about *bodies of knowledge*. Literary and cultural analyses of historical artefacts like anatomical illustrations, medical handbooks, obstetric atlases, maternal myths and forms of literature such as novels can tell us much about the history of the reproductive body and its entanglements with material discourses. With regard to science and society, studying the history of sexuality and reproduction and the control thereof will also reveal power structures relating to questions of nation. As the political scientist Joe Rollins emphasises: "Regulating sex and particularly reproduction is an essential objective of the state because, ultimately, sex and reproduction are key to how the state regulates the fundamental element of its own composition: citizenship" (Rollins 2011, 27).

In this context, what most of the previous analyses have in common is one issue in particular: the erasure of the maternal subject, either through fragmentation or absence, and the simultaneous elevation of the foetus, a phenomenon that goes hand in hand with the (power) shift from midwifery to obstetrics. It cannot be overstated that this change has had very real, material consequences for the reproductive subject, such as the pathologisation of pregnancy, the control of the birth process and of (female) reproduction in general. In my view, the greatest potential lies in those texts that allow their characters to refuse reproduction or debate the legal rights of foetuses. These questions strongly – and disturbingly – (still) resonate with modern debates about the right to abortion, from the referendum in Ireland in 2018 that legalised this medical procedure to the overturn of this right in the US in 2022.

Especially the decades from the second half of the twentieth century onwards are crucial for a new understanding of the female reproductive body. While the 1960s and 1970s witnessed significant legal progress in terms of abortion such as the (now overturned) *Roe v. Wade* landmark decision, at the same time these years experienced backlashes with regard to material representations of reproduction. Particularly noteworthy is the foetal imagery of Swedish photographer Lennart Nilsson, published in the 1965 *Life* magazine edition and titled *Drama of Life Before Birth.*[13] These iconic images display foetuses at different stages of development in extreme close-ups that seem to 'float' in front of a black background.

As Emily Martin has convincingly argued, "such fetal imagery effaces women's reproductive bodies" and has consequences that reach far beyond those of sex and gender:

> In feminist accounts, the image of a solitary fetus and the erasure of the woman's body demonstrate a certain set of social relations in which women and their bodies are subject to men – a paradigm more or less complicated by other categories, such as race, class and/or historical context.
>
> (Martin 1996, 8)

Such images have also had a major influence on the way abortion is viewed. What we see in these photographs are little *homunculi*, tiny 'living' humans, in the midst of the 'drama of *life* before birth.' As other photographers have stated, what characterises these images is their "'awesome beauty' of 'life at its beginning'"; yet, this sublime beauty, according to Martin, "depends on a distinction between the grotesque medical specimen and an aesthetic of distance or voyeurism" (Martin 1996, 15).

What most viewers do not know, remember or at least do not consider are the *material* circumstances of such foetal imagery. As Martin stresses, almost all of the photographs display "surgically removed" foetuses, in other words: abortions (Martin 1996, 11). As a result, the series does not visualise the 'drama of *life* before birth' but rather 'the drama of *death* before birth.' In order to fully grasp the meaning of such representations it thus does not suffice to remain on the level of 'language' only but to also consider their material conditions. We need to entangle meaning with matter as Martin equally seems to imply in her 1996 study:

> Not only the lead paragraph but the entire Life essay is a *tangle* of contradictions as it negotiates between its claim to represent 'life' and the various qualifications produced by the medico-technological processes, including

> backlighting, instrumental miniaturization and photographic enlargement, chemical and surgical preparation, and medical intervention, which are relegated to a series of parentheses and which continually admit of a quite different drama.
>
> (emphasis added, Martin 1996, 15)

What strikes the eye is that this fetal imagery not only mingles matter with meaning but also enables sympathy with a seemingly living autonomous foetus. As this book has carved out, such representations that focus on the foetus while erasing the mother's body have a long history and reach back to the Enlightenment and the rise of obstetrics. It is therefore essential to understand the development of childbirth and medicine to better grasp our present. Cultural artefacts like midwifery handbooks, obstetric illustrations or novels function as valuable resources to trace the history of reproduction. This study has attempted such a reconstruction by int*ra*-linking the body with its representations.

Before this chapter ends with a final emphasis on the importance of material culture, it addresses more recent developments in representations of reproductive bodies that have occurred since the late twentieth century. Ursa speaks of a "new type of pregnancy" that emerged from the generation following the baby boomers and which represented a "paradoxically holistic" form of "*trendy pregnancy*" (emphasis in the original, Ursa 2014, 140). This trend started in 1991 when the American actress Demi Moore provoked the world with an iconic photograph of her gravid body in the magazine *Vanity Fair* in an edition titled *More Demi Moore*.[14] Described as "one of the most significant photographs of its era," Moore is here displayed fully naked, covering her breast with one hand, holding her pregnant belly with the other, and gazing confidently into the camera (Tyler 2001, 69). In terms of its scholarly reception, the sociologist Imogen Tyler first laments this pivotal image's academic neglect and then continues with the question of how this representation ties in with the "history of foetal imagery" (Tyler 2001, 69).

In sum, Tyler ascribes the revolutionary nature of this photograph to the "visibility of the pregnant woman as the actual subject of gestation" as opposed to previous representations that for centuries had focussed on the "visibility of the foetus" (Tyler 2001, 79). She equally criticises Nilsson's photographs in *Life* magazine, which construct a live, vulnerable and to-be-protected foetus at the cost of female pregnant embodiment that is completely absent (Tyler 2001, 80). In this context, Tyler identifies a "political need to theorise and reframe pregnant women" not as passive objects, as obstetric birthing machines, but rather as the active "subjects of their own gestation" (Tyler 2001, 81).[15]

Only by doing this will it be possible to improve medically assisted pregnancy and childbirth, reduce (global) FOC and endow birthing subjects and their bodies with agency. Verbal as well as visual representations can function as powerful tools in this respect, as Tyler stresses by the example of this particular photograph: It "can be read as a shield against the imaging of foetal personhood and refusal of the mother/child dichotomy that monopolize discourses around reproduction" (Tyler 2001, 81). Yet, as I have demonstrated in this book, it is of utter importance not only to look at one side of the coin – representation – but also to expand this approach by mingling it with matter. The meaning of matter is, in fact, a question that has still not been solved. This is all the more surprising given the assumption that the Cartesian dualism is overcome and we today understand ourselves as inherently embodied beings.

This book ends with final remarks on the importance of matter. As Harvey reminds us: "We exist in a world of materials and matter; indeed, we ourselves are embodied and material things" (Harvey 2018, 1). As she insists in her guide to *History and Material Culture* (2018), "[h]istory is impoverished without attention to material culture," which is why she calls for "new approaches" to the past (Harvey 2018, 2). In line with scholars such as Alaimo and Hekman, Harvey recognises the value of material-centred approaches as they put matter not only centre stage but also use it as a vantage point. Matter, she continues, is "embedded in a social world and as such can provide a distinctive entry-point to that world" (Harvey 2018, 3).

By reference to the historian Henry Glassie, Harvey demands to study and contextualise "things *as well as* words" (emphasis added, Harvey 2018, 3). As she outlines, material culture addresses not only the haptic dimensions of matter, "but the myriad and shifting contexts *through* which it acquires meaning" (emphasis added, Harvey 2018, 4). Like Barad, Harvey ascribes agency to matter and outlines two implications for a materialist approach: "first, material culture is a source type that demands new research practices and skills [...] that enable us to study the matter of things; second, objects [and matter] are active [...] and not simply reflective" (Harvey 2018, 4). This statement coincides with Barad's diffraction metaphor that helps to think *through* matter or the female reproductive body. In fact, metaphors should not be underestimated or even dismissed in the scope of a materialist approach, as they play an essential role in "people's understanding of the physical world" (Harvey 2018, 5). As Harvey continues, "[m]etaphor is inextricably connected to things" and functions as a bridge to understanding the entanglement of words, things and actions (Harvey 2018, 5).

Indeed, the assumption that matter is agentive and not "merely reflective" has become central to material culture studies, although critics still vigorously debate this assertion (Harvey 2018, 6). Nevertheless, there exists broad consensus on matter and materiality "shaping experiences, identities and relationships" (Harvey 2018, 6). With reference to Bruno Latour and Tim Ingold,[16] Harvey emphasises the 'enmeshment' of humans and matter that "interact with the world" (Harvey 2018, 6–7). Generally speaking, what material culture aims at is a "re-balancing of our view" (Harvey 2018, 7). The question thus concerns not only what representations but also what matter and materiality can 'do' while avoiding the preference of one over the other.

More precisely, scholars' aim should be to investigate "how [...] matter interacts with the rest of the material environment and human society" (Harvey 2018, 8). Harvey insists on the advantages to be gained from a materialist approach to history. She stresses that "material culture is [only] one important key [of many] to unlocking the everyday lives of people in the past" (Harvey 2018, 15).

What can be said for sure is that questions of matter, including the body's materiality, are still unresolved until this day. They demonstrate the need for further investigations in this field to which this book shall offer just one of many future contributions.[17]

Notes

1 This reference is based on professor Barbara Schmidt-Haberkamp's oral introduction to the twelfth annual conference *Sex and Sexualities in the Eighteenth Century*, organised by the Bonn Group for Eighteenth-Century Studies at the University of Bonn on 6 October 2022.

2 As John Robertson points out, scholars agree that "it has become impossible to think of one Enlightenment, 'the' Enlightenment, and prefer instead to think of 'Enlightenments' in the plural": It is therefore "hard to distinguish any particular set of ideas as unique to the Enlightenment" (Robertson 2015, 12).

3 At the same time, however, twentieth-century scholarship for a long time neglected eighteenth-century novels in favour of older texts and especially dismissed "women's texts" (Hunter 1998, 11–12). As Morrissey emphasises, "contrary to the familiar literary history about the rise of the novel, many of the most popular novelists until 1740 were women, e.g., Aphra Behn [or] Eliza Haywood," only to name a few (Morrissey 2017, 218). In fact, the novel genre as such was from the very beginning rather regarded as a "female-gendered genre" (Morrissey 2017, 218).

4 Of course, this is not exactly true for narratives like *Robinson Crusoe* or *Gulliver's Travels* that surely do not take place in "familiar" settings.

5 In her view, this inability to act can especially be attributed to the way medical practitioners treated the "supine female body, whether on the delivery table or the autopsy table" (Murphey-Lawless 1998, 6, 8).

6 The term 'mid-wife,' deriving from Old English *mid* and *wif*, literally means 'with woman.'

7 As already outlined in Chapter 1.2.3., the term 'maternal imagination' describes the myth about the ability of the "pregnant woman's mind" to influence "her unborn child[s]" body, resulting in what would today be called birth defects (Buckley 2017, 19). "Classic examples" included pregnant women's emotions such as fright, anger or craving affecting the child's gestation which was then born with missing or deformed limbs (Buckley 2017, 2–3).

8 Buckley values Cody's and Lieske's research as both also briefly address the myth of the maternal imagination, but at the same time she criticizes their "tendency to downplay the complexities of its evolution" (Buckley 2017, 9). She specifically problematises the claim that the myth of maternal imagination quickly vanished and emphasises that this "discourse survived"; it "became [...] more diversely defined by medical professionals, novelists and other commentators" and "continued to be felt in debates concerning [...] the politics of gender [...] and theories of reproductive [...] creativity" (Buckley 2017, 10). Conclusively, Buckley accentuates the "multiplicity of discursive practices" that were entangled with the myth of maternal imagination (Buckley 2017, 25).

9 The attempt to control (his) reproduction becomes particularly clear when the King considers to pair Gulliver's 'monstrous' body with other 'monsters,' thus further entangling science, medicine and reproduction with eighteenth-century literature and culture: "Gulliver's categorization as an uncategorizable monster gives licence to the king to control him sexually through breeding" (Spratt 2012, 145; *Travels*, 86).

10 Ultimately, Swift's target remains unclear. What can be said for sure is that the descriptions of bodies or parts thereof in *Travels* are so detailed and complex that the reader can almost *feel* their texture, an effect that can also be ascribed to both visual and, naturally, haptic obstetrics representations of the female reproductive body.

11 See also my article on practices of abortion in nineteenth-century Britain (2024).
12 For more information and current research on obstetric violence in Europe and other parts of the world, see the eponymous project funded by the EU Horizon 2020 research and innovation programme: https://www.obstetricviolence-project.com/europe. Last access: November 2024.
13 See https://time.com/3876085/drama-of-life-before-birth-landmark-work-five-decades-later/ and https://www.lennartnilsson.com/work/drama-of-life-before-birth/. Last access: November 2024.
14 See https://archive.vanityfair.com/article/1991/8/demis-big-moment. Last access: November 2024. This trend continues into the twenty-first century with so-called 'celebrity baby bumps' being displayed in various media from magazines to social media, Beyoncé's 2017 Instagram reveal photo constituting one of the most recent and well-known examples. See for example https://www.vogue.co.uk/gallery/beyonce-pregnancy-pictures-bump-diary. Last access: November 2024.
15 Though Demi Moore's iconic photograph and the images that followed it represent a breakthrough in that they make the material-discursive maternal body *matter* again, at the same time, they also invite the viewer to voyeurism as the communication and media arts scholar Laura Tropp argues in *A Womb With a View* (2013). What is more, comparable photographs by twenty-first-century celebrities like Beyonce (2017), for example, further commoditize pregnancy and the maternal body (cf. Tropp 2013, 9).
16 Cf. Ingold's "Materials against Materiality" (2007).
17 See also my current book chapter "Matters of Interest" in the volume *Undue Burdens* (2025).

References

Abrams, Jamie. 2022. "Liability in Reproduction and Birth." In *Laws of Medicine*, edited by Amirala S. Pasha, 151–170. Cham: Springer.

Berndt, Katrin, and Alessa Johns. 2022. "Introduction." In *Handbook of the British Novel in the Long Eighteenth Century*, edited by Katrin Berndt and Alessa Johns, 1–20. Berlin; Boston, MA: De Gruyter.

Bode, Christoph. 2011. *The Novel: An Introduction*. Translated by James Vigus. Oxford: Wiley-Blackwell.

Buckley, Jenifer. 2017. *Gender, Pregnancy and Power in Eighteenth-Century Literature: The Maternal Imagination*. Basingstoke: Palgrave Macmillan.

Cleland, John. 2008. *Memoirs of a Woman of Pleasure*. Edited with an introduction by Peter Sabor. Oxford: Oxford University Press.

Cody, Lisa Forman. 2008. *Birthing the Nation: Sex, Science, and the Conception of Eighteenth-Century Britons*. Oxford: Oxford University Press.

Cressy, David. 1999. *Birth, Marriage, and Death: Ritual, Religion, and the Life Cycle in Tudor and Stuart England*. Oxford: Oxford University Press.

Defoe, Daniel. 1994. *Robinson Crusoe*. New York: W. W. Norton.

Fenwick, Eliza. 1998. *Secresy*. Edited with an introduction by Isobel Grundy. Peterborough, Ontario: Broadview Press.

Goring, Paul. 2009. *The Rhetoric of Sensibility in Eighteenth-Century Culture*. Cambridge: Cambridge University Press.

Harvey, Karen. 2018. *History and Material Culture: A Student's Guide to Approaching Alternative Sources*. London: Routledge.

Hunter, J. Paul. 1998. "The Novel and Social/Cultural History." In *The Cambridge Companion to the Eighteenth-Century Novel*, edited by John Richetti, 9–40. Cambridge: Cambridge University Press.

Ingold, Tim. 2007. "Materials against Materiality." *Archeological Dialogues* 14 (1): 1–16.
Kitson, Peter. 2017. "The Romantic Period, 1780–1832." In *English Literature in Context*, 2nd ed., edited by Paul Poplawski, 406–420. Cambridge; New York: Cambridge University Press.
Louden, Irvine. 2000. *The Tragedy of Childbed Fever*. Oxford: Oxford University Press.
Macpherson, Sandra. 2010. *Harm's Way: Tragic Responsibility and the Novel Form*. Baltimore, MD: Johns Hopkins University Press.
Mangham, Andrew, and Greta Depledge, eds. 2012. *The Female Body in Medicine and Literature*. Liverpool: Liverpool University Press.
Martin, Emily. 1996. *Fetal Positions: Individualism, Science, Visuality*. Stanford, CA: Stanford University Press.
Mena-Tudela, Desirée et al. 2023. "Experiences with Obstetric Violence among Healthcare Professionals and Students in Spain: A Constructivist Grounded Theory Study." *Women and Birth* 36 (2): 219–226.
Moers, Ellen. 2022. "From Female Gothic: The Monster's Mother." In *Frankenstein: The 1818 Text, Contexts, Criticism*, 3rd ed., edited by Mary Shelley and J. Paul Hunter, 214–219. New York: Norton.
Morrissey, Lee. 2017. "The Restoration and Eighteenth Century, 1660–1780." In *English Literature in Context*, 2nd ed., edited by Paul Poplawski, 189–273. Cambridge: Cambridge University Press.
Murphey-Lawless, Jo. 1998. *Reading Birth and Death: A History of Obstetrics Thinking*. Bloomington: Indiana University Press.
Newman, Karen. 1996. *Fetal Positions: Individualism, Science, Visuality*. Stanford, CA: Stanford University Press.
Nichols, Marcia D. 2013. "Venus Dissected: The Visual Blazon of Mid-Eighteenth-Century Medical Atlases." In *Sex and Death in Eighteenth-Century Literature*, edited by Jolene Zigarovich, 119–138. New York; London: Routledge.
Nilsson, C., E. Hessman, H. Sjöblom, A. Dencker, E. Jangsten, M. Mollberg et al. 2018. "Definitions, Measurements and Prevalence of Fear of Childbirth: A Systematic Review." *BMC Pregnancy and Childbirth* 18 (1): 28.
Porter, Roy. 2004. *Flesh in the Age of Reason*. London: Penguin.
Richetti, John, ed. 1998. *The Cambridge Companion to the Eighteenth-Century Novel*. Cambridge: Cambridge University Press.
Robertson, John. 2015. *The Enlightenment – A Very Short Introduction*. Oxford: Oxford University Press.
Rollins, Joe. 2011. "Political Science, Political Sex." *PS: Political Science and Politics* 44 (1): 27–30.
Rousseau, Jean Jacques. [1789] 1969. *Oeuvres Completes*. Vol. 4. Ed. Pierre Burgelin. Paris: Gallimard.
Shelley, Mary. 2022. *Frankenstein*. Edited with an introduction by J. Paul Hunter. New York: Norton.
Smith-Oka, Vania. 2022. "Cutting Women: Unnecessary Caesareans as Iatrogenesis and Obstetric Violence." *Social Science & Medicine* 296.
Sprang, Felix. 2013. "Let Me See the Child, and Die: The Medicalization of Childbirth in Eighteenth- and Nineteenth-Century Novels." In *The Writing Cure: Literature and Medicine in Context*, edited by Alexandra Lembert-Heidenreich and Jarmila Mildorf, 135–153. Zurich: Lit Verlag.
Spratt, Danielle. 2012. "Gulliver's Economized Body: Colonial Projects and the Lusus Naturae in the *Travels*." *Studies in Eighteenth-Century Culture* 41: 137–159.

Sterne, Laurence. 2019. *Tristram Shandy*. Edited with an introduction by Judith Hawley. New York: Norton.

Swift, Jonathan. 2002. *Gulliver's Travels*. Edited with an introduction by Albert J. Rivero. New York: Norton.

Tropp, Laura. 2013. *A Womb with a View: America's Growing Interest in Pregnancy*. Santa Barbara, CA: Praeger.

Tyler, Imogen. 2001. "Skin-tight: Celebrity, Pregnancy and Subjectivity." In *Thinking Through the Skin*, edited by Sara Ahmed and Jackie Stacy, 69–85. London: Routledge.

Ursa, Mihaela. 2014. "Giving Birth the Posthuman Way: Technology, Disembodiment, and Cyber-Progenies." *Ekphrasis: Images, Cinema, Theatre, Media* 12 (2): 131–140.

Waddington, Keir. 2011. *An Introduction to the Social History of Medicine: Europe since 1500*. London: Red Globe Press.

Watt, Ian. 2015. *The Rise of the Novel: Studies in Defoe, Richardson and Fielding*. London: Bodley Head.

Williams, Carolyn. 2012. "Difficulties, at Present in No Degree Clear'd Up: The Controversial Mother, 1600–1800." In *The Female Body in Medicine and Literature*, edited by Andrew Mangham and Greta Depledge, 16–33. Liverpool: Liverpool University Press.

Wilson, Adrian. 1995. *The Making of Man-Midwifery: Childbirth in England, 1660–1770*. Cambridge, MA: Harvard University Press.

Wollstonecraft, Mary. 2009. *Mary and the Wrongs of Woman*. Edited with an introduction by Gary Kelly. Oxford: Oxford University Press.

Woods, Robert, and Chris Galley. 2014. *Mrs Stone & Dr Smellie: Eighteenth-Century Midwives and Their Patients*. Liverpool: Liverpool University Press.

Bibliography

Abrams, Jamie. 2022. "Liability in Reproduction and Birth." In *Laws of Medicine*, edited by Amirala S. Pasha, 151–170. Cham: Springer.

Ahmed, Sara. 2010. *The Promise of Happiness*. Durham, NC: Duke University Press.

Alaimo, Stacy, and Susan Hekman, eds. 2008. *Material Feminisms,* 200–226. Bloomington: Indiana University Press.

Armintor, Deborah Needleman. 2007. "The Sexual Politics of Microscopy in Brobdingnag." *Studies in English Literature, 1500–1900* 47 (3): 619–640.

Armitage, David. 2004. "Monstrosity and Myth in Mary Shelley's *Frankenstein*." In *Monstrous Bodies/Political Monstrosities in Early Modern Europe*, edited by Laura Lunger Knoppers and Joan B. Landes. Ithaca, NY: Cornell University Press.

Baldick, Chris. 2015. *The Oxford Dictionary of Literary Terms*. 4th ed. Oxford: Oxford University Press.

Barad, Karen. 2007. *Meeting the Universe Halfway: Quantum Physics and the Entanglement of Matter and Meaning*. Durham, NC: Duke University Press.

Barad, Karen. [2003] 2008. "Posthumanist Performativity: Toward an Understanding of How Matter Comes to Matter." *Signs* 28 (3): 801–831.

Barad, Karen. 2018. "Diffracting Diffraction: Cutting Together-Apart." In *Diffracted World – Diffracted Readings: Onto-Epistemologies and the Critical Humanities*, edited by Birgit Mara Kaiser and Kathrin Thiele, 1–24. Abingdon: Routledge.

Behn, Aphra. [1688] 1997. *Oroonoko*. New York: W. W. Norton.

Benedict, Barbara M. 2016. "'Male' and 'Female' Novels? Gendered Fictions and the Reading Public, 1770–1832." In *The Oxford Handbook of the Eighteenth-Century Novel*, edited by James Alan Downie, 355–371. Oxford: Oxford University Press.

Bergès, Sandrine. 2013. *The Routledge Guidebook to Wollstonecraft's A Vindication of the Rights of Woman*. London: Routledge.

Berndt, Katrin, and Alessa Johns. 2022. "Introduction." In *Handbook of the British Novel in the Long Eighteenth Century*, edited by Katrin Berndt and Alessa Johns, 1-20. Berlin; Boston, MA: De Gruyter.

Bewell, Alan. 1988. "An Issue of Monstrous Desire: 'Frankenstein' and Obstetrics." *The Yale Journal of Criticism* 2 (1): 105–125.

Birke, Lynda. 1999. *Feminism and the Biological Body*. Edinburgh: Edinburgh University Press.

Blackwell, Bonnie. 2001. "Tristram Shandy and the Theatre of the Mechanical Mother." *ELH* 68 (1): 81–133.

Blackwell, Bonnie. 2013. "Corkscrews and Courtesans: Sex and Death in Circulation Novels." In *Sex and Death in Eighteenth-Century Literature*, edited by Jolene Zigarovich, 81–98. New York; London: Routledge.
Bleakley, Alan (ed). 2020. *Handbook of the Medical Humanities*. Abingdon: Routledge.
Bode, Christoph. 2011. *The Novel: An Introduction*. Translated by James Vigus. Oxford: Wiley-Blackwell.
Boucé, Paul-Gabriel. 2001. "Gulliver Phallophorus and the Maids of Honour in Brobdingnag." *XVII-XVIII* 53 (1): 81–98.
Boyle, Frank. 2000. *Swift as Nemesis: Modernity and Its Satirist*. Stanford, CA: Stanford University Press.
Bradford, Barbara Taylor. 2004. *Mary Wollstonecraft and the Feminist Imagination*. Cambridge: Cambridge University Press.
Braidotti, Rosi. 2013. *The Posthuman*. Cambridge: Polity.
Brown, Laura. 1990. "Reading Race and Gender: Jonathan Swift." *Eighteenth-Century Studies* 23: 424–443.
Browner, Stephanie. 1992. "Review of Thomas Laqueur, *Making Sex*." *Victorian Studies* 35: 221–222.
Buchan, William. [1769] 2014. *Domestic Medicine, Or: The Family Physician*. Cambridge Library Collection. Cambridge: Cambridge University Press.
Buckley, Jenifer. 2017. *Gender, Pregnancy and Power in Eighteenth-Century Literature: The Maternal Imagination*. Basingstoke: Palgrave Macmillan.
Burke, Meghan L. 2009. "Making Mothers Obsolete: Eliza Fenwick's *Secresy* and the Masculine Appropriation of Maternity." *Eighteenth Century Fiction* 21 (3): 357–384.
Butler, Judith. 1990. *Gender Trouble: Feminism and the Subversion of Identity*. Abingdon: Routledge.
Butler, Judith. 1993. *Bodies That Matter: On the Discursive Limits of Sex*. Abingdon: Routledge.
Cannon, Mercy. 2008. "Hygienic Motherhood: Domestic Medicine and Eliza Fenwick's *Secresy*." *Eighteenth-Century Fiction* 20 (4): 535–561.
Carter, Sophie. 2004. *Purchasing Power: Representing Prostitution in Eighteenth-Century English Popular Print Culture*. Aldershot: Ashgate.
Cervantes, Miguel de. [1605] 2020. *Don Quixote*. New York: W. W. Norton.
Chabor, Lois A. 1997. "This Affecting Subject: An 'Interested' Reading of Childbearing in Two Novels by Samuel Richardson." *The Scriblerian and the Kit-Cats* 29 (2): 169.
Cleland, John. 2005. *Memoirs of a Coxcomb*. Edited by Hal Gladfelder. Peterborough, Ontario: Broadview Press.
Cleland, John. 2008. *Memoirs of a Woman of Pleasure*. Edited by Peter Sabor. Oxford: Oxford University Press.
Close, Anne. 2004. "Into the Public: The Sexual Heroine in Eliza Fenwick's *Secresy* and Mary Robinson's *The Natural Daughter*." *Eighteenth-Century Fiction* 17 (1): 35–52.
Cody, Lisa Forman. [2005] 2008. *Birthing the Nation: Sex, Science, and the Conception of Eighteenth-Century Britons*. Oxford: Oxford University Press.
Conboy, Katie, Nadia Medina, and Sarah Stanbury, eds. 1997. *Writing on the Body: Female Embodiment and Feminist Theory*. New York: Columbia University Press.
Cook, Daniel. 2022. "Mary Shelley, *Frankenstein*, or *The Modern Prometheus* (1818)." In *Handbook of the British Novel in the Long Eighteenth Century*, edited by Katrin Berndt and Alessa Johns, 231–249. Berlin; Boston, MA: De Gruyter.
Cooper, Christine M. 2004. "Reading the Politics of Abortion: Mary Wollstonecraft Revisited." *Eighteenth-Century Fiction* 16 (4): 735–782.

Cressy, David. 1999. *Birth, Marriage, and Death: Ritual, Religion, and the Life Cycle in Tudor and Stuart England*. Oxford: Oxford University Press.

Cunningham, Andrew. 2010. *The Anatomist Anatomis'd: An Experimental Discipline in Enlightenment Europe*. Farnham: Ashgate.

Defoe, Daniel. [1719] 1994. *Robinson Crusoe*. New York: W. W. Norton.

Defoe, Daniel. [1722] 2003. *Moll Flanders*. New York: Norton.

Defoe, Daniel. [1724] 2008. *Roxana: The Fortunate Mistress*. Edited by John Mullan. Oxford World's Classics. Oxford: Oxford University Press.

Defoe, Daniel. 2011. *Moll Flanders*. Edited by George A. Starr and Linda Bree. Oxford World's Classics. Oxford: Oxford University Press.

DeMello, Margo. 2014. *Body Studies: An Introduction*. Abingdon: Routledge.

Deutscher, Penelope. 2017. *Foucault's Futures: A Critique of Reproductive Reason*. New York: Columbia University Press.

Dolan, Elizabeth A. 2008. *Seeing Suffering in Women's Literature of the Romantic Era*. Aldershot; Burlington, VT: Ashgate.

Donoghue, Denis. 1998. *The Practice of Reading*. New Haven, CT: Yale University Press.

Duden, Barbara. 1988. *The Women beneath the Skin: A Doctor's Patients in Eighteenth-Century Germany*. Cambridge, MA: Harvard University Press.

Ebenstein, Joanna. 2016. *The Anatomical Venus*. London: Thames & Hudson.

Edelman, Diana Pérez. 2021. *Embryology and the Rise of the Gothic Novel*. London; New York: Palgrave Macmillan.

Eide, Kristiane Tislevoll et al. 2019. "Maternal Reasons for Requesting Planned Cesarean Section in Norway: A Qualitative Study." *BMC Pregnancy and Childbirth* 19 (1): 1–11.

Emsley, Sarah. 1999. "Radical Marriage." *Eighteenth-Century Fiction* 11 (4): 477–498.

Fenwick, Eliza. 1795. *Secresy*. Edited by Isobel Grundy. Peterborough, Ontario: Broadview Press, 1998.

Fissell, Mary Elizabeth. 2009. *Vernacular Bodies: The Politics of Reproduction in Early Modern England*. Oxford: Oxford University Press.

Flynn, Carol H. 1990. *The Body in Swift and Defoe*. Cambridge: Cambridge University Press.

Foucault, Michel. [1976] 1978. *The History of Sexuality*. New York: Pantheon.

Foucault, Michel. [1963] 1994. *The Birth of the Clinic: An Archaeology of Medical Perception*. New York: Vintage Books.

Fournier, Marian. 1996. *The Fabric of Life: Microscopy in the Seventeenth Century*. Baltimore, MD: Johns Hopkins University Press.

Fox Keller, Evelyn. 1995. *Reflections on Gender and Science*. New Haven, CT: Yale University Press.

Fox, Sarah. 2022. *Giving Birth in Eighteenth-Century England*. London: University of London Press.

Francus, Marilyn. 2012. *Monstrous Motherhood: Eighteenth-Century Culture and the Ideology of Domesticity*. Baltimore, MD: Johns Hopkins University Press.

Furniss, Tom. 1992. "Wollstonecraft, Mary (1759–97)." In *A Handbook to English Romanticism*, edited by Jean Raimond and John Richard Watson, 284–288. Basingstoke: Macmillan.

Gautier, Gary. 2001. "Introduction: Fanny Hill's Mapping of Sexuality, Female Identity, and Maternity". John Cleland. *Fanny Hill Or, Memoirs of a Woman of Pleasure*. Notes by Audrey Bilger, xi–xxxiii. New York: The Modern Library.

George, Margaret. 1970. *One Woman's "Situation": A Study of Mary Wollstonecraft*. Urbana, Chicago, and London: University of Illinois Press.

Gilbert, Sandra M., and Susan Gubar. [1979] 2012. "Mary Shelley's Monstrous Eve." In Mary Shelley. *Frankenstein*, edited by J. Paul Hunter, 328–344. New York: Norton.

Girten, Kristi M. 2013. "Mingling with Matter: Tactile Microscopy and the Philosophic Mind in Brobdingnag and Beyond." *The Eighteenth Century* 54 (4): 497–520.

Godwin, William. [1793] 2013. *Enquiry Concerning Political Justice*. Edited by Mark Philp. Oxford: Oxford University Press.

Godwin, William. [1798] 2018. *Posthumous Works of the Author of 'A Vindication of the Rights of Woman'*. Norderstedt: Hansebooks.

Gordon, Lyndall. 2005. *Vindication: A Life of Mary Wollstonecraft*. New York: Harper.

Goring, Paul. 2009. *The Rhetoric of Sensibility in Eighteenth-Century Culture*. Cambridge: Cambridge University Press.

Gowing, Laura. 2003. *Common Bodies: Women, Touch, and Power in Seventeenth-Century England*. New Haven, CT: Yale University Press.

Greenfield, Susan C., and Carol Barash. 1999. *Inventing Maternity: Politics, Science, and Literature, 1650–1865*. Lexington: University Press of Kentucky.

Grundy, Isobel. 1998. "Introduction." In *Secresy, Or: The Ruin on the Rock*, 2nd ed., edited by Eliza Fenwick and Isobel Grundy, 7–36. Broadview Press.

Gubar, Susan. 1994. "Feminist Misogyny: Mary Wollstonecraft and the Paradox of 'It Takes One to Know One.'" *Feminist Studies* 20 (3): 452–473.

Guralnick, Elissa S. 2009. "Radical Politics in Mary Wollstonecraft's A Vindication of the Rights of Woman." In *A Vindication of the Rights of Woman: An Authoritative Text, Backgrounds, and Contexts, Criticism*, edited by Mary Wollstonecraft and Deidre S. Lynch, 309–319. New York: Norton.

Gurr, Jens Martin. 1999. *Tristram Shandy and the Dialectic of Enlightenment*. Heidelberg: Winter.

Gurr, Jens Martin. 2022. "Laurence Sterne, The Life and Opinions of Tristram Shandy, Gentleman (1759–1767)." In *Handbook of the British Novel in the Long Eighteenth Century*, edited by Katrin Berndt and Alessa Johns, 365–389. Berlin; Boston, MA: De Gruyter.

Hall, Stuart. 1997. "Introduction." In *Representation: Cultural Representations and Signifying Practices*, edited by Stuart Hall, 1–13. Thousand Oaks, CA: Sage.

Hanson, Clare. 2004. *A Cultural History of Pregnancy: Pregnancy, Medicine and Culture, 1750–2000*. Basingstoke: Palgrave Macmillan.

Haraway, Donna J. 1990. *Primate Visions: Gender, Race, and Nature in the World of Modern Science*. Abingdon: Routledge.

Haraway, Donna J. [1985] 2000. "A Cyborg Manifesto: Science, Technology and Socialist Feminism in the Late Twentieth Century." In *The Cybercultures Reader*, edited by David Bell and Barbara Kennedy, 292–324. New York: Routledge.

Haraway, Donna J. 2007. *When Species Meet*. Minneapolis and London: University of Minnesota Press.

Harries, Elizabeth W. 2009. "Words, Sex, and Gender in Sterne's Novels." In *The Cambridge Companion to Laurence Sterne*, edited by Thomas Keymer, 112–127. Cambridge: Cambridge University Press.

Harvey, Karen. 2004. *Reading Sex in the Eighteenth Century: Bodies and Gender in English Erotic Culture*. Cambridge: Cambridge University Press.

Harvey, Karen. 2010. "Visualizing Reproduction: A Cultural History of Early-Modern and Modern Medical Illustrations." *The Journal of Medical Humanities* 31 (1): 37–51.

Harvey, Karen. 2018. *History and Material Culture: A Student's Guide to Approaching Alternative Sources*. London: Routledge.

Hawes, Clement. 1991. "Three Times Round the Globe: Gulliver and Colonial Discourse." *Cultural Critique*, No. 18 (Spring). 187–214.

Hawes, Clement. 2020. "Gulliver Effects." In *The Oxford Handbook of the Eighteenth-Century Novel*, edited by Alan Downie, 523–541. Oxford: Oxford University Press.

Hawley, Judith. 2019. "The Anatomy of Tristram Shandy." In Laurence Sterne. *Tristram Shandy*, edited by Judith Hawley, 203–215. New York: Norton.

Hayles, N. Katherine. 1999. *How We Became Posthuman: Virtual Bodies in Cybernetics, Literature, and Informatics*. Chicago, IL; London: University of Chicago Press.

Henke, Jennifer S. 2018. "In the Flesh – The Politics of Abortion in Ireland." *Hard Times* 102 (2): 114–126. In *Gender Today*, edited by Anke Bartels, Irmgard Maassen, and Ingrid von Rosenberg. Potsdam: Universität Potsdam, Institut für Anglistik und Amerikanistik.

Henke, Jennifer S. 2022. "Mary Wollstonecraft, *Maria: or, The Wrongs of Woman* (1798)." In *Handbook of the British Novel in the Long Eighteenth Century*, edited by Katrin Berndt and Alessa Johns, 449–466. Berlin; Boston, MA: De Gruyter.

Henke, Jennifer S. 2023. "Contesting Spaces of Knowledge: Reproduction, Medicine and Literature." In *Contradiction Studies: Mapping the Field/Inaugural Conference on Concepts of Contradiction in the Humanities*, edited by Kerstin Knopf, Gisela Febel, and Martin Nonhoff, 233–256. Heidelberg: Springer.

Henke, Jennifer S. 2024. "'Fruits which that unknown orchard bore': Practices of Abortion in the 19th Century." *Journal for the Study of British Cultures* 31 (2). Edited by Sarah Wegener and Wolfgang Funk. Heidelberg: Winter, 219–236.

Henke, Jennifer S. 2025. "Matters of Interest: Entangling the Maternal Body." In *Undue Burdens: Reproductive Rights and Bodily Autonomy in the Long Eighteenth Century*, edited by Fiona Brideoake, Ula Lukszo Klein, and Nicole Garret. University of Virginia Press.

Hillman, David, and Ulrika Maude, eds. 2015. *The Cambridge Companion to the Body in Literature*. New York: Cambridge University Press.

Homans, Margaret. 1994. "Feminist Fictions and Feminist Theories of Narrative." *Narrative* 2 (1): 3–16.

Hoppe, Katharina, and Thomas Lemke. 2015. "Die Macht der Materie: Grundlagen und Grenzen des agentiellen Realismus von Karen Barad." *Soziale Welt* 66 (3): 261–280.

Hoyert, Donna L. 2022. *Maternal Mortality Rates in the United States*. www.cdc.gov/nchs/data/hestat/maternal-mortality/2022/maternal-mortality-rates-2022.htm. Last access: July 2023.

Huet, Marie Hélène. 1993. *Monstrous Imagination*. Cambridge, MA: Harvard University Press.

Hunter, William. 1774. *The Anatomy of the Human Gravid Uterus Exhibited in Figures*. London: D. Wilson.

Hunter, J. Paul. 1998. "The Novel and Social/Cultural History." In *The Cambridge Companion to the Eighteenth-Century Novel*, edited by John Richetti, 9–40. Cambridge: Cambridge University Press.

Hunter, J. Paul. 2012. "Introduction." In Mary Shelley [1818]. *Frankenstein*, 2nd ed., edited by J. Paul Hunter, ix–xviii. New York: Norton.

Hunter, J. Paul. 2022. "Introduction." In Mary Shelley [1818]. *Frankenstein*, 3rd ed., edited by J. Paul Hunter, vii–xix. New York: Norton.

Ingold, Tim. 2007. "Materials against Materiality." *Archeological Dialogues* 14 (1): 1–16.

Ingram, Allan. 1986. *Intricate Laughter in the Satire of Swift and Pope*. Basingstoke: Macmillan.

Ingram, Allan. 2012. "Introduction." In *Gulliver's Travels*, edited by Allan Ingram, 1–12. Peterborough, ON: Broadview Press.

Ingram, Allan. 2022. *Swift, Pope and the Doctors: Medicine and Writing in the Early Eighteenth Century*. Leiden, Netherlands: Brill Fink.

Isaac, Janice A. 1999. "*Secresy, or: The Ruin on the Rock*." Review of *Secresy*, by Eliza Fenwick. *ESC: English Studies in Canada* 25 (1): 114–116.

Jeffares, A. Norman, (ed.) 1992. *Jonathan Swift: The Selected Poems*. London: Kyle Cathie Limited.

Johnson, Claudia L., ed. 2002. *The Cambridge Companion to Mary Wollstonecraft*. Cambridge: Cambridge University Press.

Jones, Vivien. 1997. "Placing Jemima: Women Writers of the 1790s and the Eighteenth-Century Prostitution Narrative." *Women's Writing* 4 (2): 201–220.

Jong, Erica. 1978. *Introduction to Fanny Hill*. New York: Erotic Art Book Society.

Jordanova, Ludmilla J. 1989. *Sexual Visions: Images of Gender in Science and Medicine between the Eighteenth and Twentieth Centuries*. Madison: University of Wisconsin Press.

Joseph, K. S. et al. 2021. "Maternal Mortality in the United States." *Obstetrics and Gynecology* 137 (5): 763–771.

Jouhki, Maija-Riitta, Tarja Suominen, and Päivi Åstedt-Kurki. 2017. "Giving Birth on Our Own Terms: Women's Experience of Childbirth at Home." *Midwifery* 53: 35–41.

Kantorowicz, Ernst H. 2016. *The King's Two Bodies: A Study in Medieval Political Theology*. Princeton, NJ: Princeton University Press.

Kaplan, Cora. 2009. "From *Wild Nights: Pleasure/Sexuality/Feminism*." In Mary Wollstonecraft [1792]. *A Vindication of the Rights of Woman: An Authoritative Text, Backgrounds, and Contexts, Criticism*, edited Deidre S. Lynch, 335–349. New York: Norton.

Keag, O. E., J. E. Norman, and S. J. Stock. 2018. "Long-Term Risks and Benefits Associated with Caesarean Delivery for Mother, Baby, and Subsequent Pregnancies: Systematic Review and Meta-Analysis." *PLOS Medicine* 15 (1): e1002494.

Kelly, Gary. 2009. "Introduction." In *Mary and The Wrongs of Woman*, by Mary Wollstonecraft. Oxford World's Classics, ix–xxxi. Oxford: Oxford University Press.

Keymer, Thomas. 2018. "Sterne and the New Species of Writing." In Laurence Sterne [1759] *Tristram Shandy*, edited by Judith Hawley, 89–101. New York: Norton.

King, Helen. 2007. *Midwifery, Obstetrics and the Rise of Gynaecology: The Uses of a Sixteenth-Century Compendium*. London: Routledge.

King, Helen. 2013. *The One-Sex Body on Trial: The Classical and Early Modern Evidence*. London; New York: Routledge.

Kipp, Julie. 2009. *Romanticism, Maternity, and the Body Politic*. Cambridge: Cambridge University Press.

Kitson, Peter. 2017. "The Romantic Period, 1780–1832." In *English Literature in Context*, 2nd ed., edited by Paul Poplawski, 406–420. Cambridge; New York: Cambridge University Press.

Knellwolf, Christa, and Jane Goodall, eds. 2016. *Frankenstein's Science: Experimentation and Discovery in Romantic Culture, 1780–1830*. London; New York: Routledge.

Knight, Charles. 2004. *The Literature of Satire*. Cambridge: Cambridge University Press.

Knight, Richard Payne. 1974. *A Discourse on the Worship of Priapus, and Its Connection with the Mystic Theology of the Ancients: To Which Is Added an Essay on the Worship of the Generative Powers During the Middle Ages of Western Europe*. New Foreword by O. V. Garrison. New York: University Books.

Knoppers, Laura Lunger, and Joan B. Landes, eds. 2004. *Monstrous Bodies/Political Monstrosities in Early Modern Europe.* Ithaca, NY: Cornell University Press.

Kristeva, Julia. 1982. *Powers of Horror: An Essay on Abjection.* New York: Columbia University Press.

La Mettrie, Julien Offray de. 1996. *Machine Man and Other Writings.* Edited by Ann Thomson. Cambridge: Cambridge University Press.

Lamb, Jonathan. 1998. "Sterne and Irregular Oratory." In *The Cambridge Companion to the Eighteenth-Century Novel*, edited by John Richetti, 147–163. Cambridge: Cambridge University Press.

Lanser, Susan S. 1992. *Fictions of Authority: Women Writers and Narrative Voice.* Ithaca, NY: Cornell University Press.

Laqueur, Thomas, and Catherine Gallagher, eds. 1987. *The Making of the Modern Body: Sexuality and Society in the Nineteenth Century.* Berkeley: University of California Press.

Laqueur, Thomas. [1990] 1992. *Making Sex: Body and Gender from the Greeks to Freud.* Cambridge, MA: Harvard University Press.

Laqueur, Thomas. 2012. "The Rise of Sex in the Eighteenth Century: Historical Context and Historiographical Implications." *Signs: Journal of Women in Culture and Society* 37 (4): 802–813.

Latour, Bruno. 2004. "How to Talk About the Body? The Normative Dimension of Science Studies." *Body & Society*, 10(2–3): 205–229.

Latour, Bruno. 2015. *Science in Action: How to Follow Scientists and Engineers through Society.* Cambridge, MA: Harvard University Press.

Lewis, Ann, and Markman Ellis, eds. 2016. *Prostitution and Eighteenth-Century Culture: Sex, Commerce, and Morality.* Oxfordshire/New York: Routledge.

Lewis, Matthew G. [1796] 2016. *The Monk.* Oxford: Oxford University Press.

Lieske, Pam, ed. 2008. *Eighteenth-Century British Midwifery, Volume 5: The State of Midwifery Considered, William Smellie and His Critics.* London: Pickering and Chatto.

Lieske, Pam. 2012. "'Made in Imitation of Real Women and Children': Obstetrical Machines in Eighteenth-Century Britain." In *The Female Body in Medicine and Literature*, edited by Andrew Mangham and Greta Depledge, 16–33. Liverpool: Liverpool University Press.

Linnaeus, Carl. [1735] 1964. *Systema Naturae.* London: Coronet Books.

Louden, Irvine. 2000. *The Tragedy of Childbed Fever.* Oxford: Oxford University Press.

Lynall, Gregory. 2012. *Swift and Science: The Satire, Politics, and Theology of Natural Knowledge, 1690–1730.* New York: Palgrave Macmillan.

Macpherson, Sandra. 2010. *Harm's Way: Tragic Responsibility and the Novel Form.* Baltimore, MD: Johns Hopkins University Press.

Malory, Thomas. [1485] 2008. *Le Morte d'Arthur: The Winchester Manuscript.* Oxford: Oxford University Press.

Mangham, Andrew, and Greta Depledge, eds. 2012. *The Female Body in Medicine and Literature.* Liverpool: Liverpool University Press.

Marcus, Steven, ed. 2009. *The Other Victorians: A Study of Sexuality and Pornography in Mid-Nineteenth-Century England.* New York/London: Routledge.

Marshall, Ashley. 2013. *The Practice of Satire in England, 1658–1770.* Baltimore, MD: Johns Hopkins University Press.

Martin, Emily. 1991. "The Egg and the Sperm: How Science Has Constructed a Romance Based on Stereotypical Male-Female Roles." *Signs* 16 (3): 485–501.

Martin, Emily. 1996. *Fetal Positions: Individualism, Science, Visuality.* Stanford, CA: Stanford University Press.

Massey, Lyle. 2005. "Pregnancy and Pathology: Picturing Childbirth in Eighteenth-Century Obstetrical Atlases." *The Art Bulletin* 87 (1): 73–91.

McCormick, Ian. 2013. "Sex, Sodomy, and Death Sentences in the Long Eighteenth Century." In *Sex and Death in Eighteenth-Century Literature*, edited by Jolene Zigarovich, 42–67. New York; London: Routledge.

McGrath, Roberta. 2002. *Seeing Her Sex: Medical Archives and the Female Body*. Manchester: Manchester University Press.

Mellor, Anne K. 1988. *Mary Shelley: Her Life, Her Fiction, Her Monsters*. New York: Routledge.

Mellor, Anne K. 1996. "Righting the Wrongs of Woman: Mary Wollstonecraft's *Maria*." *Nineteenth-Century Contexts* 19: 413–424.

Mellor, Anne K. 2003. "Making a 'Monster': An Introduction to Frankenstein." In *The Cambridge Companion to Mary Shelley*, edited by Esther Schor, 9–25. Cambridge: Cambridge University Press.

Mena-Tudela, Desirée et al. 2023. "Experiences with Obstetric Violence among Healthcare Professionals and Students in Spain: A Constructivist Grounded Theory Study." *Women and Birth* 36 (2): 219–226.

Miller, Nancy K. 1980. *The Heroine's Text: Readings in the French and English Novel, 1722-1782*. New York: Columbia University Press.

Milton, John. [1667] 2014. *Paradise Lost*. London: Penguin.

Moers, Ellen. [1974] 2012. "Female Gothic: The Monster's Mother." In Mary Shelley [1818]. *Frankenstein*, edited by J. Paul Hunter, 213–218. New York: Norton.

Moers, Ellen. [1974] 2022. "From Female Gothic: The Monster's Mother." In Mary Shelley [1818]. *Frankenstein*, 3rd ed., edited by J. Paul Hunter, 214–219. New York: Norton.

Moore, Jane. 2012. *Mary Wollstonecraft*. Farnham: Ashgate.

Morrissey, Lee. 2017. "The Restoration and Eighteenth Century, 1660–1780." In *English Literature in Context*, 2nd ed., edited by Paul Poplawski, 189-273. Cambridge: Cambridge University Press.

Morton, Timothy. 2016. "Frankenstein and Ecocriticism." In *The Cambridge Companion to Frankenstein*, edited by Andrew Smith, 143–157. Cambridge: Cambridge University Press.

Moscucci, Ornella. [1990] 1993. *The Science of Woman. Gynaecology and Gender in England, 1800–1929*. Cambridge: Cambridge University Press.

Mossmann, Mark. 2001. "Acts of Becoming: Autobiography, Frankenstein, and the Postmodern Body." In *Mary Shelley's Fictions: From 'Frankenstein' to 'Falkner'*, edited by Michael Eberle-Sinatra, 197–210. New York: Macmillan.

Mottolese, William C. 2007. "Tristram Cyborg and Toby Toolmaker: Body, Tools, and Hobbyhorse in *Tristram Shandy*." *SEL Studies in English Literature 1500–1900* 47 (3): 679–701.

Mulvey-Roberts, Marie, and Roy Porter, eds. 1993. *Literature and Medicine during the Eighteenth Century*. London: Routledge.

Murphey-Lawless, Jo. 1998. *Reading Birth and Death: A History of Obstetrics Thinking*. Bloomington: Indiana University Press.

Neumann, Birgit and Barbara Schmidt-Haberkamp, eds. 2015. *Emotionen, Wissen und Aufklärung: Gefühlskulturen im Großbritannien des 18. Jahrhunderts/Emotions, Knowledge and Enlightenment: Cultures of Emotion in 18th-Century Britain*. Ed. by Carsten Zelle. Special Issue *Das 18. Jahrhundert* 39 (2).

Newman, Karen. 1996. *Fetal Positions: Individualism, Science, Visuality*. Stanford, CA: Stanford University Press.

Newnham, Elizabeth C. et al. 2021. "Comparison of Labour and Birth Outcomes between Nulliparous Women Who Used Epidural Analgesia in Labour and Those Who Did Not: A Prospective Cohort Study." *Women and Birth* 34: 435–441.

Nichols, Marcia D. 2013. "Venus Dissected: The Visual Blazon of Mid-Eighteenth-Century Medical Atlases." In *Sex and Death in Eighteenth-Century Literature*, edited by Jolene Zigarovich, 119–138. New York; London: Routledge.

Nilsson, C., E. Hessman, H. Sjöblom, A. Dencker, E. Jangsten, M. Mollberg et al. 2018. "Definitions, Measurements and Prevalence of Fear of Childbirth: A Systematic Review." *BMC Pregnancy and Childbirth* 18 (1): 28.

Noggle, James. 2018. "Introduction." In *The Norton Anthology of English Literature – The Restoration and the Eighteenth Century*, 10th ed., edited by Stephen Greenblatt, 3–31. New York: Norton.

Pallister, Janis L. 1983. "Introduction." In *On Monsters and Marvels*, by Ambroise Paré, xi–xxii. Chicago, IL: University of Chicago Press.

Paré, Ambroise. 1983. *On Monsters and Marvels*. Translated by Janis L. Pallister. Chicago, IL: University of Chicago Press.

Park, Katharine, and Robert A. Nye. 1991. "Destiny is Anatomy." *New Republic:* 53–57.

Paul, Lissa. 2019. *Eliza Fenwick: Early Modern Feminist*. Newark: University of Delaware Press.

Peakman, Julie. 2012. *Mighty Lewd Books: The Development of Pornography in Eighteenth-Century England*. Houndmills, Basingstoke, Hampshire: Palgrave Macmillan.

Peakman, Julie. 2016. *Amatory Pleasures: Explorations in Eighteenth-Century Sexual Culture*. London; New York: Bloomsbury Academic.

Pickering, Andrew. 1995. *The Mangle of Practice: Time Agency, and Science*. Chicago, IL: University of Chicago Press.

Plumb, John H. 1965. "Introduction." In *Memoirs of Fanny Hill*, by John Cleland, v–xv. New York: Signet.

Poovey, Mary. 1984. *The Proper Lady and the Woman Writer: Ideology as Style in the Works of Mary Wollstonecraft, Mary Shelley, and Jane Austen*. Chicago, IL: University of Chicago Press.

Poovey, Mary. 1998. *A History of the Modern Fact: Problems of Knowledge in the Sciences of Wealth and Society*. Chicago, IL: University of Chicago Press.

Poovey, Mary. 2009. "*A Vindication of the Rights of Woman* and Female Sexuality." In Mary Wollstonecraft [1792]. *A Vindication of the Rights of Woman*, edited by Mary Wollstonecraft, 349–363. New York: Norton.

Porter, Roy. 2001. *Enlightenment: Britain and the Creation of the Modern World*. London: Penguin.

Porter, Roy. 2004. *Flesh in the Age of Reason*. London: Penguin.

Porter, Roy. 2021. *Bodies Politic: Disease, Death and Doctors in Britain, 1650–1900*. London: Reaktion.

Rabb, Melinda. 2006. "The Secret Memoirs of Lemuel Gulliver: Satire, Secrecy, and Swift." *ELH* 73 (2): 325–354.

Rauch, Alan. 1995. "The Monstrous Body of Knowledge in Mary Shelley's 'Frankenstein'." *Studies in Romanticism* 34 (2): 227–253.

Richards, Cynthia. 2018. "History without Trauma: Recovering Bodily Loss in the Eighteenth Century." In *The Future of Feminist Eighteenth-Century Scholarship: Beyond Recovery*, edited by Robin Runia, 132–145. New York: Routledge.

Richardson, Samuel. [1740] 2008. *Pamela: Or, Virtue Rewarded*. edited by Thomas Keymer and Alice Wakely. Oxford World's Classics. Oxford: Oxford University Press.

Richardson, Samuel. [1748] 2010. *Clarissa: Or, The History of a Young Lady*. Edited by Toni Bowers and John Richetti. Peterborough, ON: Broadview Press.

Richetti, John, ed. 1998. *The Cambridge Companion to the Eighteenth-Century Novel*. Cambridge: Cambridge University Press.

Rigby, Mair. 2009. "'Do you Share my Madness?' Frankenstein's Queer Gothic." In *Queering the Gothic*, edited by William Hughes and Andrew Smith, 36–54. Manchester: Manchester University Press.

Rivero, Albert J. 2002. "Preface." In *Gulliver's Travels*, by Jonathan Swift, edited by Albert J. Rivero, vii–xii. New York: Norton.

Robertson, John. 2015. *The Enlightenment – A Very Short Introduction*. Oxford: Oxford University Press.

Rollins, Joe. 2011. "Political Science, Political Sex." *PS: Political Science and Politics* 44 (1): 27–30.

Rosenthal, Laura J. 2006. *Infamous Commerce: Prostitution in Eighteenth-Century British Literature and Culture*. Ithaca, NY: Cornell University Press.

Ross, Ian Campbell. 2009. "Introduction." In *The Life and Opinions of Tristram Shandy*, edited by Laurence Sterne and Ian Campbell Ross, ix–xxviii. Oxford: Oxford University Press.

Rousseau, Jean Jacques. [1789] 1969. *Oeuvres Completes*. Vol. 4. Ed. Pierre Burgelin. Paris: Gallimard.

Runia, Robin, ed. 2018. *The Future of Feminist Eighteenth-Century Scholarship: Beyond Recovery*. New York: Routledge.

Runia, Robin. 2018. "Introduction." In *The Future of Feminist Eighteenth-Century Scholarship: Beyond Recovery*, edited by Robin Runia, 1–10. New York: Routledge.

Sabor, Peter. [1985] 2008. "Introduction." In *Memoirs of a Woman of Pleasure,* edited by John Cleland, vii-xxxiii. Oxford: Oxford University Press.

Salvaggio, Ruth. 1988. "Swift's Disruptive Woman." In *Enlightened Absence: Neoclassical Configurations of the Feminine*, edited by Ruth Salvaggio, 77–102. Urbana: University of Illinois Press.

Saunders, John B., and Charles O'Malley. 1973. *The Illustrations from the Works of Andreas Vesalius of Brussels*. New York: Dover Publications.

Schabert, Ina. 2017. "Gender and Class." In *Handbook of British Romanticism*, edited by Ralf Haekel, 49–66. Berlin; Boston, MA: De Gruyter.

Schäfer-Althaus, Sarah. 2020. "Dissecting Birth: Obstetrics, Bodily Transience, and the Anatomist's Gaze in Eighteenth-Century Medical Atlases." In *Transient Bodies in Anglophone Literature and Culture*, edited by Sarah Schäfer-Althaus and Sara Strauß, 15–36. Vol. 91 of *Anglistik und Englischunterricht*. Heidelberg: Winter.

Schama, Simon. 2004. "Foreword." In *Flesh in the Age of Reason*, by Roy Porter, vii–xiii. London: Penguin.

Schiebinger, Londa. 1987. "Skeletons in the Closet: The First Illustrations of the Female Skeleton in Eighteenth-Century Anatomy." In *The Making of the Modern Body: Sexuality and Society in the Nineteenth Century*, edited by Thomas Laqueur and Catherine Gallagher, 42–82. Berkeley: University of California Press.

Schiebinger, Londa. 1996. "Gender and Natural History." In *Cultures of Natural History*, edited by Nicholas Jardine, James A. Secord, and Emma C Spary, 163–177. Cambridge: Cambridge University Press.

Schiebinger, Londa. 2004. *Nature's Body: Gender in the Making of Modern Science*. New Brunswick, NJ: Rutgers University Press.

Schwennesen, Nete, and Lene Koch. 2009. "Visualizing and Calculating Life: Matters of Fact in the Context of Prenatal Risk Assessment." In *Contested Categories: Life Sciences in Society*, edited by Susanne Bauer and Ayo Wahlberg, 69–87. New York: Routledge.

Seager, Nicholas. 2022. "Jonathan Swift, Gulliver's Travels (1726)." In *Handbook of the British Novel in the Long Eighteenth Century*, edited by Katrin Berndt and Alessa Johns, 279–301. Berlin; Boston, MA: De Gruyter.

Seidel, Michael. 1998. "Samuel Richardson: Fiction and Knowledge." In *The Cambridge Companion to the Eighteenth-Century Novel*, edited by John Richetti, 131–150. Cambridge: Cambridge University Press.

Seijmonsbergen-Schermers, A. E., T. van den Akker, E. Rydahl, K. Beeckman, A. Bogaerts, L. Binfa et al. 2020. "Variations in Use of Childbirth Interventions in 13 High-Income Countries: A Multinational Cross-Sectional Study." *PLOS Medicine* 17 (5): e1003103.

Sheehan, Paul. 2015. "Posthuman Bodies." In *The Cambridge Companion to the Body in Literature*, edited by David Hillman and Ulrika Maude, 45–59. New York: Cambridge University Press.

Shelley, Mary. 1818. *Frankenstein.* Edited by J. Paul Hunter. 3rd ed. New York: Norton, 2022.

Shilling, Chris. 2016. *The Body: A Very Short Introduction.* Oxford: Oxford University Press.

Smellie, William. 1754. *A Set of Anatomical Tables, with Explanation and an Abridgement of the Practice of Midwifery, with a view to illustrate a treatise on that subject, and collection of cases.* London: D. Wilson.

Smith, Andrew, and Diana Wallace. 2004. "The Female Gothic. Then and Now." *Gothic Studies* 6 (1): 1–7.

Smith-Oka, Vania. 2022. "Cutting Women: Unnecessary Caesareans as Iatrogenesis and Obstetric Violence." *Social Science & Medicine* 296 (4).

Sommers, Sheena. 2012. "Transcending the Sexed Body: Reason, Sympathy, and 'Thinking Machines' in the Debates over Male Midwifery." In *The Female Body in Medicine and Literature*, edited by Andrew Mangham and Greta Depledge, 89–106. Liverpool: Liverpool University Press.

Sontag, Susan. 1979. *Illness as Metaphor.* New York: Random House.

Speck, William A. 2016. "Social Structure, Class and Gender: 1770–1832." In *The Oxford Handbook of the Eighteenth-Century Novel*, edited by Alan Downie, 339–354. Oxford: Oxford University Press.

Spivak, Gayatri Chakravorty. 1985. "Three Women's Texts and a Critique of Imperialism." *Critical Inquiry* 12 (1): 235–261.

Sprang, Felix. 2008. "Tristram Shandy und die *Anthropologia Nova*: Systematik in Literatur und Medizin." In *Medizinische Schreibweisen: Ausdifferenzierung und Transfer zwischen Medizin und Literatur (1600–1900)*, edited by Nicolas Pethes and Sandra Richter, 135–153. Tübingen: Niemeyer.

Sprang, Felix. 2013. "Let Me See the Child, and Die: The Medicalization of Childbirth in Eighteenth- and Nineteenth-Century Novels." In *The Writing Cure: Literature and Medicine in Context*, edited by Alexandra Lembert-Heidenreich and Jarmila Mildorf, 135–153. Zurich: Lit Verlag.

Spratt, Danielle. 2012. "Gulliver's Economized Body: Colonial Projects and the *Lusus Naturae* in the Travels." *Studies in Eighteenth-Century Culture* 41: 137–159.

Sterne, Laurence. [1749] 2019. *Tristram Shandy.* Edited with an introduction by Judith Hawley. New York: Norton.

Stretser, Thomas. 1932. *Merryland.* New York: Robin Hood House.

Stone, Sarah. 1737. *A Complete Practice of Midwifery: Consisting of Upwards of Forty Cases or Observations in that valuable Art, [...]. Recommended to All Female*

Practitioners in an Art so important to the Lives and Well-Being of the Sex. London: printed for T. Cooper, at the Globe, Paternoster Row.

Sussman, Charlotte. 2004. "The Colonial Afterlife of Political Arithmetic: Swift, Demography, and Mobile Populations." *Cultural Critique* 56 (1): 96–126.

Swift, Jonathan. 2002. *Gulliver's Travels*. Edited by Albert J. Rivero. New York: Norton.

Tauchert, Ashley. 2002. *Mary Wollstonecraft and the Accent of the Feminine*. Basingstoke; New York: Palgrave.

Taylor, Barbara. 2003. *Mary Wollstonecraft and the Feminine Imagination*. Cambridge: Cambridge University Press.

Tegan, Mary Beth. 2011. "Mocking the Mothers of the Novel: Mary Wollstonecraft, Maternal Metaphor, and the Reproduction of Sympathy." *Studies in the Novel* 42 (4): 357–376.

Todd, Janet. 1980. *Women's Friendship in Literature: The Eighteenth-Century Novel in England and France*. New York: Columbia University Press.

Todd, Janet. 1989. "Introduction." In *Secresy, Or: The Ruin on the Rock*, by Eliza Fenwick, vii–x. Norfolk/UK: Pandora.

Todd, Janet. 2000. *Mary Wollstonecraft: A Revolutionary Life*. London: Phoenix Press.

Tomalin, Claire. 2012. *The Life and Death of Mary Wollstonecraft*. London: Penguin.

Tropp, Laura. 2013. *A Womb with a View: America's Growing Interest in Pregnancy*. Santa Barbara, CA: Praeger.

Tyler, Imogen. 2001. "Skin-Tight: Celebrity, Pregnancy and Subjectivity." In *Thinking Through the Skin*, edited by Sara Ahmed and Jackie Stacy, 69–85. London: Routledge.

Ursa, Mihaela. 2014. "Giving Birth the Posthuman Way: Technology, Disembodiment, and Cyber-Progenies." *Ekphrasis: Images, Cinema, Theatre, Media* 12 (2): 131–140.

Vanderbeke, Dirk. 2006. "Winding up the Clock: The Conception and Birth of Tristram Shandy." In *Fashioning Childhood in the Eighteenth Century: Age and Identity*, edited by Anja Müller, 179–188. Aldershot: Ashgate.

Waddington, Keir. 2011. *An Introduction to the Social History of Medicine: Europe since 1500*. London: Red Globe Press.

Wahrman, Dror. 2008. "Change and the Corporeal in Seventeenth-and Eighteenth-Century Gender History: Or, Can Cultural History Be Rigorous?" *Gender and History* 20: 584–602.

Walpole, Horace. 2014. *The Castle of Otranto*. Oxford: Oxford University Press.

Watt, Ian. [1957] 2015. *The Rise of the Novel: Studies in Defoe, Richardson and Fielding*. London: Bodley Head.

Wertz, Richard W., and Dorothy C. Wertz. 1977. *Lying-In: A History of Childbirth in America*. New York: Free Press.

Whitehead, Anne, and Angela Woods, eds. 2016. *The Edinburgh Companion to the Critical Medical Humanities*. Edinburgh: Edinburgh University Press.

Whiteley, Rebecca. 2023. *Birth Figures: Early Modern Prints and the Pregnant Body*. Chicago, IL; London: University of Chicago Press.

Williams, Carolyn. 2012. "Difficulties, at Present in No Degree Clear'd Up: The Controversial Mother, 1600–1800." In *The Female Body in Medicine and Literature*, edited by Andrew Mangham and Greta Depledge, 16–33. Liverpool: Liverpool University Press.

Wilson, Adrian. 1995a. *The Making of Man-Midwifery: Childbirth in England, 1660–1770*. Cambridge, MA: Harvard University Press.

Wilson, Catherine. 1995b. *The Invisible World: Early Modern Philosophy and the Invention of the Microscope*. Princeton, NJ: Princeton University Press.

Wollstonecraft, Mary. 2008. *A Vindication of the Rights of Men*. Edited with an introduction by Janet Todd. Oxford: Oxford University Press.

Wollstonecraft, Mary. [1792] 2009. *A Vindication of the Rights of Woman: An Authoritative Text, Backgrounds, and Contexts, Criticism*. Edited by Deidre S. Lynch. New York: Norton.
Wollstonecraft, Mary. [1798] 2009. *Mary and the Wrongs of Woman*. Edited with an introduction by Gary Kelly. Oxford: Oxford University Press.
Woods, Robert, and Chris Galley. 2014. *Mrs Stone & Dr Smellie: Eighteenth-Century Midwives and Their Patients*. Liverpool: Liverpool University Press.
Zigarovich, Jolene, ed. 2013. *Sex and Death in Eighteenth-Century Literature*. New York; London: Routledge.

Further Reading

Allen, Dennis W. 1985. "Sexuality/Textuality in *Tristram Shandy*." *Studies in English Literature,* 1500-1900 25 (3): 651–664.
Andreolle-Spalding, Donna, and Veronique Molinari. 2011. *Women and Science, 17th Century to Present: Pioneers, Activists, and Protagonists*. Newcastle upon Tyne: Cambridge Scholars Publishing.
Armitage, David. 2004. "Monstrosity and Myth in Mary Shelley's *Frankenstein*." In *Monstrous Bodies/Political Monstrosities in Early Modern Europe*, edited by Laura Lunger Knoppers and Joan B. Landes, 200–226. Ithaca, NY: Cornell University Press.
Armstrong, Nancy, and Leonard Tennenhouse, eds. 2014. *The Ideology of Conduct: Essays in Literature and the History of Sexuality*. London: Routledge.
Aune, Ingvild, Mari A. Hoston, Nora J. Kolshus, and Christel E. G. Larsen. 2017. "Nature Works Best When Allowed to Run Its Course: The Experience of Midwives Promoting Normal Births in a Home Birth Setting." *Midwifery* 50: 21–26.
Bates, Victoria, Alan Bleakley, and Sam Goodman, eds. 2015. *Medicine, Health and the Arts: Approaches to the Medical Humanities*. London: Routledge.
Beauvoir, Simone de, and Martine Reid, eds. 2015. *Extracts from the Second Sex*. London: Vintage Books.
Benedict, Barbara M. 1992. "Dear 'Madam': Rhetoric, Cultural Politics, and the Female Reader in Sterne's *Tristram Shandy*." *Studies in Philology* 89 (4): 485–498.
Berndt, Katrin. 2016. *Narrating Friendship and the British Novel*. London: Routledge.
Blondel, B., B. Coulm, C. Bonnet, F. Goffinet, and C. Le Ray. 2017. "Trends in Perinatal Health in Metropolitan France from 1995 to 2016: Results from the French National Perinatal Surveys." *Journal of Gynaecology, Obstetrics and Human Reproduction* 46 (10): 701–713.
Bordo, Susan. 1993. *Unbearable Weight: Feminism, Western Culture, and the Body*. Berkeley/Los Angeles/London: University of California Press.
Bowers, Toni. 2005. *The Politics of Motherhood: British Writing and Culture, 1680–1760*. Cambridge: Cambridge University Press.
Bradford, Barbara Taylor. 2004. *Mary Wollstonecraft and the Feminist Imagination*. Cambridge: Cambridge University Press.
Braudy, Leo. 1970. "Fanny Hill and Materialism." *Eighteenth-Century Studies* 4 (1): 21–40.
Brownstein, Rachel M., and Susan Sniader Lanser. 1993. "Fictions of Authority: Women Writers and Narrative Voice." *Eighteenth-Century Studies* 27 (1): 161–170.
Bruce, Susan. 1988. "The Flying Island and Female Anatomy: Gynaecology and Power in *Gulliver's Travels*." *Genders* 2: 60–76.
Chabor, Lois A. 1997. "'This Affecting Subject': An 'Interested' Reading of Childbearing in Two Novels by Samuel Richardson." *The Scriblerian and the Kit-Cats* 29 (2): 169–180.

Cisney, Vernon W., and Nicolae Morar, eds. 2016. *Biopower: Foucault and Beyond*. Chicago, IL: The University of Chicago Press.

Clarke, Bruce, and Manuela Rossini, eds. 2011. *The Routledge Companion to Literature and Science*. 1st ed. London: Routledge.

Cleland, John. 2018. *Titus Vespasian: A Tragedy*. Gale ECCO.

Cole, Thomas R., Nathan S. Carlin, and Ronald A. Carson. 2015. *Medical Humanities: An Introduction*. New York: Cambridge University Press.

Conboy, Katie, Nadia Medina, and Sarah Stanbury, eds. 1997. *Writing on the Body: Female Embodiment and Feminist Theory*. New York: Columbia University Press.

Condren, Conal. 2012. "Satire and Definition." *Humor* 25 (4): 375–399.

Crasnow, Sharin, and Kristen Inteman. 2020. *The Routledge Handbook of Feminist Philosophy of Science*. Abingdon: Routledge.

Creed, Barbara. 1986. "Horror and the Monstrous-Feminine: An Imaginary Abjection." *Screen* 27 (1): 44–71.

Dahlen, Hannah G. et al. 2013. "Rates of Obstetric Intervention during Birth and Selected Maternal and Perinatal Outcomes for Low-Risk Women Born in Australia Compared to Those Born Overseas." *BMC Pregnancy and Childbirth* 13: 1–10.

Descargues-Grant, Madeleine. 2006. "The Obstetrics of *Tristram Shandy*." *Études anglaises* 59 (4): 401–413.

Duffin, Jacalyn. 2010. *History of Medicine: A Scandalously Short Introduction*. 2nd ed. Toronto: University of Toronto Press.

Federico, Annette R., and Sandra M. Gilbert, eds. 2011. *Gilbert & Gubar's The Madwoman in the Attic after Thirty Years*. Columbia: University of Missouri Press.

Foucault, Michel. 1970. *The Order of Things: An Archaeology of the Human Sciences*. New York: Vintage Books.

Foucault, Michel. 1972. *The Archaeology of Knowledge and the Discourse on Language*. Translated by A. M. Sheridan Smith. New York: Pantheon Books.

Ford, Thomas. 2009. "Mary Wollstonecraft and the Motherhood of Feminism." *Women's Studies Quarterly* 37 (3–4): 189–205.

Friedman, Susan Stanford. 1987. "Creativity and the Childbirth Metaphor: Gender Difference in Literary Discourse." *Feminist Studies* 13 (1): 49–82.

Gautier, Gary. 1995. "Fanny Hill's Mapping of Sexuality, Female Identity, and Maternity." *Studies in English Literature, 1500-1900* 35 (3): 473–491.

George, Margaret. 1970. *One Woman's "Situation": A Study of Mary Wollstonecraft*. Urbana, Chicago, and London: University of Illinois Press.

Gerard, William B. 2006. *Laurence Sterne and the Visual Imagination*. Florence: Taylor and Francis.

Gordon, Lyndall. 2005. *Vindication: A Life of Mary Wollstonecraft*. New York: Harper.

Graham, Rosemary. 1997. "The Prostitute in the Garden: Walt Whitman, *Fanny Hill*, and the Fantasy of Female Pleasure." *ELH* 64 (2): 569–597.

Grundy, Isobel. 1998. "Introduction." In *Secresy*, by Eliza Fenwick, edited by Isobel Grundy. 2nd ed. Peterborough, ON: Broadview Press.

Haekel, Ralf, ed. 2017. *Handbook of British Romanticism*. Berlin; Boston, MA: De Gruyter.

Haekel, Ralf, and Sabine Blackmore. 2013. *Discovering the Human: Life Science and the Arts in the Eighteenth and Early Nineteenth Centuries*. Göttingen: V & R Unipress.

Harol, Corrinne. 2006. *Enlightened Virginity in Eighteenth-Century Literature*. New York: Palgrave Macmillan US.

Harvey, Graham. 2013. *Eternal Eve: The History of Gynaecology and Obstetrics*. Whitefish, MT: Literary Licensing.

Haslam, Fiona. 1996. *Medicine in Art in Eighteenth-Century Britain: From Hogarth to Rowlandson*. Liverpool: Liverpool University Press.

Haslanger, Andrea. 2011. "What Happens When Pornography Ends in Marriage: The Uniformity of Pleasure in *Fanny Hill*." *ELH* 78 (1): 163–188.

Hayden, Judy A. 2011. *The New Science and Women's Literary Discourse: Prefiguring Frankenstein*. New York: Palgrave Macmillan.

Henke, Jennifer S. 2025. "Matters of Interest: Entangling the Maternal Body." In *Undue Burdens: Reproductive Rights and Bodily Autonomy in the Long Eighteenth Century*, edited by Fiona Brideoake, Ula Lukszo Klein, and Nicole Garret. University of Virginia Press.

Hentschel, Klaus. 2015. *Visual Cultures in Science and Technology: A Comparative History*. Oxford: Oxford University Press.

Hitchcock, Tim. 1996. "Redefining Sex in Eighteenth-Century England." *History Workshop Journal* 41: 72–90.

Holmes, Thomas A. 2009. "Sexual Positions and Sexual Politics: John Cleland's *Memoirs of a Woman of Pleasure*." *South Atlantic Review* 74 (1): 124–139.

Hurley, Kelly. 1996. *The Gothic Body: Sexuality, Materialism, and Degeneration at the Fin de Siècle*. Cambridge: Cambridge University Press.

Jagose, Annamarie. 2007. "Critical Extasy: Orgasm and Sensibility in *Memoirs of a Woman of Pleasure*." *Signs* 32: 2459–2482.

Juengel, Scott J. 2009. "Doing Things with *Fanny Hill*." *ELH* 76 (2): 419–446.

Kaplan, Cora. 2002. "Mary Wollstonecraft's Reception and Legacies." In *The Cambridge Companion to Mary Wollstonecraft*, edited by Claudia L. Johnson, 246–270. Cambridge: Cambridge University Press.

Keymer, Tom, and Jon Mee, eds. 2004. *The Cambridge Companion to English Literature, 1740–1830*. Cambridge: Cambridge University Press.

Knoppers, Laura Lunger, and Joan B. Landes, eds. 2004. *Monstrous Bodies/Political Monstrosities in Early Modern Europe*. Ithaca, NY; London: Cornell University Press.

Korte, Barbara. 1990. "In Sorrow Thou Shalt Bring Forth Children: On Childbirth in Literature." *Orbis Litterarum* 45 (1): 30–48.

Landry, Donna, and Gerald MacLean. 1990. "Of Forceps, Patents, and Paternity: *Tristram Shandy*." *Eighteenth-Century Studies* 23 (4): 522–543.

Laqueur, Thomas. 1986. "Orgasm, Generation, and the Politics of Reproductive Biology." *Representations* 14: 1–41.

Latour, Bruno. 2017. *Die Hoffnung der Pandora: Untersuchungen zur Wirklichkeit der Wissenschaft*. 6th ed. Frankfurt am Main: Suhrkamp.

Lembert-Heidenreich, Alexandra, and Jarmila Mildorf, eds. 2013. *The Writing Cure: Literature and Medicine in Context*. Zurich: Lit Verlag.

Lieske, Pam. 2003. "Procreation, Impotency, and the Nature of Desire in Enlightenment Fiction and Culture." *Eighteenth-Century Studies* 36 (2): 275–282.

Louden, Irvine. 2003. "Maternal Mortality: 1880–1950: Some Regional and International Comparisons." *Social History of Medicine* 1 (2): 183–228.

Mannheimer, Katherine. 2012. *Print, Visuality, and Gender in Eighteenth-Century Satire: The Scope in Ev'ry Page*. Hoboken: Taylor & Francis.

Marsh, Sarah. 2015. "Romantic Medicine, the British Constitution, and *Frankenstein*." *Keats-Shelley Journal* 64: 105–122.

Mauriceau, François. 1985. *The Diseases of Women with Child, and in Child-Bed*. New York: Garland.

Müller, Anja, ed. 2006. *Fashioning Childhood in the Eighteenth Century: Age and Identity*. Aldershot: Ashgate.

Mulvey-Roberts, Marie, and Roy Porter, eds. 1993. *Literature and Medicine during the Eighteenth Century*. London: Routledge.

Muri, Allison. 2010. "Imagining Reproduction: The Politics of Reproduction, Technology, and the Woman Machine." *The Journal of Medical Humanities* 31 (1): 53–67.

Oliver, Kelly. 2010. "Motherhood, Sexuality, and Pregnant Embodiment: Twenty-Five Years of Gestation." *Hypatia* 25 (4): 760–777.

Osterman, Michelle J. K., and Joyce A. Martin. 2008. "Epidural and Spinal Anaesthesia Use During Labor." *National Vital Statistics Reports*.

Owens, Deirdre Benia Cooper. 2017. *Medical Bondage: Race, Gender, and the Origins of American Gynecology*. Athens: University of Georgia Press.

Peritz, Janice H. 2010. "Necessarily Various: Body Politics and Discursive Ethics in Wollstonecraft's *The Wrongs of Woman*." *European Romantic Review* 21 (2): 251–266.

Pietrzak-Franger, Monika. 2017. *Syphilis in Victorian Literature and Culture: Medicine, Knowledge and the Spectacle of Victorian Invisibility*. Cham: Palgrave Macmillan.

Poovey, Mary. 1982. "Mary Wollstonecraft: The Gender of Genres in Late Eighteenth-Century England." *NOVEL: A Forum on Fiction* 15 (2): 111–126.

Poovey, Mary. 1985. *The Proper Lady and the Woman Writer: Ideology as Style in the Works of Mary Wollstonecraft, Mary Shelley, and Jane Austen*. Paperback ed. Chicago, IL: University of Chicago Press.

Porter, Roy. 2001. *Enlightenment: Britain and the Creation of the Modern World*. London: Penguin.

Resnik, David B. 2005. *The Ethics of Science: An Introduction*. London: Routledge.

Reynalde, Thomas. 2009. *The Birth of Mankind: Otherwise Named, the Woman's Book*. Farnham; Burlington: Ashgate.

Rosenberg, Ingrid v. 2013. "Childbirth—Women's Very Own Topic? Imaginations of the Female Birth Experience in Male Authors' Novels." *Anglistik: International Journal of English Studies* 24 (1): 19–28.

Rosenthal, Laura Jean, ed. 2008. *Nightwalkers: Prostitute Narratives from the Eighteenth Century*. Peterborough, ON: Broadview Press.

Rossi, A. Cristina, and Federico Prefumo. 2018. "Planned Home versus Planned Hospital Births in Women at Low-Risk Pregnancy: A Systematic Review with Meta-Analysis." *European Journal of Obstetrics, Gynaecology, and Reproductive Biology* 222: 102–108.

Ruston, Sharon. 2013. *Creating Romanticism: Case Studies in the Literature, Science, and Medicine of the 1790s*. Houndmills, Basingstoke, Hampshire; New York: Palgrave Macmillan.

Schlegel, Johannes. 2017. "Mary Shelly, *Frankenstein* (1818)." In *Handbook of British Romanticism*, edited by Ralf Haekel, 523–539. Berlin; Boston, MA: De Gruyter.

Schwanebeck, Wieland. 2016. "The Womb as a Battlefield: Debating Medical Authority in the Renaissance Midwife Manual." *Journal for the Study of British Cultures* 23 (2): 101–114.

Sharp, Jane, and Elaine Hobby, eds. 1999. *The Midwives Book, or the Whole Art of Midwifery Discovered*. New York: Oxford University Press.

Sill, Geoffrey. 2016. "Developments in Sentimental Fiction." In *The Oxford Handbook of the Eighteenth-Century Novel*, edited by Alan Downie, 426–439. Oxford: Oxford University Press.

Smith, Andrew. 2016. *The Cambridge Companion to Frankenstein*. Cambridge: Cambridge University Press.

Smith, Andrew, and Diana Wallace. 2004. "The Female Gothic: Then and Now." *Gothic Studies* 6 (1): 1–7.

Spencer, Jane. 2005. *Literary Relations: Kinship and the Canon, 1660–1830*. Oxford; New York: Oxford University Press.
Staley, Kent W. 2014. *An Introduction to the Philosophy of Science*. Cambridge: Cambridge University Press.
Taylor, Anne Robinson. 1981. *Male Novelists and Their Female Voices: Literary Masquerades*. New York: Troy.
Todd, Dennis. 1982. "Three Characters in Hogarth's *Cunicularii* and Some Implications." *Eighteenth-Century Studies* 16 (1): 26–40.
Todd, Janet. 1986. *Sensibility: An Introduction*. London: Routledge.
Walker, James Johnston. 2017. "Planned Home Birth." *Best Practice & Research Clinical Obstetrics and Gynaecology* 43: 76–86.
Weed, David. 1997. "Fitting Fanny: Cleland's *Memoirs* and the Politics of Male Pleasure." *NOVEL: A Forum on Fiction* 31 (1): 7–20.

Index

Note: *Italic* page numbers refer to figures and page numbers followed by "n" denote endnotes.

FSC
www.fsc.org
MIX
Papier | Fördert gute Waldnutzung
FSC® C083411

Kolibri 360 GmbH
Ferdinand-Jühlke-Straße 7
99095 Erfurt, Deutschland
produktsicherheit@kolibri360.de